Marma Points of Ayurveda

Other Publications by Vasant D. Lad

Ayurveda: The Science of Self-Healing. 1985

The Complete Book of Ayurvedic Home Remedies. 1998

The Textbook of Ayurveda: Fundamental Principles.
Volume One. 2002

Strands of Eternity: A Compilation of
Mystical Poetry and Discourses. 2004

The Textbook of Ayurveda: A Complete Guide
to Clinical Assessment. Volume Two. 2006

Secrets of the Pulse: The Ancient Art
of Ayurvedic Pulse Diagnosis. 2nd ed., 2006

Pranayama for Self-Healing. DVD, 2010.

The Textbook of Ayurveda: General Principles of Management
and Treatment, Volume Three. 2012

Ayurvedic Perspectives on Selected Pathologies. 2nd ed., 2012

Applied Marma Therapy Cards. 2013

The Yoga of Herbs: An Ayurvedic Guide to Herbal Medicine. 1986
by Vasant Lad and David Frawley

Ayurvedic Cooking for Self-Healing. 2nd ed., 1997
by Usha and Vasant Lad

Ayuryoga: VPK Basics. 2014
by Vasant Lad and Maria Garre

Marma Points of Ayurveda

The Energy Pathways for Healing Body, Mind and Consciousness with a Comparison to Traditional Chinese Medicine

by **Vasant D. Lad, B.A.M.&S., M.A.Sc.**
and **Anisha Durve, M.S.O.M., Dipl. Ac., A.P.**

Sonam Targee
Traditional Chinese Medicine Reviewer

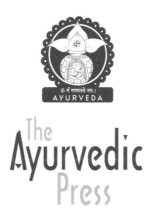

AYURVEDA

The Ayurvedic Press

Albuquerque, New Mexico

The Ayurvedic Press, Albuquerque 87112

Although the information contained in this book is based on Ayurvedic principles practiced for thousands of years, it should not be taken or construed as standard medical treatment. For any medical condition, always consult with a qualified health care practitioner.

This book is printed on acid-free paper.
Edited by Jack Forem.

Cover design by Michael Quanci.
Illustrations by Yvonne Wylie Walston, CMI, of Creative Imagery, Inc.
Layout design by Laura Humphreys.
Project manager: Laura Humphreys.

Printed in Malaysia.

10 9 8 7 6 5 4 3 2

Library of Congress Cataloging-in-Publication Data

Lad, Vasant, 1943-
  Marma points of ayurveda : the energy pathways for healing body, mind, and consciousness with a comparison to traditional Chinese medicine / by Vasant D. Lad, B.A.M.S., M.A.Sc. and Anisha Durve, M.S.O.M., Dipl. Ac., A.P.; Sonam Targee, traditional Chinese medicine reviewer. -- First paperback edition.
       p. cm.
  Summary: "Presents healing energetics of Ayurvedic marma points and compares them with Chinese system of acupuncture. Based on traditional medicine system from India, provides commentaries of diagnostic and therapeutic scope for each marma point including techniques for massage, detoxification, acupressure, aromatherapy, yoga and meditation"--Provided by publisher.
  Includes bibliographical references and index.
  1. Acupuncture points. 2. Medicine, Ayurvedic. I. Durve, Anisha. II. Targee, Sonam. III. Title.
  RM184.5.L32 2015
  615.8'92--dc23
                      2014028809

For more information on Ayurveda contact: The Ayurvedic Institute, 11311 Menaul Blvd NE, Albuquerque, N.M. 87112-0008. Phone (505) 291-9698 or www.ayurveda.com.

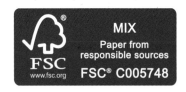

Dedication

This book is dedicated with all my heart to my most loving wife, Usha,
my children, Pranav and his wife, Yesurani, and Aparna and her husband Manjit,
and their children, Charan Jyot and Verneet.   ~ Vasant Lad

Dedication

To my loving parents and younger sisters, Anuja and Namita, for your infinite
dedication, support and patience. You have allowed strength and inspiration to flow
within me and within the writing of this book.   ~ Anisha Durve

Table of Contents

List of Illustrations vii

Foreword ix

Preface xi

The Use of Sanskrit xiii

Introduction 1

INTRODUCTION TO PART ONE 5

1 Introduction to Āyurveda 7
The Five Elements 9
The Three Doshas 11
Vāta 11
Pitta 12
Kapha 13
The Seven Dhātus (Bodily Tissues) 14
The Prakruti/Vikruti Paradigm in Āyurvedic Medicine 14

2 Introduction to Marmāni 17
The History of Marmāni 17
Mechanisms of Action 18
Functions of Marmāni 19
Communication 19
Diagnostic Indicators 19
Therapeutic Influences 19
Mechanism of Pain Relief 20
Stimulation of Agni and Detoxification of Āma 20
Calming the Mind and Balancing Emotions 20
Enhancing Awareness 20
Preventative Care and Rejuvenation 20
Classification of Marmāni 21
Location 21
Elemental Associations 21
Marmāni and Doshic Subtypes 21
Corresponding Organs And Srotāmsi 22
Degrees Of Vitality of Marmāni 22
Sadyah Prānahara Marmāni 22
Conclusion 22

3 The Spiritual Dimension of Marmāni 25
The Spiritual Value of Touch 25
Mahad: Innate Intelligence of the Body – and the Universe 25
Universal Mind and Particular Mind: Opening to Infinity 26
Marmāni and Mind/Body Medicine 26
Chakra System 28

    Emotions: Origin, Expression and Healing 29
    Go With the Flow: Marmāni and the Art of Calming the Mind 31

4   Āyurveda and Traditional Chinese Medicine 33
    The Creation Model in Traditional Chinese Medicine 33
      Yin and Yang 33
      The Five Principles of Yin and Yang 34
      The Five Elements in TCM 36
    Comparing the Philosophies of TCM and Sānkhya 37
      Unity 37
      Duality 37
      Qualities 37
      Qi and Prāna 38
      The Five Elements 38
      Individual Constitution 39
    Health and Disease in Āyurveda and TCM 40
      Etiology and Pathogenesis in Āyurveda 40
      TCM Etiology 40
      TCM Pathology and Diagnosis 41
      Diagnosis in Āyurveda 41
      Diagnosis in Āyurveda and TCM 42
    Models of Pain 42
      Pain in TCM 42
      Pain in Āyurveda 43

5   Channels, Energy Points and Measurements in Āyurveda and Traditional Chinese Medicine 45
    Channels 45
      Channels in TCM 46
      Channels in Āyurveda: Srotāmsi and Nādī 50
      Nādīs 50
      Srotas 51
      Functions of Srotāmsi and Nādīs 52
      Comparison 52
    Energy Points 52
      Classification of Acupuncture Points 52
      Classification of Marmāni 53
    Measurements 53

6   Samprāpti: Pathogenesis and Disturbance of Marmāni 57
    Etiological Factors 57
    Samprāpti (Pathogenesis) 58
      Vyadhi Mārga, the Three Pathways of Disease 60
    Vikruti, the Present Imbalance 61
      Role of Marmāni in Relation to Samprāpti and Pathways of Disease 61
      Marmāni as Khavaigunya 62
      Marmāni in Relation to Āma and Agni 62

7   Introduction to Chikitsā, Āyurvedic Therapy 65
    Types of Chikitsā and the Role of Marmāni 65
      Shodhana, Cleansing through Marmāni 65
      Shamana, Palliation of Doshas via Marmāni 66
      Rasāyana, Rejuvenation via Marmāni 66

Apunarbhava Chikitsā, Preventive Therapy through Marmāni 66
Sadyah Phaladai Chikitsā, Marmāni as First Aid Therapy 67
Tanmātrā, Five Element Chikitsā 67
Shabda (Sound) 67
Sparsha (Touch) 68
Rūpa (Vision) 68
Rasa (Taste) 68
Gandha (Smell) 69
Context of Marma Chikitsā within Āyurvedic Therapy 69

8 Techniques of Marma Stimulation – Guidelines for the Practitioner 71
Techniques of Marma Chikitsā – 10 Methods of Stimulating Marma Points 71
Snehana (Oleation) 71
Svedana (Sudation) 72
Mardana (Deep Connective Tissue Massage) 72
Pīdana (Deep, Dry Pressure) 72
Veshtana (Binding or Holding) 72
Lepana (Application of Paste) 72
Agni Karma (Application of Heat) 73
Sūchi Bharana (Puncturing with Needles) 73
Trasana (Irritation) 73
Rakta Moksha (Bloodletting) 74
Guidelines for Practitioners of Marma Chikitsā 74
Clinical Knowledge 74
Meditation and Breath Awareness 74
Guidelines for Touch and Pressure 75

INTRODUCTION TO PART TWO 77

9 Mukha (Face) and Shiro (Head) Marmāni 81
Mūrdhni or Adhipati   82
Brahmarandhra   84
Shivarandhra   86
Kapāla   88
Ājñā or Sthapanī   89
Shankha   91
Bhrūh Antara / Bhrūh Madhya / Bhrūh Agra   92
Ashrū Antara / Ashrū Madhya / Ashrū Agra   94
Kanīnaka   95
Apānga   96
Antara Vartma / Madhya Vartma / Bāhya Vartma   97
Nāsā Mūla   99
Nāsā Madhya   100
Nāsā Agra   101
Nāsā Puta   102
Ūrdhva Ganda   103
Adhah Ganda   104
Kapola Nāsā   105
Kapola Madhya   106
Oshtha   107
Hanu   108

Chibuka 110
Marma Head and Facial Massage 111

10 Shiro (Head), Grīvā (Neck) and Karna (Ear) Marmāni 115
Manyāmūla 116
Vidhuram 118
Krikātikā 120
Grīvā (4) 121
Manyāmani 122
Kantha 123
Kanthanādī 124
Mantha 125
Sirāmantha 126
Akshaka 127
Jatru 128
Karnapālī 130
Karnapāla or Karna Ūrdhva 131
Karnamūla (2) 132
Marma Massage for Back of the Head and Neck 133

11 Antaradhi (Chest and Trunk) Marmāni 135
Kakshadhara or Skandadhara 136
Apastambha 137
Hrid Marmāni (3) 138
Hridayam 140
Agra Patra 141
Stanya Mūla 142
Stanya or Chuchuka 143
Stanya Pārshva 144
Pārshva Sandhi 145
Vankri 146
Yakrut 147
Plīhā 148
Sūrya or Āmāshaya 149
Nābhi Marmāni (5) 150
Basti 152
Bhaga 153
Vankshana 154
Lohita 155
Marma Massage for the Trunk 156

12 Prushtha (Back) Marmāni 159
Amsa Phalaka 160
Prushtha or Antar Amsa (3) 161
Bruhatī 162
Vrukka 163
Kukundara 164
Kati 165
Trik 166
Marma Massage for the Back 167

13 Ūrdhva Shakhah (Upper Extremities) Marmāni 169
Ūrdhva Skandha 170

Amsa   171
Adhah Skandha   172
Kaksha   173
Bāhu Ūrvī   174
Ānī   175
Bāhū Indrabasta   176
Kūrpara   178
Bāhya Kūrpara   179
Angushtha Mūla   180
Bāhya Manibandha   181
Manibandha   182
Kūrcha Shira   183
Tala Hrida   184
Kūrcha   185
Hasta Kshipra   186
Tarjani   187
Kanīshthika   188
Marma Massage for the Arms and Hands 189

14 Adha Shakha (Lower Extremities) Marmāni 191
Sphij   193
Ūrū (2)   194
Lohitāksha   195
Medhra and Yoni Jihvā   196
Vrushana and Yoni Oshtha   197
Sakthi Ūrvī (2)   198
Jānu (2)   199
Charana (2)   200
Indrabasta (2)   202
Gulpha (2)   203
Pāda Charana   204
Pāda Kshipra   205
Pārshni   206
Pāda Madhya   207
Marma Massage for the Legs And Feet 208

INTRODUCTION TO PART THREE 209

15 Aromatherapy, Essential Oils and Attars in Āyurveda 211
16 Marmāni that Treat Channel Disturbance 219
Introduction to Srotāmsi 219
Disturbance and Treatment of Srotāmsi 220
Prāna Vaha Srotas 220
Ambu/Udaka Vaha Srotas 221
Anna Vaha Srotas 221
Rasa Vaha Srotas 222
Rakta Vaha Srotas 223
Māmsa Vaha Srotas 224
Meda Vaha Srotas 224
Asthi Vaha Srotas 225
Majjā Vaha Srotas 225

Shukra/Ārtava Vaha Srotas 226
Purīsha Vaha Srotas 227
Mūtra Vaha Srotas 227
Sveda Vaha Srotas 228
Mano Vaha Srotas 228

17 Management of Specific Disorders with Marma Chikitsā 231
Sadyah Phaladai Chikitsā – Āyurvedic First Aid 231

18 Yoga Therapy and Marmāni 239
Āsana and Marmāni 241

Appendix A ~ Specialized Āyurvedic Information 251

Appendix B ~ Specialized TCM Information 263

Appendix C ~ Marma Illustrations 269

Appendix D ~ Marmāni and Acupoints: Correspondences, Locations and Lists 291

Glossaries: Āyurvedic, Chinese and Medical 299

Bibliography and References 315

Acknowledgments 316

Index 317

List of Illustrations

Sānkhya Philosophy 8
The Five Elements at the Cellular Level 9
The Five Elements and Their Manifestation in the Body 10
Doshas, Elements and Gunas 11
Regions of the Five Subtypes of Vāta 12
Regions of the Five Subtypes of Pitta 13
Regions of the Five Subtypes of Kapha 13
Five Elements and Regions of the Body 20
Sadyah Prānahara Marmāni 23
The Koshas of the Body 27
The Seven Chakras 28
Flow of Awareness 30
Meditation 31
TCM Creation Model 34
TaiJi Symbol 35
Yin and Yang Qualities 35
TCM Promoting Cycle and Controlling Cycle 36
Sānkhya Creation Model 37
20 Gunas and Their Relationship with Yin and Yang 38
Comparison of Five Elements 39
Ayurvedic Picture of Tongue 42
TCM Picture of Tongue 42
Jingluo Meridians and Collaterals 47
TCM Organ Clock 49
Ayurveda Organ Clock 49
Īdā, Pingalā and Sushumnā Nādīs and the Seven Chakras 50
The Five Shu Points of the Pericardium Meridian 53
Cun Measurement Using the Hands 53
Angula Measurement Using the Hands 54
Anterior, Posterior and Lateral Acupuncture Points 55
Samprāpti, the Process of Disease 58
Vyādhi Mārga 60
Qualities of Āma and Agni 63
Bīja Mantras for the Seven Chakras 67
Color Therapy 68
Colors and Their Healing Effects on the Doshas 69
Bīja Mantras for the Organs 70
"So-hum" Meditation 75
The Flame of Awareness 90
The Eight Limbs of Yoga 241
TCM Pulse Diagram 256, 265
Ayurvedic Pulse Diagram 257

With more than 300 illustrations in the book, it is not practical to list each one. The beginning pages of **chapters 9 – 14** contain illustrations of the marma points for that region of the body, with focused illustrations of the individual points. For convenience, **appendix C** has full illustrations of the marma points on the whole body as well as the illustrations grouped according to the regions of the body, e.g., head and neck, trunk, arms, legs, etc. These grouped illustrations are duplicates of illustrations that begin each chapter in chapters 9 – 14. **Chapter 16,** beginning on page 219, contains all of the srotāmsi illustrations and their page numbers are listed in the Table of Contents. Finally, **chapter 18** has photos of the yogāsanas.

Foreword

Āyurveda is the mother of healing systems. As every good mother, she instills core values in her offspring and then takes pride in their development and accomplishments. This exceptional book on marma therapy is a tribute to the mother science.

Life is evolutionary. As the science of life, Āyurveda is an evolutionary system that perpetually renews itself as each generation interprets and applies its profound principles. Its core insights into life and health are as relevant to modern Western society as they are to Āyurveda's ancient native India, in the same way that the laws of physics as revealed by Isaac Newton in England remain universally applicable today. As our contemporary culture explores the importance of body, mind, and spirit in health and illness, it is reassuring that we can access the wisdom of ancient healing systems for guidance.

Human beings are multidimensional. We live simultaneously on physical, emotional, and spiritual levels. As the insights of our greatest scientists slowly permeate our collective awareness, the materialistic view of people as physical machines secreting thoughts and feelings is giving way to the recognition that human beings are networks of intelligence, inextricably interwoven into the fabric of the cosmos. With this expanded view of life, new opportunities for healing and transformation emerge. This book is an expression of this expanded perspective.

Marmas are portals into the multidimensionality of life. As junction points between consciousness and physiology, they provide a window into the interchangeability of energy and matter. According to Āyurveda, if we want to understand a person's past experiences, we only need to examine his or her body today, for every impulse of life is metabolized into physiology. Our choices become our biology. Every thought in the mind is accompanied by a corresponding shift in the body. From this viewpoint, we can see the body as the subconscious mind. Applying healing interventions to the body can have a deeply therapeutic effect on emotional as well as physical levels, just as healing interventions directed to the mind can profoundly influence the body.

Marma points can be used both diagnostically and therapeutically. In addition to serving as junction points between mind and body, they can be connecting points between patient and healer. Attentively listening to the subtle information the body offers, an Ayurvedic healer gains access to the state of balance or imbalance of a person. This can occur even when the patient and healer are the same person, for bringing attention to marma points can catalyze a self-referral healing process. Activating these vital energy-rich marma points support the body's perpetual quest for balance and healing.

This remarkable treatise on marma is destined to become a classic for generations to come, for it fulfills several important needs. Its detailed descriptions of the 117 marma points and their relationship to the fundamental mind body principles of Āyurveda is unprecedented, as are the potential therapeutic benefits of marma activation. Correlating marma therapy with the more widely recognized traditional Chinese medical system of acupuncture establishes clear channels of communication between these ancient sister healing systems. The well explained guidance on the appropriate use of essential oils and the relationship of marma therapy to yoga creates a work that is worthy of the attention of health practitioner regardless of training or orientation. With this work, Vasant Lad and Anisha Durve have given Āyurveda, and the healing arts a gift of inestimable value.

David Simon, M.D.
Co-Founder and Medical Director,
The Chopra Center for Well Being
Carlsbad, California
1951 – 2012

Preface

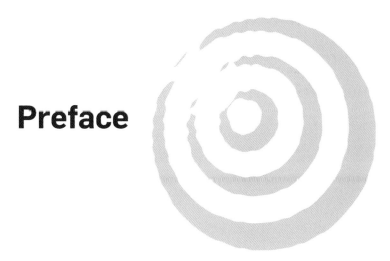

In the heart of every student burns the desire to pursue knowledge and bring it into fruition in his or her daily life. In the heart of every guru burns the flame of awareness and compassion. From this meeting of *guru* (teacher) and *shishya* (disciple), flowers greater understanding. This book is the creation of this meeting point.

Through our journey of delving deeper into the Ayurvedic system of marma points arose the desire to do a comparative study with the energetics of acupoints within the Chinese medical system. We were fascinated by the multifaceted nature of these energy points and how this knowledge flourished within both cultures. Combining our diverse backgrounds of almost forty years of clinical work in the Ayurvedic and acupuncture fields, we were able to create a unique integrated work pooling our clinical observations and insights. This project culminated in a desire to share this wealth of information with practitioners and students of both traditions in the form of a book.

About Vasant Lad

When I was a student of Āyurveda, I studied the ancient scriptures of Sushruta, Charaka and Vagbhata. These teachings were a springboard for me to further develop marma chikitsā. After commencing my practice in private clinics and hospitals, I developed the art of utilizing marmāni as diagnostic and therapeutic tools. I collected my own database of clinical observations and taught the wisdom from my personal experience to students in both India and America.

This book comes out of my years as a clinical practitioner and from Anisha's training and enthusiasm for these two beautiful systems of healing. Anisha was a very talented, sincere and dedicated student of Āyurveda who was greatly inspired by these teachings because of her background in Traditional Chinese Medicine. Then the thought arose in her heart to write an integrated book for practitioners, students and laypersons alike.

About Anisha Durve

Through the journey of my medical training, I pursued the vast healing traditions of Acupuncture and Āyurveda simultaneously. I believed the integration of both medical systems provided a truly rich understanding of the human body/mind/spirit complex as a vehicle to develop our fullest creative and energetic potential. Within both traditions, the energetic points especially fascinated me, particularly in the ways this knowledge thrived in both cultures. I felt compelled to deeply explore the energy points by organizing a comparative study of their personal development within both medical traditions.

This heart-felt desire took shape with the blessings of my Ayurvedic mentor, Dr. Vasant Lad. I fashioned a project over a two-year period to discuss each marma individually in its myriad facets and compare it to the energetics of the acupoints within the Chinese medical tradition. Then we collaborated on comparing the two systems with this book being the wonderful result. This collaboration culminates in a resource book that will hopefully bring expanded knowledge, awareness and healing into the lives of all who read and practice the wisdom in its pages.

The Use of Sanskrit

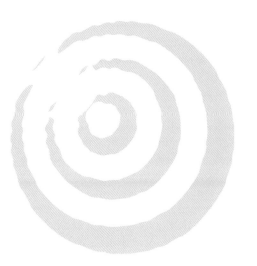

Knowledge of Āyurveda originates in the Sanskrit language. Sanskrit is a precise phonetic language that uses a set of written symbols not familiar to most Westerners. The phonetic representation of Sanskrit words using the English alphabet is called transliteration. We can transliterate Sanskrit to English characters, but not every sound translates directly. There are quite a few sounds that do not exist in the English language, requiring special characters to represent them accurately.

One example is वात ,which translates to vāta. The first 'a' in vāta is a 'long a', as in "father"; it is held for two beats. The second 'a' is a 'short a', as in "what." Another example is a sound somewhere between an 'i', a 'u' and an 'r' that occurs in the word प्रकृति. This word is transliterated as prakṛti. The 'ṛ' is pronounced as the 'ri' in the English spelling of the word Krishna. To make things even more complicated, among those who use Sanskrit the 'ṛ' is pronounced in northern India as the 'i' in "it" and in southern India as the 'u' sound in "root." Because of the regional variations in pronunciation, in this book both ru and ri are found in place of the technically correct 'ṛ'.

Another consideration is that the trailing 'a' in Sanskrit words is sometimes omitted because of the influence of the Hindi language. It is included in many of the words in this book. The trailing 'a' is also subject to grammatical changes depending on the letters that follow it and, for simplicity's sake, we generally ignore these rules. For example, the word *meda* (fat) can be transliterated as *medo, medas* and meda, depending on the word following it. Ordinarily, we use the most common form, meda, so that you, the reader, will have to learn only the one word. Of course, it would be wonderful if all our readers began the study of Sanskrit, inspired by the knowledge available in these ancient texts, but it is not our purpose here to teach that language.

In this book we have chosen to use transliteration characters only for long vowels, denoted by an overscore or macron character, and for the 'nya' sound denoted by 'ñ'. The pronunciations of the vowels are:

a as in about; **ā** as in father

i as in ink; **ī** as in fee

u as in put; **ū** as in food

e as in pay; **ai** as in I

o as in corn; **au** as in loud

Editor's Note

I so enjoyed working with Dr. Vasant Lad on creating his book, *The Complete Book of Ayurvedic Home Remedies,* and I learned so much from this living encyclopedia of knowledge, that I was thrilled when I got a call from Wynn Werner, the Administrator of the Ayurvedic Institute, asking me to edit the final version of this book. Once again I got to spend many delightful hours with Dr. Lad, listening to him recount spiritual stories and recite sutras packed with knowledge, sharing gales of laughter. As before, we sat on the floor of his living room as I read through the material for his approval and corrections, while his wife Usha cooked or prepared Ayurvedic concoctions and their young grandson played and explored around us. It was an honor and a privilege to be there. And though my knowledge is like a thimbleful of water compared to Dr. Lad's ocean, he always treated me with great respect, listened with openness to my remarks, and replied with patience and thoroughness to my questions.

In the course of our conversations, which I recorded in order not to miss any important points or nuances, Dr. Lad occasionally went off on interesting tangents, telling stories, expounding spiritual principles, elucidating subtleties of Ayurvedic knowledge. Then he'd stop, look at me and say, "But – probably that won't go into the book!" And we'd both break into laughter. Students of Dr. Lad, and those who have heard him lecture or teach, are familiar with these poetic flights of insight and how wonderful they are. With the permission of the authors, I have included a few of these in sidebars throughout the book. They go beyond the matter-of-fact, clinical tone of this marvelous textbook of Marma Therapy, but I believe they will enrich your experience and understanding as they have enhanced my own.

~ Jack Forem

Introduction

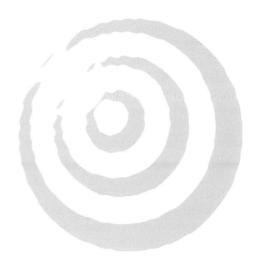

Over the past several decades, the concept of complementary medicine has increasingly taken root among Western health care professionals, bringing a growing awareness of the many existing medical traditions both ancient and new. While these traditions were at first marginalized and tended to be viewed as "alternatives" to mainstream medical practice, it is now clear that each tradition has its place in health care and its own unique contribution to make to our collective understanding of health and disease. More and more, the strengths and insights from these traditions are being integrated into a richer, more whole vision of healing. Both practitioners and patients benefit from the broadened perspectives, deeper insights and augmented array of therapeutic modalities.

Āyurveda, literally the "science of life," is known to have existed 5000 years ago, and is generally considered by many scholars and historians as the oldest living system of medicine and health care in the world. Its eight principal branches (gynecology and obstetrics, pediatrics, ophthalmology, otolaryngology, toxicology, geriatrics, surgery and internal medicine) encompass the many specialties and subspecialties of medicine as it is practiced today. As the "science of life," the focus of Āyurveda has always been on creating a balanced, vibrant state of healthy mind, body and spirit: life lived with vitality, expanded awareness and in harmonious relationship with the environment, the laws of nature and the cosmos, and our fellow beings on our beautiful planet. Āyurveda has much to offer modern medicine, which, despite its remarkable achievements, sometimes lacks this holistic perspective.

This state of total health can be achieved through the vast array of preventative and rejuvenative teachings and practices of Āyurveda: lifestyle and dietary recommendations, herbal tonics, detoxification regimens, exercise methods such as yoga postures,[1] meditation and more. Whether for prevention, healing or rejuvenation, all of these are *individually tailored* for maximum benefit, according to a person's *prakruti* or individual constitution. This is perhaps the greatest contribution of Āyurveda to the field of medicine.

Indeed, Āyurveda's sophisticated analysis and depth of insight regarding an individual's unique constitution is without parallel in the world of medicine. Because every individual is different, all diagnosis and treatment are specific to the individual and cannot be standardized.

Traditional Chinese Medicine (TCM) has also flourished for thousands of years. Remarkably, many of the principles within the two traditions are strikingly common. Both these ancient Eastern healing traditions are rooted in the understanding that we are connected to the cosmos and that our health or illness is inherently related to living in harmony with nature. Both systems view the individual as an energetic entity who functions through the harmonious interaction of body, mind and spirit.

In this paradigm, the more concrete layers of the body are suffused by a subtler life energy, known in Āyurveda as *prāna* and in TCM as *qi* or *chi*. The body is seen less as a collection of limbs, organs and physical systems, and more as a network of energy pathways, a living, constantly changing flow.

---

1. Called yogāsanas. In Sanskrit, this is the correct combined form of the two terms yoga and āsanas.

Smooth, harmonious, balanced flow brings health and vitality; blocked flow and stagnant energy bring sluggishness, mental dullness and disease.

Many of the practices of both TCM and Āyurveda aim to keep the channels of energy open and flowing. This is particularly true of the use of energy points, known as *marmāni* or marma points in Āyurveda and acupoints or acupuncture points in TCM.

The primary focus of this book is on Āyurveda and the system of marmāni[2]. Information about TCM and its system of acupoints has been included along with the Āyurvedic material to demonstrate both parallels and differences and to stimulate in-depth study and research.

The acceptance and use of acupuncture has grown in many countries and cultures. In the West, it is perhaps best known for its now well-documented usefulness in pain management. By contrast, Āyurveda's marma system has not shared in this popular acclaim, and has been until recently a lost treasure, now experiencing a revival in the modern day practice of Āyurveda. The authors hope that this book will play a role in the revival of this valuable science, and will provide a medium for both systems to learn from each other. It is also their sincere wish that this book will open more doors for an integrated multi-disciplinary approach to healing.

No medical system is complete in itself. Every system has its limitation. Modern medicine verges on the miraculous for emergencies and acute conditions, but offers less help for chronic ailments. Similarly, Āyurveda offers comprehensive strategies for prevention and excellent care and management for chronic illnesses, but its expertise is not in critical, acute care. The ideal medical model will integrate ancient wisdom with the modern medical approach, so that the combined strengths of each will provide the best possible care for every patient.

This book is divided into three main sections, as described below.

Part One

Part 1 begins with an introduction to Āyurveda and marma therapy in the context of ancient Indian philosophy. We then introduce TCM and begin our exploration of some of its similarities to Āyurveda, as well as some significant differences. The Āyurvedic view of the origin and development of disease is briefly explained, followed by a discussion of Āyurvedic treatment modalities in general and marma therapy in particular. Part 1 closes with guidelines for health practitioners for the proper – and most effective – practice of marma therapy.

✳ Chapter 1 introduces Sāṅkhya, one of the principal branches of Indian philosophy, and how it informs the Āyurvedic medical tradition. Some of the basic concepts that constitute the framework of Āyurvedic language are defined and discussed, including dosha theory, constitution, disease and treatment.

✳ Chapter 2 presents an overview of the marmāni in their development, historical use, mechanism of action and myriad classifications: function, location, elements, doshas and doshic subtypes, organs, srotāmsi (energetic and bodily pathways) and vitality.

✳ Chapter 3 portrays the relationship between the energy points and the mind, emotions, perception and consciousness.

✳ Chapter 4 introduces Traditional Chinese Medicine (TCM) and compares it to Āyurveda starting with their creation models, moving on to their views of health, disease and pain, and briefly touching upon their methods of treatment.

✳ Chapter 5 continues the comparative study between Āyurveda and TCM by closely examining the understanding of channels, energy points and measurement methods in both systems.

✳ Chapter 6 discusses the Āyurvedic view of the pathogenesis or origin of disease, pathways and stages of disease development, and various etiological factors. The relevance of marmāni at each stage of the disease process is introduced.

✳ Chapter 7 introduces the fundamentals of Āyurvedic *chikitsā* or therapy, including marma therapy.

✳ Chapter 8 offers various techniques for marma stimulation, along with practitioner guidelines.

---

2. Marma points are Ayurvedic energy points. Marma (technically, marman) is singular, marmāni is the plural form.

Part Two

Part 2 provides a schematic presentation of the 117 marmāni of Āyurveda and the role of each one in treatment and healing.

* An important, detailed introduction to this section is provided on page 77.

* Chapters 9–14 discuss each one of the 117 marmāni individually, organized by six body regions: head and face, neck and ears, chest and abdomen, back, upper extremities, lower extremities.

* The energetics of each marma is discussed in relation to anatomical location, associated doshic subtypes, actions, indications, treatment and corresponding acupoint.

Part Three

Part 3 demonstrates how marma therapy supports and complements other Āyurvedic therapies, and discusses in some detail a variety of health conditions the use of energy points can help to relieve.

* Chapter 15 explains the art of aromatherapy and the use of essential oils in relation to the energy points.

* Chapter 16 discusses the fourteen principal channels (srotāmsi) and the energy points that regulate their function and treat their disturbances.

* Chapter 17 considers a number of medical conditions organized into broad categories and the energy points associated with them.

* Chapter 18 illustrates yoga therapy in the context of Āyurveda and how particular yoga postures stimulate the energy points.

This work is our humble effort to systematically organize the marma points of Āyurveda, and to present detailed information about their diagnostic and therapeutic scope. It is the first book to begin a comparative study of Āyurveda and the Chinese medical system, with regard to the energy points. It is the intention of the authors to inspire students and practitioners alike, from all backgrounds and medical systems including Āyurveda, Traditional Chinese Medicine, allopathy, osteopathy, massage, chiropractic, yoga and so on, to put this knowledge to use in their own development as clinicians. It is our desire that this book may serve as a practical guidebook for both students and practitioners.

Through the fertile ground of this knowledge, may the seeds of wisdom and compassion bloom within the heart of every practitioner.

Introduction to Part One

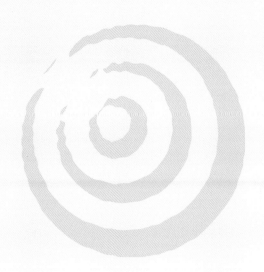

Every science has two aspects: the theoretical and the practical or applied. In every discipline from Astronomy to Zoology, and certainly in medicine and the healing professions, the day-to-day practical work rests on a body of knowledge, a foundation of solid principles. Part 1 of this book presents the theoretical knowledge at the heart of Āyurveda, the information needed in order to apply the practical information contained in parts 2 and 3 most effectively. Marma chikitsā—Āyurvedic marma therapy—is essentially a hands-on practice. But, it is based upon ancient, field-tested knowledge that must be absorbed, digested and assimilated in order for the clinical work to bring the desired healing.

The knowledge contained in part 1 includes:

* An introduction to the principles and philosophical framework of Āyurveda, placed within the context of the Vedic knowledge of India.

* An introduction to the marma points of Āyurveda—their history, mechanisms of action, therapeutic uses including for pain relief, and more.

* The spiritual dimension: how marma chikitsā can assist in emotional healing and spiritual unfoldment.

* A two-chapter comparison of Āyurveda and Traditional Chinese Medicine (TCM), with special regard to the channels (meridians in TCM, srotāmsi and nāḍīs in Āyurveda) and energy points (acupoints and marmāni). We point out that TCM and Āyurveda are embedded in a similar world view that places the individual in intimate relationship with nature and the cosmos, and that both view the human body more as fields of ever-flowing and shifting energy than as solid material structures.

* A discussion of the precisely delineated Āyurvedic understanding of how disease develops through distinct stages, and the importance of this knowledge for the clinician, helping to determine how far the disease has progressed and what is needed at each stage for an effective cure.

* An overview of Āyurvedic chikitsā, the various types of therapy in Āyurveda and how knowledge of marmāni can be employed within and alongside each of these healing modalities

* An introduction to marma chikitsā; techniques and guidelines to help the practitioner achieve maximum results.

Introduction to Āyurveda

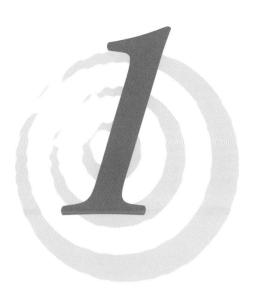

Āyurveda, literally translated as the "Science of Life," is a 5,000 year old system of medicine that originated in India. It is a profound union of holistic medicine, philosophy and spirituality. The wisdom of this ancient tradition of healing offers a comprehensive understanding of body, mind and soul and teaches us how to live in harmony with ourselves, our environment, and each other. Its deep insight into living each moment fully, experiencing the sweet nectar that life has to offer, is the jewel of Āyurveda.

Āyurveda embraces Sānkhya (one of the six classical systems of Indian philosophy) as the foundation of its concept of the body. Said to be formulated by the legendary sage Kāpila, Sānkhya describes the process of creation and the journey of consciousness as it evolves into matter. Before creation, there is neither light nor darkness, neither form nor name. There is only an expansive state of pure existence called *Avyakta* (the unmanifest), also known as *Brahma*. (*Bra* is the Sanskrit root meaning expansion.) This parallels the view in modern science that we live in an ever-expanding universe.

From Brahma emerge both *Purusha* (unbounded pure consciousness, considered by Sānkhya as masculine) and *Prakruti* (the infinite creative potential, the Divine Mother). Both Purusha and Prakruti are eternal, timeless, immeasurable, and divine.

Purusha is pure, undifferentiated, silent consciousness, an ocean without waves. It is pure existence, transcendental being, choiceless, passive awareness that does not take part in creation. It is termed *sākshin*—the witnessing awareness. Prakruti is the creative will that expresses herself through the form, color, name, shape and attribute of every object. Purusha is being; Prakruti is becoming. Purusha is silent and unmoving; Prakruti is active and dynamic. Before the creation of the universe, Purusha and Prakruti are merged together in wholeness. Then the perfect equilibrium is disturbed; Prakruti starts to vibrate, throb and pulsate. Within the core of her pulsation, there is an intense cosmic will that has the notion,

"I am one, I want to become many." Hence, Prakruti becomes the womb of all creation, from which springs forth the birth of a beautiful child, the universe.

In her process of becoming, the first expression of Prakruti is *Mahad*—the supreme cosmic intelligence, which is conscious of consciousness. This intelligence permeates every aspect of creation. Mahad manifests into *Ahamkāra* (the I-former), which gives all things an identity. Otherwise known as the ego, ahamkāra exists even at the cellular level and provides each cell with a form that distinguishes it from other cells. From Ahamkāra evolve the three *gunas* or three distinct qualities that pervade all creation and are used to describe Prakruti. These are *sattva*—the principle of purity and equilibrium, *rajas*—the principle of movement and activity, and *tamas*—the principle of inertia and manifestation.

Both on the cosmic scale and within individual awareness, when the three gunas are perfectly balanced, Prakruti and Purusha merge together in Avyakta, the unmanifest state. The moment this balance is disturbed, Prakruti differentiates from Purusha, leading to the creation of the universe. Every aspect of creation can be described in terms of the gunas. For example, each guna is involved in the simple process of looking. Sattva is the observer; it is purity, clarity and perception. Rajas is the act of observation or movement that bridges the observer and the object. Tamas is the object of perception. When the observer is conscious of being separate from the observation, ahamkāra is involved. In its self-perceived separateness, the ego tends toward judgment and viewpoint, assessing every experience as good or bad, satisfactory or unsatisfactory, pleasurable or painful. At the moment when the observer merges with the object of observation, judgment and conflict dissolve. There is only awareness of awareness, or being conscious of consciousness. *Samādhi* (equilibrated consciousness) is the supreme bliss experienced when awareness transcends

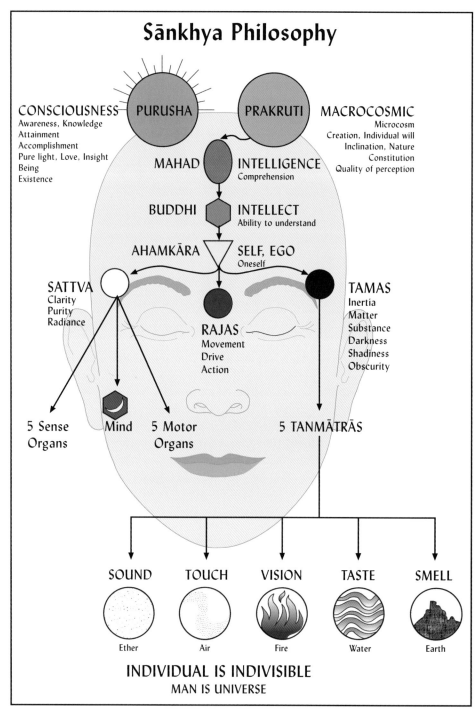

Sānkhya Philosophy

CONSCIOUSNESS
Awareness, Knowledge
Attainment
Accomplishment
Pure light, Love, Insight
Being
Existence

PURUSHA

PRAKRUTI

MACROCOSMIC
Microcosm
Creation, Individual will
Inclination, Nature
Constitution
Quality of perception

MAHAD — INTELLIGENCE
Comprehension

BUDDHI — INTELLECT
Ability to understand

AHAMKĀRA — SELF, EGO
Oneself

SATTVA
Clarity
Purity
Radiance

TAMAS
Inertia
Matter
Substance
Darkness
Shadiness
Obscurity

RAJAS
Movement
Drive
Action

5 Sense Organs   Mind   5 Motor Organs   5 TANMĀTRĀS

SOUND	TOUCH	VISION	TASTE	SMELL
Ether	Air	Fire	Water	Earth

INDIVIDUAL IS INDIVISIBLE
MAN IS UNIVERSE

ual mahad or intellect (*buddhi*). Likewise, there is a cosmic Ahamkāra and individual ahamkāra, a cosmic Mind and an individual mind, a cosmic Soul (*Paramātman*) and an individual soul (*jīvātman*).

It is fascinating to view modern physiology through the lens of Sānkhya philosophy. Within the body, every cell is a center of awareness, of Brahma. Likewise, every cell has cellular intelligence, mahad. Through that cellular intelligence, cellular choice is exercised, and the cell selects the appropriate nutrients. For example, plasma cells "choose" plasma protein. Red blood cells "choose" hemoglobin or iron molecules. Muscle cells "choose" muscle protein. The cells of the bones "choose" calcium-magnesium-zinc molecules. The ceaseless intercommunication that takes place between two cells is the flow of intelligence or cellular *prāna*. Prāna is the flow of communication between purusha, prakruti, mahad, ahamkāra and physiology, according to the Sānkhya scheme of creation.

In this flow, from Mahad the three gunas further differentiate themselves. Sattva generates the mind, the five motor organs and the five cognitive organs. The five motor organs, *karmendriyāni*, include the hands, feet, vocal cord, genitals and excretory organs. The five sensory faculties and their cogni-

the three gunas and merges into the oneness that is beyond these three qualities.

Sānkhya's description of creation is intimately connected to the manifestation of the individual being. The term Purusha denotes both a cosmic being and an individual. The individual is indivisible and an energetic focal point of the universe. Each individual is a unique expression of cosmic consciousness. Hence, Prakruti is the individual constitution, while Purusha is the individual soul (*ātman*). According to Sānkhya, there exists a cosmic Mahad or universal intelligence and an individ-

tive organs, *jñānendriyāni*, perceive sound, touch, sight, taste and smell. The cognitive organs are related to their respective organs of perception and the objects of perception. In the act of touching, for example, the skin, which is the organ of perception, is sattva, the process of touching that gives rise to the tactile sensation is rajas, and the object being touched is tamas. Each and every sensory experience exemplifies the functional integrity between sattva, rajas and tamas, which are perpetually interacting.

Sattva guna expresses itself in the creation of the organic universe. Tamas manifests the inorganic universe. Tamas guna includes the five gross elements, termed *pañcha mahābhūta*, and the five subtle elements, termed *tanmātrā*. The pañcha mahābhūta are *ākāsha* (space[1]), *vāyu* (air), *tejas* (fire), *āpa* (water) and *pruthivī* (earth). Each gross element (pañcha mahābhūta) has a subtle element (tanmātrā) that corresponds to it: *shabda* (sound/space), *sparsha* (touch/air), *rūpa* (vision/fire), *rasa* (taste/water) and *gandha* (smell/earth). Rajas guna expresses itself through the interaction between sattva and tamas; that is, by linking the mind and the cognitive and motor organs with the five elements and five tanmātrā. For sattva guna to express itself through the cognitive and motor organs, the action of rajas guna is required; without rajas there is no creation to move from the unmanifest state (sattva) to the manifest state (tamas).

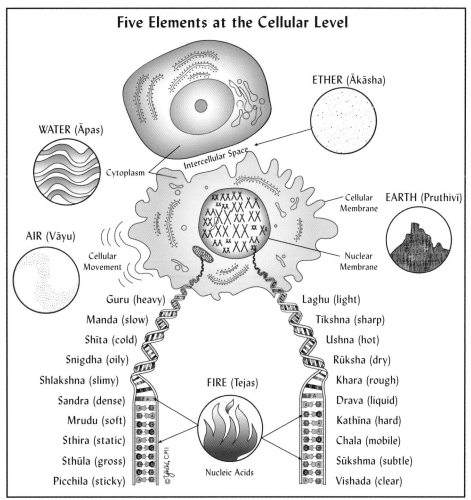

Five Elements at the Cellular Level

ETHER (Ākāsha)

WATER (Āpas)

Intercellular Space

Cytoplasm

Cellular Membrane

EARTH (Pruthivī)

AIR (Vāyu)

Cellular Movement

Nuclear Membrane

Guru (heavy)
Manda (slow)
Shīta (cold)
Snigdha (oily)
Shlakshna (slimy)
Sandra (dense)
Mrudu (soft)
Sthira (static)
Sthūla (gross)
Picchila (sticky)

Laghu (light)
Tīkshna (sharp)
Ushna (hot)
Rūksha (dry)
Khara (rough)
Drava (liquid)
Kathīna (hard)
Chala (mobile)
Sūkshma (subtle)
Vishada (clear)

FIRE (Tejas)

Nucleic Acids

The Five Elements

• •

Equivalent to the modern scientific theory of the big bang, the ancient Vedic philosophy of India attributes the origin of creation to the vibration of the eternal cosmic sound, *aum*. The first subtle element to arise is sound (*shabda*), and through its powerful vibrations, it gives birth to cosmic space. Thus, there is an intrinsic connection between etheric space and the tanmātrā (measurement) of sound.

Each element, in turn, precipitates from its preceding element. As we trace this sequential unfoldment, it is helpful to keep in mind that the elements, the processes by which they are generated, and the dynamics of their actions and interactions are nothing but the transformations and permutations of consciousness, as waves are simply the shapes and movements of water.

Within the field of space, the vibration or pulsation of the air element (sparsha) is created. The pulsation of air in space generates radiant heat. This is fire (rūpa).

Because of the radiant heat of fire, consciousness is melted into water (rasa). In turn, water "crystallizes" into solid earth (gandha). Each gross element is related to a specific subtle element and to the tanmātrā of the elements that precede it. Thus, air is affiliated with two tanmātrā, sound and touch, although touch is prevalent. And so on, to the level of earth, which contains all five tanmātrā, with smell as its principal tanmātrā.

The five elements of creation are manifestations of consciousness and represent specific types of energy. Space is expansive, omnipresent consciousness that is comparable to nuclear energy. Air is electrical energy; fire is hot, penetrating consciousness and is radiant energy; water is chemical energy, because water is a universal chemical solvent. Finally, earth is physical, mechanical energy. Each of these in turn has specific classifications as shown in table 45 on page 251 in appendix A and table 52 on page 263 in appendix B.

The pañcha mahābhūta (five elements) are all present in the structure and physical formation of the human body. Each structure is imbued with the properties of its corresponding element. Even at the microscopic level, one can observe the relationships between the elements and the structure of a single cell. Ether is the space occu-

---

1. Ether is the literal translation of ākāsha. We use the equivalent but more familiar term "space."

Five Elements and Their Manifestation in the Body

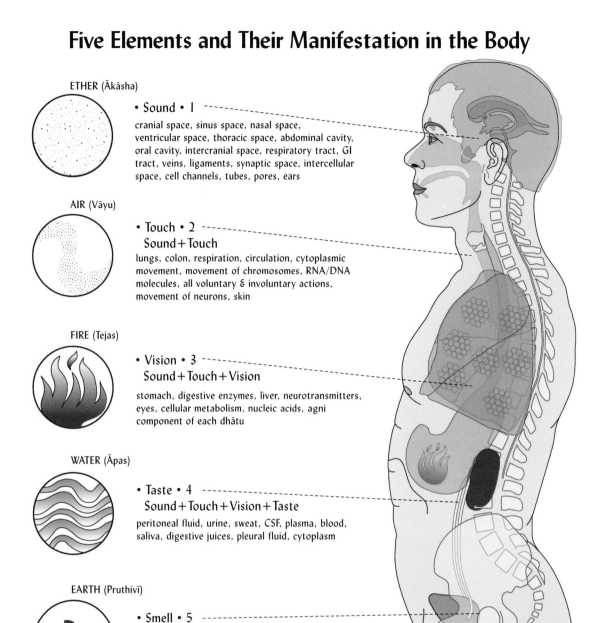

ETHER (Ākāsha)

• Sound • 1

cranial space, sinus space, nasal space, ventricular space, thoracic space, abdominal cavity, oral cavity, intercranial space, respiratory tract, GI tract, veins, ligaments, synaptic space, intercellular space, cell channels, tubes, pores, ears

AIR (Vāyu)

• Touch • 2
Sound + Touch

lungs, colon, respiration, circulation, cytoplasmic movement, movement of chromosomes, RNA/DNA molecules, all voluntary & involuntary actions, movement of neurons, skin

FIRE (Tejas)

• Vision • 3
Sound + Touch + Vision

stomach, digestive enzymes, liver, neurotransmitters, eyes, cellular metabolism, nucleic acids, agni component of each dhātu

WATER (Āpas)

• Taste • 4
Sound + Touch + Vision + Taste

peritoneal fluid, urine, sweat, CSF, plasma, blood, saliva, digestive juices, pleural fluid, cytoplasm

EARTH (Pruthivī)

• Smell • 5
Sound + Touch + Vision + Taste + Smell

pelvic bone, skeletal structure, bones, cartilage, muscle, tendons, nails, hair, teeth, flesh, skin, feces

pied by the cell, air carries out cellular movement, fire is responsible for cellular metabolic activity, water is the cytoplasm, and earth is represented by the cellular and nuclear membranes that provide structure and support.

Ākāsha (space) offers the space and freedom for each cell and organism to exist. Without space, there is no possibility of communication among the cells. Ākāsha predominates in all spaces and cavities of the body including channels, joints, tubes, pores, arteries and veins. It is present in the thoracic space, abdominal space, intracranial space, synaptic space and intercellular space. It is also the primary element in the respiratory tract, gastrointestinal tract and oral cavity, as these are

usually hollow passageways. All the open systems in the body, the respiratory or gastrointestinal system, are defined spaces created by etheric space, ākāsha.

Vāyu or air is the principle of movement that governs all sensory stimuli and motor responses, voluntary and involuntary actions, respiration and circulation. It governs all subtle cytoplasmic and microscopic movement, including that of RNA and DNA molecules. The major sites of air in the body are within the colon and lungs.

Tejas or fire governs body temperature. It is the psycho-physiological radiant heat energy, directing all transformative processes of life. Described as the light of knowledge, it is the energy for understanding, comprehension and intelligence. It is responsible for creation of hunger and thirst, and guides the process of digestion, absorption, and transformation of food into energy and energy into consciousness. All digestive enzymes of the stomach, liver and pancreas function through the fire element. Tejas also manifests as the perception of color, vision, form, luster and illumination. It is responsible for color in skin complexion and luster of the eyes. At the cellular level, fire transforms sensory input into intelligence.

Āpas or water appears in the human body as liquid, aqueous, unctuous, soft and slimy substances. Water predominates in all bodily secretions and excretions, including cerebrospinal fluid, glandular secretions, pleural fluid and digestive juices. It is also a significant part of plasma, blood, sweat, saliva and urine.

Finally, pruthivī, the earth element, is responsible for all physical embodiment. It creates body parts that are thick, stable, massive, heavy and coarse. It manifests in all solid substances, such as bones, cartilage, tendons and nails. Earth is a substantial part of hair, teeth, skin, flesh and feces. The earth element plays an important role in all structural aspects of the body. All bodily structures are created by earth.

The Three Doshas

. . . .

As the five elements govern the physical structure of the human body, so the three *doshas* influence its function. Each of the three doshas is derived from a unique permutation and combination of the five elements. All five elements are present in each dosha, but the predominance of space and air creates vāta, the principle of movement. The predominance of fire and water constitute pitta, the principle of transformation. Likewise, the predominance of water and earth precipitates *kapha*, the principle of substance. The three doshas are an elegant description of biological, physiological and psychological organization. When this organization is disturbed, Ayurvedic clinicians focus on restoring doshic balance.

The three doshas are present in every cell, organ, tissue, system and organism, and at all levels of consciousness. The salient features of the doshas are:

❋ They have functional integrity amongst themselves, between doshic subtypes and between organs.

❋ They are a protective mechanism or barrier that responds to internal and external changes.

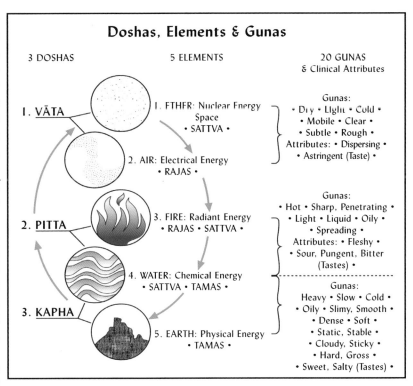

❋ They play a critical role in the creation of an individual's constitution.

Though the doshas have different or even opposite qualities, still they work together harmoniously, in functional integrity. And they control and balance each other. For example, if *pitta* is high, vāta and kapha, by their cold qualities, will balance pitta. If vāta is high, pitta and kapha will balance the vāta, in order to maintain a unique psychophysiology.

Each *dosha* has specific qualities, functions and locations to describe its nature. These qualities are termed gunas and describe most phenomena. The gunas are: *guru* (heavy), *laghu* (light), *manda* (slow), *tīkshna* (sharp), *shīta* (cold), *ushna* (hot), *snigdha* (oily), *rūksha* (dry), *shlakshna* (slimy), *khara* (rough), *sandra* (dense), *drava* (liquid), *mrudu* (soft), *kathīna* (hard), *sthira* (static), *chala* (mobile), *sthūla* (gross), *sūkshma* (subtle), *picchila* (sticky), *avila* (cloudy) and *vishada* (clear).

In reality, there is only one vāta, one pitta and one kapha dosha, and they are present throughout the body. But because of changing structures and functions, each dosha is also differentiated into five subtypes—related to the five elements—as described below.

Vāta

Vāta, the principle of movement, is formed from the combination of the space and air elements. Its primary qualities are dry, light, cold, subtle, mobile, rough and clear. It is present in the colon, pelvic girdle, bones and thighs. It also has an affinity for the ears, nose and lungs. Vāta governs all biological movement, including inhala-

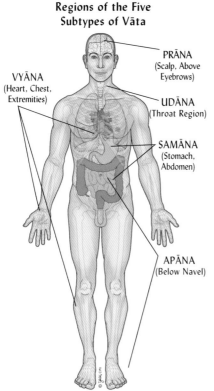

Regions of the Five
Subtypes of Vāta

PRANA
(Scalp, Above
Eyebrows)

VYANA
(Heart, Chest,
Extremities)

UDANA
(Throat Region)

SAMANA
(Stomach,
Abdomen)

APANA
(Below Navel)

tion, exhalation, ingestion, ejection, absorption, assimilation and elimination as well as circulation. It governs the expression of thoughts, feelings, and the whole range of emotions. It is responsible for *tantra*—the mechanisms of the body, and *yantra*—the entire engineering of the body. Vāta is the active force in an organism. All the bodily *dhātus* (tissues) as well as pitta and kapha dosha are static, in the sense that vāta is responsible for their movements and activities within the body.

Vāta is classified according to five subtypes (*vāyus*): *prāna, udāna, samāna, apāna* and *vyāna*. In health, all five of these vāyus function harmoniously.

Prāna vāyu is present principally in the cranial cavity and governs higher cerebral activity. It rules the functions of the mind such as looking, listening, breathing, thinking and feeling. It is responsible for stimulating the flow of optical and auditory perception into sensation, sensation into feelings, feelings into emotion, and emotion into thought. Prāna stimulates transformation and then experience through tejas.

Udāna vāyu resides predominantly in the diaphragm and moves upwards into the respiratory and thoracic cavity, the nose and throat, and the brain. It is responsible for respiratory function, coughing, spitting, vomiting, and sneezing. It governs all effort and upward movement such as rising, standing, climbing and jumping. Udāna also has a role in color complexion, memory, and self-awakening.

Samāna vāyu is present in the umbilical area, and has an affinity for the stomach, duodenum, small intes-

tine and solar plexus area. It governs digestion, absorption, assimilation and transformation of food into chyme. Food is brought from the mouth to the stomach by prāna but samāna vāyu churns and processes the chyme. Two to three hours after food enters the stomach, samāna vāyu opens the pyloric valve, allowing the food to progress to the duodenum, jejunum, and ileum. Samāna vāyu is a form of *agni*, the digestive energy.

Apāna vāyu is present mostly in the pelvic cavity and is responsible for creation of the natural urges of urination, defecation, and flatulence. It governs the movement of the colon, ejection of flatus, and elimination of urine and feces. It is present in the sacroiliac plexus (second *chakra* or *svādhishthāna*) and influences the function of the testicles, ovaries and fallopian tubes. It rules menstruation, ejaculation and ejection as well as expulsion of the fetus during delivery.

Vyāna vāyu resides in the heart and governs arterial and venous circulation, lymphatic circulation and heart rate. It is responsible for all physical activity, facilitates movement of the joints and controls all voluntary and involuntary movements.

Pitta

Pitta dosha, the biological fire component, is a combination of the fire and water elements. Its predominant qualities are hot, sharp, light, oily, liquid and spreading. It has an affinity for the stomach, intestines, liver and gallbladder. It is also present in the skin, eyes, gray matter of the brain, blood (*rakta*), heart (*hrid*), sebaceous secretion (*lasīkā*), and sweat (*sveda*). Pitta is primarily responsible for digestion, absorption and assimilation. It governs body temperature, color complexion and the higher mental functions of comprehension, recognition, discrimination, justification and evaluation. The five subtypes are: *pāchaka, rañjaka, sādhaka, ālochaka* and *bhrājaka*. All these *subdoshas* of pitta have functional coordination.

Ālochaka pitta, present in the eyes, absorbs light and facilitates color perception. It governs the function of the retina, optic disc, lens, cornea and the color of the eyes. It regulates sight and optical perception. Ālochaka pitta enhances visual acuity and maintains the luster of the eyes. It is responsible for three-dimensional visual perception.

Sādhaka pitta is present in the heart, gray matter of the brain, and the synaptic space. It maintains normal functions of the mind—memory, intellect and ego. It governs cognition, comprehension, concentration and awareness. Sādhaka pitta in the brain processes sensory perception into intellectual understanding, while sādhaka pitta in the heart processes thoughts and emotions into love and compassion. Sādhaka pitta in the heart is the seat of devotion (*bhakti*).

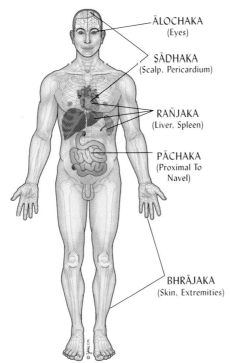

Regions of the Five
Subtypes of Pitta

ĀLOCHAKA
(Eyes)

SĀDHAKA
(Scalp, Pericardium)

RAÑJAKA
(Liver, Spleen)

PĀCHAKA
(Proximal To Navel)

BHRĀJAKA
(Skin, Extremities)

Rañjaka pitta resides primarily in the liver, spleen and blood. It controls the production, preservation, destruction and smooth consistency of blood. It also produces bile, hemoglobin, liver enzymes and cholesterol and aids in the metabolism of fat, sugars and alcohol. Rañjaka pitta also gives color to the eyes, blood, urine and feces.

Pāchaka pitta resides mainly in the small intestine, stomach and other digestive organs. It differentiates foodstuff into essential (*sāra*) and non-essential (*kitta*) components. It digests, absorbs and assimilates nutrients from the diet into one's consciousness.

Lastly, *bhrājaka pitta* is located in the skin and subcutaneous tissue. It regulates skin temperature, complexion, luster and texture. It stimulates capillary circulation and absorbs medicated oils, pastes and ointments. It also maintains a barrier that offers protection from the external environment. Bhrājaka pitta in the skin also has the important function of stereognosis—three dimensional tactile perception—which is why a blind person can recognize, through touch, the difference between a chair, table, coin, pencil, and so on.

Kapha

Kapha is the protoplasmic biological substance, plasma, derived mainly from the earth and water elements. Its qualities include heavy, slow, liquid, cold, oily, sticky, slimy/smooth, dense, hard, static, cloudy, soft, and gross. It is the constructing, cementing material that gives structure and stability to the body. Any new tissue

or cell is created by kapha. It maintains growth, nutrition and nourishment, providing the body with strength and energy. The repair, rehabilitation and reconstruction of all body parts and tissues are facilitated by this dosha. It provides oleation and lubrication to nourish joints and tissues. Kapha is responsible for the retention of psychological and cellular memory. It has an affinity for the stomach, chest, lungs and lymphatic system. It also exists in the kidneys, pancreas, adipose tissue and bodily fluids. Kapha has a slow sustained action compared to the other doshas. It is present in all connective tissues, where subconscious memories are stored.

The five subtypes of kapha are: *tarpaka, bodhaka, avalambaka, kledaka* and *shleshaka*. These five subdoshas work in conjunction with each other as one kapha principle.

Tarpaka kapha is located largely in the white matter of the brain, the cerebrospinal fluid, interstitial fluid, and nasal and auditory canals. It lubricates, protects, and nourishes the nervous system. It also lubricates the sinus and nasal cavities. Tarpaka is responsible for nourishing sensory perception and storing neurological experience as memory in the brain cells.

Bodhaka kapha resides in the oral cavity and saliva. Its principal function is to lubricate the oral cavity and throat and to govern taste perception. It aids in mastication, swallowing and maintaining proper oral temperature. Bodhaka kapha plays a very important role in the gustatory reflex (the sensation of taste), facilitating perception of the six tastes—sweet, sour, salty, bitter, pungent and astringent.

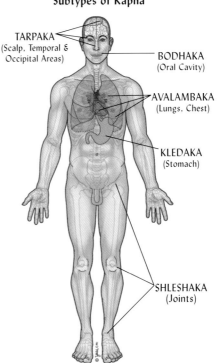

Regions of the Five
Subtypes of Kapha

TARPAKA
(Scalp, Temporal & Occipital Areas)

BODHAKA
(Oral Cavity)

AVALAMBAKA
(Lungs, Chest)

KLEDAKA
(Stomach)

SHLESHAKA
(Joints)

Avalambaka kapha is present in the chest, lungs and pleural fluid. It maintains lubrication and moisture of the alveoli, and supports the gaseous exchange between alveoli and capillaries through mucus secretions and membranes. It supports the heart and cardiovascular system.

Kledaka kapha is mainly present in the stomach and upper part of the intestines. Its primary function is to liquefy food, aiding in the process of digestion. It accomplishes this by breaking down the bigger molecules of food into smaller molecules. Kledaka kapha forms the mucous lining that protects the gastrointestinal (GI) tract; it helps to create a new lining every second or third day, thus protecting the stomach and intestines from burning due to pitta. Kledaka serves as an effective medium to carry the molecules of different enzymes into close contact with the molecules of food. It maintains acid-base equilibrium. It also maintains blood sugar. An hour after taking food, kledaka kapha sustains balanced blood sugar.

Shleshaka kapha is found in the joints, synovial fluid, and periosteum. It lubricates the joints, preventing friction and enabling freedom of movement. It nourishes the bones and prevents decay.

For a more extensive description and discussion of the three doshas, see *The Textbook of Ayurveda,* volume 1, chapter 3, pages 45–79.

The Seven Dhātus (Bodily Tissues)

In addition to the three doshas that govern function and the five elements that influence structure, the seven dhātus (tissues) play an important role in both the structural and functional aspects of human anatomy and physiology. The seven dhātus are *rasa* (plasma), *rakta* (blood), *māmsa* (muscle), *meda* (adipose), *asthi* (bone), *majjā* (nerve and blood marrow) and *shukra/ārtava* (male/female reproductive) tissues. A dhātu is the tissue formed by cells of the same function joining together. Each dhātu precipitates and nourishes its subsequent; hence rasa precipitates and nourishes rakta, rakta builds māmsa dhātu, and so forth, through shukra/ārtava. This is their natural, sequential order for nourishment. This refining or distillation of bodily dhātus ultimately generates *ojas*, the superfine juice of bodily immunity. Ojas is the pure essence of all bodily tissue. It is the supreme end-product of dhātu nourishment. When the tissues are depleted, the immune system becomes compromised.

Rasa dhātu is plasma and has the important function of *prīnanan* (nutrition). This tissue creates and nourishes the entire lymphatic system. It produces the lymph fluid, which has both nutritive and protective function. Rakta dhātu is the blood and hematopoietic system. It main-

tains life function, called *jīvana*. Māmsa dhātu or muscle has the role of *lepana*, which involves plastering, protection and movement. Adipose tissue or meda dhātu acts as insulating material to maintain body heat. It also provides lubrication and protection to the other tissue. Asthi dhātu comprises the skeletal system, whose function is *dhārana,* to give support, structure and form to the body. The bone marrow and nervous tissue constitute majjā dhātu, whose function is *pūranam,* to fill the spaces within the bones to accomplish communication. Lastly, shukra and ārtava dhātus are the reproductive tissue in the male and female respectively, which govern *prajananam* (procreation).

Each dhātu (tissue) has an *upadhātu* (by-product) and a *mala* (waste product) formed in the process of nutrition. These are summarized in table 46 on page 254 in appendix A. The three malas—urine, feces and sweat—are impurities that must be eliminated from the body. Each has a unique function. The function of urine is to carry excess kleda out of the system and maintain normal kleda (water-electrolyte balance). Feces or stool has the function of giving support to the wall of the colon, which absorbs fluid into the body. Sveda has the function of retaining optimum kleda under the skin, for lubrication.

Thus Āyurveda reveals the central importance of the doshas, dhātus and malas as the constituents which maintain the individual's unique psychophysiology in daily life.

The Prakruti/Vikruti Paradigm in Āyurvedic Medicine

At the time of conception, the predominant doshas in both the male seed (sperm) and female egg (ovum) determine an individual's doshic constitution (prakruti). Prakruti encompasses one's mental and physical nature. It is our home base, our point of equilibrium or homeostasis; it governs our behavior and our response to internal and external challenges.

Although every individual has a unique constitution, in which all three doshas are present to some extent, there are seven basic constitutional types:

* mono-doshic prakruti (primarily vata, pitta, or kapha)

* dual doshic prakruti (primarily vata-pitta, pitta-kapha, or vata-kapha)

* triple doshic prakruti (a more or less equal combination of vata, pitta, and kapha)

These are the seven main prakruti types. However, because the quality and quantity of the doshas will differ from individual to individual, there are in actuality innumerable prakrutis. As many human beings as exist, that many unique prakrutis will also be found. This is one of the most beautiful and profound contributions of Āyurveda to the understanding of health and medicine in the modern world: that every individual is unique. The ramifications of this are enormous, calling for subtlety of diagnosis, sensitivity in treatment, and awareness of a broad range of factors (physiological, psychological, environmental, etc.) in recommending preventive measures and lifestyle choices. Āyurveda is not a "one size fits all" health care system!

Knowledge of one's prakruti or constitution is extremely valuable for good health as well as for self-understanding. Appropriate dietary and lifestyle choices, proper yoga postures and breathing exercises, and even the type and dosage of medicine depend on this knowledge. Table 51 on page 261 in appendix A lists specific characteristics of each dosha to enable a preliminary assessment of a person's prakruti, though a far more accurate and in-depth evaluation can be made by a trained Ayurvedic practitioner.

Prakruti is one's essential constitution, formed at conception and continuing through life. Nevertheless, at any specific moment in a lifespan, the doshic balance may differ from prakruti. The body's responses to external fluctuations in diet, environment, weather, seasons, work, or relationships, or to internal variations in thoughts, emotions, or degrees of stress, disturb the baseline doshic equilibrium. This present altered state of imbalance is called *vikruti*. Vikruti reflects the ever-changing current qualitative and quantitative balance of the doshas. Vikruti may not be disease, but it can create a potential bed for future disease to appear and develop.

The prakruti/vikruti paradigm is the foundation for treatment in Ayurvedic medicine. Health, according to Āyurveda, is defined as a person at ease, with all doshas balanced. (Balanced does not mean equal, but rather, in accordance with the doshic proportions of one's prakruti.) When this condition of ease and balance is disturbed, it can become *dis-ease*. If vikruti, the body's constellation of responses to internal and external change, is not set back into balance, illness can result, for doshic disturbances significantly influence the body. For example, excess hot quality, from ingesting hot and spicy food, or from high temperatures in the environment, can produce fever, acne, rash or anger. Measures must be taken to pacify the heat and cool down the system, before symptoms that are more serious develop.

Vikruti does not necessarily lead to disease. When the system falls out of balance, the body's innate intelligence can counteract the changes and restore homeostasis. A very simple example is that when cold increases in the environment, a vāta person may spontaneously shiver in order to generate heat in the short term and restore balance. Conscious choices, such as eating moist, warming foods or sipping a cup of hot tea, can also help restore balance. Only when a dosha is continuously excessive does it affect the tissues and create serious physiological disturbance.

The journey from health to disease, that process by which balance is lost and imbalance progressively increases, is called *samprāpti* (pathogenesis). As discussed in chapter 6, Āyurveda delineates several distinct stages in this process, and the type of remedies that are effective at each stage.

Prakruti determines one's disease proneness. Individuals with a vāta prakruti have a predilection towards vāta diseases, such as arthritis, osteoporosis, emaciation and sciatica. They are also more prone to constipation, insomnia, nervousness and anxiety. Pitta prakruti tends toward hyperacidity, diarrhea and inflammatory changes such as bronchitis, gastritis and colitis. Individuals of kapha constitutional predominance have more tendencies toward congestion, cough, slow metabolism, weight gain and diabetes.

Although prakruti is an indicator of disease proneness, doshic imbalances are not restricted to individuals of that constitution. If an etiological factor is strongly pitta aggravating, such as extreme environmental heat, any individual may acquire a pitta imbalance. However, it is relatively easier to cure a pitta imbalance in a vāta or kapha individual. In general, when the prakruti and vikruti of an individual are of the same doshic pattern, treatment is likely to be more challenging. Thus, the prognosis and management of a disease depend upon the prakruti/vikruti paradigm.

This book presents *marma chikitsā* (treatment) as a practical and effective vehicle to influence body, mind, and soul. However, marma chikitsā is only one therapeutic modality under the larger umbrella of treatment possibilities in the Ayurvedic repertoire, including internal medicine, cleansing and detoxification regimens, herbal medications, yoga postures, lifestyle recommendations, and more. Treatment in Āyurveda is rarely, if ever, a single "magic bullet" but rather a combination of therapies designed for this particular individual with this particular set of conditions. Thus, marma therapy is most effective when used in conjunction with other Ayurvedic therapies and with an understanding of the doshas, prakruti, vikruti and samprāpti.

Introduction to Marmāni

A *marma* is a vital energy point located on the surface of the body.[1] Like modern quantum physics (and Traditional Chinese Medicine, as we shall soon see), Āyurveda holds that a human being is not a solid, stable material structure but an ever-changing, dynamic collection of energy and intelligence in the larger field of energy and intelligence that is the universe. As the body is alive and pulsating with energy, there can be innumerable "energy points" within it and upon the surface, but Āyurveda texts have described 117 major marmāni. These points are "vital" because they are infused with prāna, the life force, and imbued with consciousness. Consciousness expresses itself in lively, concentrated form at these points. Thus, marmāni serve as a bridge or doorway between the body, mind and soul.

The Sanskrit word marma actually means mortal or vulnerable point, suggesting access to areas that may be tender, weak or sensitive. They are located at anatomical sites where veins, arteries, tendons, bones or joints intersect. Marma also derives from the etymological root *mar,* which means "to kill," and certain marmāni related to the heart, trachea, and testicles are so vital that damage to them can cause instant death. *Varman* is another term synonymous with marma. It is translated as secretive, hidden or delicate point.

The History of Marmāni

The science of marmāni developed in Vedic times. In ancient India, martial arts schools emphasized the use of energy points for therapeutic purposes, to recover from bodily injuries, as well as to inflict serious injuries upon their opponents. The Kalari martial arts school, Dhanurveda (Vedic archery), Malla Purana (wrestling) and Vajra Mushti (boxing) are traditional settings that developed this science.

Sushruta was a renowned Ayurvedic surgeon whose contributions to medicine were well known at least as long ago as the time of Buddha (ca. sixth century BCE). Sushruta applied the knowledge of marmāni to surgery and further developed the science of energy points as a healing art. Heralded as the father of surgery, Sushruta believed surgical incisions at or near a marma point diminished local vitality because prāna and consciousness were highly concentrated at these points. He taught that an understanding of marmāni was critical in surgery, to avoid injury and to inflict minimum damage. His work, set down in the *Sushruta Samhitā,* a core text of Ayurvedic medicine, describes surgical interventions and methods for treating acute conditions. Sushruta documented marmāni locations and their influences in the section of his work on anatomy. He laid a solid and enduring foundation for a science of marmāni that propagated and evolved with each generation of practitioners who studied the therapeutic influences of the marmāni and correlated these to the doshas, elements, tissues, organs and channels.

Sushruta's wisdom and practical teachings, like most of the ancient Vedic literature, are recorded in verses known as *sūtras.* Sūtras are like compressed packets of knowledge, musically poetic verses containing vital information in concentrated form. The poetic form aids memorization in learning, and later, in practice, the clinician can call the sūtras to mind, bringing back a wealth of knowledge.

It was in the context of *pañchakarma* that Ayurvedic clinicians truly integrated the knowledge of marmāni with other Ayurvedic therapies. Pañchakarma is a detoxification and rejuvenative process designed to balance the doshas and harmonize body, mind and spirit. Pañchakarma includes many subspecialties, with one of the cardinal techniques being daily therapeutic massage using specially medicated oils. During massage, trained practitioners may give emphasis to certain marma points, helping the patient to experience deeper states of relaxation

---

1. Marman is the singular form and marmāni the plural. In day-to-day use, people use the word "marma" as the singular form.

and healing. Marma therapy continues to be utilized in pañchakarma massage today. Modern practitioners have adapted and further developed Sushruta's knowledge and methodology based on their clinical experience.

Mechanisms of Action

From the perspective of Western science, the mechanism of how marmāni function is not completely understood, nor do we know from any historical record how they were discovered, nor how clinicians began to work with them in treatment. Nor, to our knowledge, have there been, up to this time, any well-designed, controlled trials to examine the mechanism of marmāni. Yet, thousands of Ayurvedic clinicians have used the knowledge of marma for centuries, bringing relief and healing to millions of their patients. It is a time-tested empirical science, verified through extensive clinical practice.

Some historians postulate that the knowledge was discovered through clinical insight and observation, and through experimentation—applying pressure, pastes, needles, or heat to various points on the body, observing the results, and recording them.

However, the Ayurvedic tradition is stated clearly in a beautiful sūtra: "This knowledge dawns in the heart of *rishis* in a deep, silent state of meditation." A rishi is a seer, one whose pure consciousness is open to receive profound insight and intuitive understanding. Those who "see" present their insights; those who follow after try it, observe the results, and pass on the knowledge to their students. Thus, a tradition is born and carried on from guru to disciple.

Interestingly, nearly 75 of the 117 principal marmāni correspond exactly to principal acupoints in Chinese medicine. Perhaps a similar mechanism exists in both systems. Research (G. Stux, B. Pomeranz 1987) on acupuncture points suggests the following:

* Energy points are located at sites richly supplied by nerves and blood vessels.

* Treatment here often restores balance to the autonomic nervous system, harmonizing sympathetic and parasympathetic functions.

* Stimulating points can release endorphins (opioids) and neurotransmitters (such as serotonin and melatonin) in the brain that results in pain modulation and mood enhancement.

* Stimulating points can have a therapeutic effect locally as well as distally from the point. This may be due to the transmission of neural impulses along nerve pathways to the brain, and from the brain to the organ or area of the body being treated.

Another perspective comes from the yogic tradition, which speaks of 72,000 *nādīs* (energy pathways) with access on the surface of the skin. Stimulating energy points on the skin in marma therapy allows prāna from that local point to move from the surface energy through the nādīs to the target organ where it balances prāna, tejas and ojas to unfold healing energy.

In the language of Āyurveda, the vital points are integral components of majjā dhātu, the nervous system. Prāna governs the entire nervous system, all neurological responses, and the sensation of touch and pressure. Through the harmonious interaction of prāna vāyu (the flow of cellular intelligence), sādhaka pitta (present especially in the gray matter of the brain) and tarpaka kapha (the white matter covering the brain), communication between marmāni is facilitated.

Based on his experience of using marma therapy over the past three decades in clinical practice, Dr. Lad has developed his own theory about the mechanism of marma. At the terminal ending point of the marma, many factors—ojas-tejas-prāna molecules, sattva-rajas-tamas qualities, and the prānic pathways related to specific srotāmsi and their associated vital organs—are all intimately connected by the body's neuroelectrical energy. So, when a physician or healer touches the marma by applying, according to the situation, either gentle or deep pressure, that touch is a complex biochemical and neuroelectrical impulse. The energy of that touch, enhanced by the vibration of the mantra uttered by the physician or healer, passes through the gateway of the marma to the respective srotas and their organs and starts balancing the prāna, tejas and ojas of the dhātus (tissues), srotāmsi (channels) and organs.

Pain or tenderness at the site of the marma is the body's way of conveying that there is some weakness, impurity or imbalance in one or more aspects of the body associated with that marma point. Pressure applied to the marma kindles dhātu agni, burns cellular *āma* (toxicity), and breaks down crystals of unresolved emotions. This clears the pathways and improves the structural and functional integrity of the srotāmsi. That is why marma chikitsā (marma therapy) can quickly relieve many conditions, such as migraine headaches, joint pain, and muscle spasm; it brings immediate relaxation and eases pain.

The mechanism of marma therapy can be further explained by the sensitivity of marmāni to stimuli such as temperature, touch, pressure, light, sound and smell. In chromotherapy, marmāni respond to light transmitted at various color frequencies. Marmāni are responsive to the biochemistry of essential oils utilized in aromatherapy, and to sound used in sound therapy. Sensitivity to temperature is expressed in the heating or cooling energetics of essential oils and herbal pastes. Cold pacifies pitta dosha and stimulates vāta and kapha. Heat stimulates pitta, but pacifies vāta and kapha dosha. Heat also facilitates the movement of prāna and unblocks stagnation. *Agni karma* (known as moxibustion in Traditional Chinese Medicine) stimulates the marmāni with heat. These therapies and their influence on the marmāni are discussed in chapter 8.

Functions of Marmāni

• •

The energy points have a wide range of functions that affect body, mind and spirit. As described below, marmāni facilitate cellular communication, serve as diagnostic indicators, and have a virtually unlimited number of therapeutic applications, including relief of pain, detoxification, and more. Marmāni also cleanse, pacify, rejuvenate, calm the mind and emotions, enhance awareness, and serve as vehicles of preventative care.

Communication

Marmāni are the vehicles for communication between cells, serving to maintain their functional activity and coordination. As prāna flows through the energy points and the prānic pathways (nādīs) within the entire body, it transmits information linking the internal and external realms and body and mind. Marmāni facilitate communication between the deeper internal organs and tissues and the more superficial structures and skin. Marma treatment can help to calm and settle the mind, leading to increased clarity of perception and more effective communication.

Diagnostic Indicators

Sensitivity of a marma point is indicative of imbalance locally or deeply. Sensitivities can reflect disturbance of the doshas, dhātus, upadhātus, srotāmsi and organs. For example, a pain response on initial pressure that disappears soon thereafter is suggestive of vāta imbalance. When a marma remains tender throughout the application of pressure, pitta may be affected. If a marma is tender only with the application of deep pressure, kapha may be imbalanced. Similarly, tenderness at Hrid marmāni (located in the center of the chest) may indicate cardiac problems or emotional disturbances. Sensitivity at Yakrut, Plīha or Vrukka marmāni may suggest liver, spleen and kidney dysfunction respectively. Pressure on marmāni can be used as a simple diagnostic tool.

Therapeutic Influences

The same marmāni that are pressed for diagnostic purposes may also be used in treatment. Marma therapy addresses the following conditions:

Doshic Imbalances. Marma therapy can either pacify or stimulate a dosha. For example, stimulating Pāda Kshipra marma on the big toe helps to pacify kapha dosha, which is responsible for sinus headaches. Marma therapy can promote the functions of the dosha or its subtypes. It also balances prakruti and vikruti and restores normal *dosha gati* (vector). Each of the five vāyus has a correct direction or vector of movement for normal function. If the direction is disrupted, disturbance occurs in that dosha and subdosha.

Dhātu Disturbances. Stimulating a marma related to a particular tissue helps to maintain the tissue's normal functions and treats specific disorders that are present. For example, rasa dhātu marmāni will enhance the functions of nutrition and immunity; rakta marmāni improve oxygenation and vitality; māmsa marmāni increase functions of movement and strength; meda marmāni augment lubrication and insulation; asthi marmāni provide support and protection; majjā marmāni improve coordination; and finally shukra and ārtava marmāni may activate sex energy and stimulate ojas (immunity).

Srotāmsi Disturbances. Marmāni associated with specific dhātu also communicate internally with the corresponding srotāmsi and regulate their functions. Srotāmsi are the network of channels within the body, related to each tissue. For example, rasa marmāni affect rasa dhātu, rasa vaha srotas, and the heart. Marma therapy can regulate channel disturbances such as overflow and stagnation. Chapter 5 describes the channels in detail, while chapter 16 discusses channel disturbances.

Organ Dysfunctions. Every marma is not necessarily related to an organ, but every organ is affiliated with one or more marmāni. Sensitive marmāni may reflect disturbances of an organ. The strength and function of each organ is governed by prāna and can be detected from the pulse by an experienced clinician. Stimulating marmāni facilitates prānic flow to the organ via the prānic pathways (or we could say it restores or enlivens cellular communication, the flow of intelligence), thus enhancing organ functions and promoting healing. This contact improves circulation and elimination, promotes optimal secretions and excretion, decreases congestion, and relieves organ stress. For example, if the heart pulse is weak, indicating disturbance, gentle pressure on the heart marmāni improves cardiac function. As the heart begins to function more normally, the patient will typically experience relaxation, stillness of mind and resolution of emotional disturbance. These subjective experiences are quite common in patients with cardiovascular disorders. The clinician can assess the therapeutic effect on the organ by examining the pulse before and after marma therapy.

Prāna, Tejas and Ojas Imbalances. Marma therapy balances the subtle doshic essences. Prāna is the pure essence of vāta and is responsible for the flow of cellular intelligence. Tejas is the subtlest form of pitta that governs cellular metabolism. Ojas, the superfine form of kapha, influences cellular immune function. Stimulation of marmāni can enhance communication at the cellular level, affecting cellular intelligence, metabolism and immune function via the media of prāna, tejas and ojas.

Mechanism of Pain Relief

Pain is generated by an impeded flow of prāna resulting from tension and stagnation. It is a reflection of doshic imbalance. Marma therapy alleviates pain by stimulating the flow of prāna, thus pacifying the doshas. For example, arthritis is pain in the joints and can involve all three doshas. Vāta is the primary dosha involved because it has an affinity for the joints. Increased pitta in a joint leads to inflammation. Diminished shleshaka kapha results in stiffness, because there is insufficient lubrication. Treating local marmāni at the joint can balance vāta, pitta, and kapha and enhance the flow of prāna at the site.

Stimulation of Agni and Detoxification of Āma

Agni, the fire principle in the body, governs digestion, absorption, and nutrition of the tissue. Healthy agni can maintain a natural resistance of the tissue, which is a protective function. Agni is present in every bodily structure—each of the tissues, channels, organs and cells. Whenever agni is low, then unprocessed metabolic wastes increase; that is called *āma.* Marma therapy activates agni and effectively detoxifies and cleanses all bodily structures. Marma stimulation can improve metabolism, circulation, nutrition and rejuvenation of the tissues. Healthy systemic agni is also promoted in Āyurveda through proper diet, regular exercise, optimal lifestyle, and pañchakarma. Refer to chapter 6 for further discussion of agni.

Calming the Mind and Balancing Emotions

Contact with marmāni can significantly calm the mind and reduce stress through their ability to influence the nervous system (majjā dhātu), of which they are essentially a part. These energy points may also trigger the release of unexpressed or unresolved emotions, which are viewed as imbalances of the dosha. Chapter 3 examines emotional balance in more detail.

Enhancing Awareness

The most effective spiritual function of marma therapy is to access consciousness at a deep level. Treatment unfolds cellular awareness that spreads to related tissues, organs and channels. Marmāni are the doorways to process the unprocessed thought, feeling, and emotion stored in majjā dhātu (nervous system) and *mano vaha srotas* (channels of the mind), unblocking the flow of prāna (cellular intelligence). Chapter 3 discusses these concepts more specifically.

Preventative Care and Rejuvenation

A central component of Āyurveda is prevention, with its focus on living a healthy lifestyle in harmony with nature. Āyurvedic diet and recommended daily routine, herbal tonics, purification practices, and so on, all aim to maintain good health and prevent the birth of illness. Marma chikitsā can contribute a great deal to this effort to enhance vitality and promote health and balance. Marma stimulation performed with a gentle oil massage nourishes ojas, tejas and prāna at a subtle level and revitalizes the body, mind and spirit. It allows for rejuvenation at the cellular level.

Effective marma therapy can be performed not only by deliberate pressure with the fingers on specific energy points. For example, when we perform *abhyanga* (oil massage), we stimulate numerous marma points on the body. Whenever we do *āsanas* (yoga postures) on a hard surface, we are using the body's weight to press directly on marma points. When we do *prānāyāma* (yogic

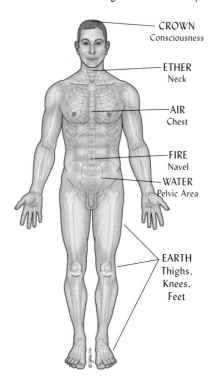

Five Elements and Regions of the Body

CROWN
Consciousness

ETHER
Neck

AIR
Chest

FIRE
Navel

WATER
Pelvic Area

EARTH
Thighs,
Knees,
Feet

breathing), the pressure of our fingers stimulates marmāni near the nose. These are practical, highly effective preventive measures we can easily employ, using marma points.

Classification of Marmāni

The primary 117 marmāni are further classified according to location, elemental associations, associations of dosha, dhātu, mala, corresponding organs and srotāmsi and degrees of vitality.

Location

Marmāni locations are organized according to their region of the body and their relationship to internal and external features, doshas and subdoshas. In the classical literature, Sushruta describes marmāni according to the six major body parts: four extremities, trunk, head and neck. He also divides the energy points according to five principal tissue structures: *māmsa* (muscles), *sira* (veins), *snāyu* (ligaments), *asthi* (bone) and *sandhi* (joints).

Marmāni located on the scalp are immediately connected to the brain and distally to other organs as well. They are connected on the chest and upper back with the heart and lungs, on the lower back with the kidneys, on the abdomen with the digestive organs and on the gluteal area with the pelvic cavity. Locations of the marmāni related to the doshas and their subtypes are found in the section below titled Marmāni and Doshic Subtypes. Large-size illustrations of the marmāni are located in appendix C.

Table 1: Relationship of Marmāni and the Elements

Element	Type of Energy	Associated Body Region	Examples of Marmāni
Space	Nuclear	Head and Neck	Mūrdhni, Ajñya
Air	Electrical	Lungs and Heart	Jatru, Apastambha, Kakshadhara
Fire	Radiant	Navel region	Nābhi, Yakrut, Plīhā
Water	Chemical	Pelvic area	Basti, Bhaga, Nābhi 3
Earth	Mechanical/ physical	Legs and Feet	Ūrū, Jānu, Pāda Madhya

Elemental Associations

Each of the five elements—Space, Air, Fire, Water and Earth—is associated with a particular region of the body. Each marma located in these regions activates the energy of its associated element. For example, by stimulating Ājñā marma (third eye), a guru may transmit spiritual energy to the disciple through the medium of ether. Hrid marmāni enhance the energy of love to the heart via the air element. Pressure at Nābhi marmāni directly enkindles the gastrointestinal energy of agni, through the radiant energy of fire. Basti marma can unfold chemical energy by working through the water element. Pāda Madhya works through the earth element and can help a person to be grounded, stable and centered. Table 1 summarizes the relationship of the marmāni and the elements.

Marmāni and Doshic Subtypes

The language of the doshas is central to the Ayurvedic understanding of health and disease. Knowing how key energy points affect a dosha is crucial to achieving excellent therapeutic results. Marmāni are classified according to a dosha's home site. For example, chest and lung energy points stimulate kapha. Umbilical marmāni affect pitta. Colon points influence vāta dosha. All marmāni below the umbilical area of the trunk stimulate vāta. We have discussed the five subtypes of each dosha in chapter 1. Table 2 shows their locations.

Table 2: Marma Locations According to Subdoshas

Subtypes Of Vāta	Marma Locations
Prāna	Scalp, Above eyebrows
Udāna	Throat
Samāna	Stomach, Abdomen
Apāna	Below Navel
Vyāna	Heart, Chest, Extremities
Subtypes Of Pitta	**Marma Locations**
Pāchaka	Proximal To Navel
Rañjaka	Liver, Spleen
Sādhaka	Scalp, Pericardium
Ālochaka	Eyes
Bhrājaka	Skin, Extremities
Subtypes Of Kapha	**Marma Locations**
Kledaka	Stomach
Avalambaka	Lungs, Chest
Bodhaka	Oral Cavity, Mouth
Tarpaka	Scalp, Temporal and Occipital areas
Shleshaka	Joints

Corresponding Organs And Srotāmsi

Many marmāni are associated with specific organs and channel systems. Table 33 on page 234 lists organs and their corresponding marmāni. Similarly, the relationship of marmāni to specific channel systems is covered in chapter 16.

Degrees Of Vitality of Marmāni

Sushruta, an expert surgeon, differentiated marmāni into five categories according to the degrees of vitality of the marmāni and the effect on the person if specific points are injured. He described how marma injuries, whether superficial or deep, can disrupt the prānic energy flow and decrease vitality. The five classifications of vitality are based somewhat on the complexity of underlying structures, such as muscles, veins, ligaments, bones and joints. *Sadyah prānahara* marmāni are marma points located at the union of these five structures—muscles, veins, ligaments, bones and joints—and are considered to have the most vitality. This classification includes the eight *mahā* (great) marmāni listed below. Illustrations of the sadyah prānahara marmāni are shown on page 23.

Sadyah Prānahara Marmāni

✳ Sadyah marmāni (the Eight Great Marmāni)
  Mūrdhni (crown)
  Brahmarandhra (anterior to crown)
  Shivarandhra (posterior to crown)
  Ājñā (third eye)
  Shanka (right and left temple)
  Hridayam (heart)
  Nābhi (umbilicus)
  Guda (anus)

✳ Special or Extra Vital Marmāni, those that can cause death or serious injury when traumatized.
  Kantha (trachea)
  Grīvā (back of neck)
  Basti (bladder)
  Vrushana (testicles)
  Yoni Jihvā (clitoris)

Sushruta further classified marmāni according to qualitative classes. Sadyah prānahara marmāni are considered fatal within 24 hours if injured; *kalāntara prānahara* marmāni cause death within two to four weeks of an injury; *vaikalyakāra prānahara* marmāni are fatal as soon as any foreign object embedded within one of these marmāni is extracted; *vishalya prānahara* marmāni result in maiming or deformity when injured; and *ruja-*

kara prānahara marmāni create persistent prolonged pain when injured.

Conclusion

Marmāni have been explored with regard to their historical use, mechanisms of action, functions, and classifications. Their relationship to doshas, dhātus, srotāmsi and organs has been examined, and their similarity to the acupoints of Traditional Chinese Medicine has been hinted at and will be elaborated in chapter 4. The vitality of marmāni is intimately related to ojas, tejas and prāna, because they are the basic support, the vital essence of life.

Now we will turn our attention to the spiritual dimension of marmāni in the following chapter.

Sadyah Prānahara Marmāni

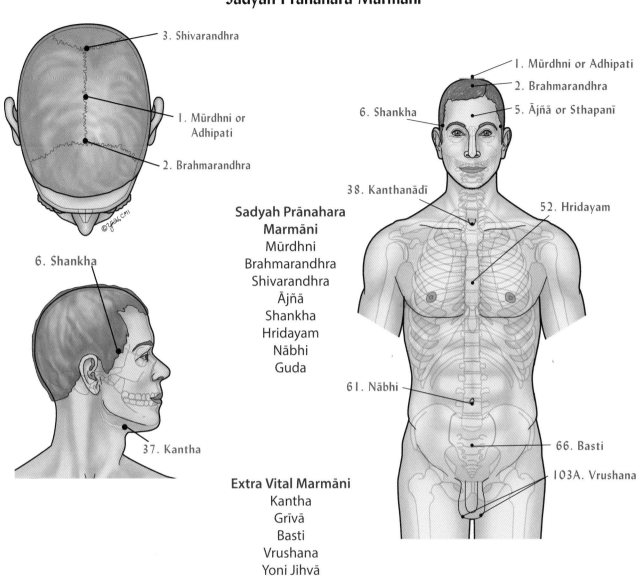

3. Shivarandhra

1. Mūrdhni or Adhipati

2. Brahmarandhra

6. Shankha

37. Kantha

1. Mūrdhni or Adhipati

2. Brahmarandhra

6. Shankha

5. Ājñā or Sthapanī

38. Kanthanādī

52. Hridayam

61. Nābhi

66. Basti

103A. Vrushana

Sadyah Prānahara Marmāni
Mūrdhni
Brahmarandhra
Shivarandhra
Ājñā
Shankha
Hridayam
Nābhi
Guda

Extra Vital Marmāni
Kantha
Grīvā
Basti
Vrushana
Yoni Jihvā

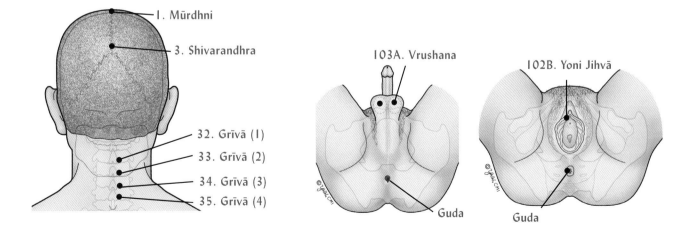

1. Mūrdhni

3. Shivarandhra

32. Grīvā (1)

33. Grīvā (2)

34. Grīvā (3)

35. Grīvā (4)

103A. Vrushana

Guda

102B. Yoni Jihvā

Guda

The Spiritual Dimension of Marmāni

Marma chikitsā is the precise art of touching an individual in exactly the right place at a critical moment in time, for the purpose of healing. Marmāni serve as points of access to the body's innate intelligence, opening the doorway to health and well-being. They are vehicles to reach the ultimate goal of Āyurveda: perfect health, firmly rooted in a vibrantly alive body and fully awakened mind.

In this chapter, we discuss the rich and significant spiritual dimensions of marmāni. Because marmāni are intimately connected to thoughts, perceptions and emotions as well as to the entire fabric of the physical body, marma chikitsā can be a powerful ally on the spiritual path, helping to settle the mind and enhance awareness in such practices as meditation, prānāyāma (breath control) and yogāsana, and to free the mind and body of the accumulated stresses and toxins that limit consciousness and burden the heart.

The Spiritual Value of Touch

Touch begins on the physical level, but it can go much deeper, traversing the media of thoughts, feelings, and emotions. Touch—the skilled touch of a sincere practitioner of the healing arts—can convey its message of love through prāna into the manas, buddhi, smruti. It can penetrate ahamkāra and speak its silent message through chitta into the soul.[1] Along the way, and especially at this deepest level, touch can engender radical change in the neurochemistry. The human body is a unique chemical laboratory; a touch through the energy points of marmāni can open new pathways that affect our inner pharmacy.

Certain marma therapies can not only enhance thinking, feeling, and perception, they also have the potential to evoke a state of choiceless, passive awareness and transform it into a transcendental state of samādhi. Thus, the total healing of body, mind and spirit can happen through marma chikitsā.

Mahad: Innate Intelligence of the Body – and the Universe

In Sānkhya philosophy, mahad or cosmic intelligence creates order in the universe. It permeates every aspect of creation from the gross to the subtle and from the macrocosm to the microcosm, from the order governing the vast galactic universe to the infinitesimal genetic code guiding the unfoldment of life within every living cell.

On the physical level, the body is shaped by mahad to reflect the perfect harmony of structure and function. The five elements govern structure, the three doshas rule function, and the seven dhātus (bodily tissues) influence both structure and function. This microcosmic mahad is evident in the precise locations of the marmāni mapped within the matrix of majjā dhātu, the nervous system.

On the mental level, cosmic intelligence manifests as individual consciousness, which expresses itself as the principal mental faculties: *manas* (sensory mind) and buddhi (intellect). The marmāni are intimately connected to the mind via majjā dhātu and mano vaha srotas (channels of the mind).

On the spiritual level mahad, which on the cosmic scale is the flow of consciousness or intelligence that facilitates harmony among all aspects of creation, is given voice in the body through the flow of prāna. Prāna is the breath that animates the organism and allows its spirit to reside in the body. The entry of consciousness into the marmāni allows communication within and

---

1. We have discussed these levels and facets of the mind in chapter 1, in outlining the Sānkhya philosophy. In brief, mind is generally referred to as manas, the mental faculty that regulates perception, thought and emotion. A subtler aspect of mind is buddhi, the individual intellect and faculty of discrimination and recognition. Buddhi in turn has three subdivisions: *dhī*—cognition, *dhruti*—retention, and *smruti*—memory. Ahamkāra is ego, the sense of "I."

between the body and mind via the flow of prāna. Marmāni are especially relevant to the development of spirituality because of their close association with the chakra system (see below). Thus, they support the integration of all three levels of being: body, mind and spirit.

Universal Mind and Particular Mind: Opening to Infinity

According to the Sānkhya philosophy of creation, there is universal mind, called *vibhu,* and individual mind, called *anu.* Universal mind is the ground mind, and individual mind is particular mind. Universal mind is vast, unbounded, infinitely creative and eternally pure, unclouded consciousness. Particular mind is conditioned mind, based upon its stockpile of thoughts, feelings, and emotions stored in memory. Memory is the background to all we think, feel and perceive, and imposes itself upon the foreground of pure, direct experience. The more the particular mind fails to apprehend the ground mind, the more life becomes suffering. The root cause of suffering is this division between the ground mind and the particular mind. Through marma therapy, new pathways are opened within the mano vaha srotas, which allow particular mind to transcend its conditioned state and expand into universal mind. This unity of individual mind and universal mind brings radical transformation and total healing in the life of the individual.

Ground mind belongs to all. It operates through the sun, the moon, rivers, mountains, oceans, the flowers and the trees. In our daily perception, particular mind creates division in which "you" become the observer and "that" becomes the object, the thing to be observed. When the observer is unaware of both the pure essence of ground mind and its all-permeating presence within all things, our powers of observation are very limited. This limited observation creates judgment, criticism, like and dislike and so on, based upon our particular background. The more our background dominates our experience, the more we lose the ground.

Particular mind freezes our perception. And because of our frozen perception, we see our world as we see it now. Marma therapy has the capacity to help us unfreeze this perception, via the media of majjā dhātu and mano vaha srotas. In this way marma chikitsā can improve the quality of perception. It brings clarity. Clarity of perception becomes compassion; and compassion is love.

Marmāni and Mind/Body Medicine

Within one month, we have totally new skin, as far as the atoms and cells are concerned. Our superficial self dies and a new one takes shape. In the space of four days, we have a completely new gastro-mucous lining. In a period of six months, all the atoms of the liver are replaced and we have an entirely new liver. Like these constant changes in the body, everything in the universe is changing. There is nothing permanent in this world. Only change itself is permanent. These changes are happening on the vast screen of awareness, which is eternal, timeless existence, the unchanging ground upon which all change occurs.

At this time in history, important changes are taking place in the Western scientific understanding of mind and body, and of the nature of life itself. The old paradigm, which held that mind lives in the brain, is giving way to a new paradigm that says the brain lives in the mind. The old paradigm assumed that mind is within the body. The new paradigm asserts that the body is in the mind. According to the old paradigm, mind and body are separate and distinct, the concrete, solid, material body being "real" and the abstract, non-physical mind grudgingly accorded a shadowy sort of existence. The new paradigm says that we cannot separate body from mind. The body is crystallized mind, and mind is the energy aspect of the body. To speak of mind and body as two distinct entities is simply not true, and creates confusion and separation. That is why we speak today of mind-body medicine.

Āyurveda has always recognized this. From the Āyurvedic perspective, going back thousands of years, we really should speak of mind-body or bodymind, because they are one. Anything that happens in mind influences the body, and vice versa. Mind is a flow of thought, as a river is a flow of water. As the water, so the river. If the water is clear, the river is clear. If the water is polluted, the river is polluted. Likewise, as the thought, so the mind. If our thoughts breathe fear, mind becomes fearful. If angry thoughts flow or flood through the mind, the mind *becomes* anger. On the other hand, if thought is clear, mind is clear. As a change in the water is a change in the river, a change in the nature of our thoughts is a change in the mind. Moreover, every change in our mental state is instantaneously reflected in the chemistry and functioning of the body.

On the cutting edge of this newly emerging model, in which the ancient understanding is being corroborated by extensive research, mind and body are no longer considered two different vehicles of experience. Mind is not a localized entity, to be sought somewhere in the electro-chemical activity of the brain, but rather it pervades the entire physical body from every cell to every fiber. Mind and body are not just interconnected, but are one cohesive entity with both physical and mental manifestations.

The term mano vaha srotas means "the pathway of the mind." *Mano* means mind, *vaha* implies carrying, and *srotas* means pathway or channel. To describe the mind as a lively channel of energy captures its reality as fluid movement. Mano vaha srotas is not a "thing" but a continuous flow or stream of consciousness. It is one of the fourteen principal channels described in more detail in chapter 16. Each channel is a network comprised of a root, a pathway and an opening.

Mano vaha srotas has its root in the heart, brain and chakra system. The mind originates through these three centers. The pathway of mano vaha srotas encompasses the entire person, through what the Vedanta school of Indian philosophy calls the five *koshas*—auric fields representing five planes or sheaths of existence of varying density. Ranging from subtle to gross, these are:

* *ānandamaya kosha* (bliss body)
* *vijñānamaya kosha* (wisdom body)
* *manomaya kosha* (mental body)
* *prānamaya kosha* (breath body)
* *annamaya kosha* (physical or food body)

The koshas are discussed extensively in Sanskrit texts but the subject is too vast for this presentation. (H.H. Adi Shankaracharaya 1999)

The "opening" of mano vaha srotas is where the energy flourishes and can be accessed. There are three principal openings for the channel of the mind: the synaptic space between neurons, the sense organs and the marmāni. Thus, marmāni provide direct access to the mind, bridging it with the physical body.

Majjā dhātu, nervous tissue, is the medium through which the marmāni express themselves. It acts as an intermediary between prāna vāyu, which governs sensory stimuli, and apāna vāyu, which governs motor response. Each dhātu is associated with a channel system. *Majjā vaha srotas* is the channel of the nervous system. Its roots are the brain, spinal cord and bone marrow; its passage is the entire central nervous system, including the sympathetic and parasympathetic nervous systems;

The Koshas of the Body

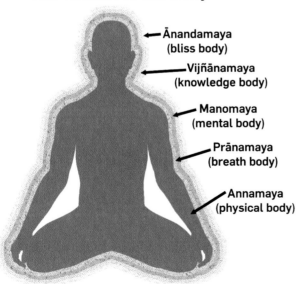

Ānandamaya
(bliss body)

Vijñānamaya
(knowledge body)

Manomaya
(mental body)

Prānamaya
(breath body)

Annamaya
(physical body)

and its opening is the synaptic space and neuromuscular cleft. Majjā vaha srotas includes structures such as the cerebrum, cerebellum, spinal nerves, and sensory and motor nerves.

Majjā dhātu and majjā vaha srotas are intimately related, function together harmoniously, and are the substratum of mano vaha srotas. Majjā provides the structure, while mano vaha srotas is the function. Majjā dhātu forms the cable wires through which the electric current of mano vaha srotas passes. Together, they govern all the basic cognitive functions of the mind: comprehension, recognition, memory storage and communication. They facilitate the capacity to perceive clearly, concentrate and meditate. These mental functions operate based on three subdoshas: tarpaka kapha is responsible for memory, sādhaka pitta for cognition and prāna vāyu for sensory perception.

Deeper examination of the mind reveals its presence at the marma sites. Each energy point is related to manas, the sensory mind, and directly communicates perception, thought and emotion. Every marma is also related to buddhi, via cognition, retention and memory, because marmāni are doorways to the nervous system and related mental faculties. The subconscious memories mentioned above in our discussion of ground mind and particular mind are stored in the deep connective tissue of majjā dhātu. These memories can be directly accessed by stimulating the marmāni, as they are a part of majjā dhātu. Marmāni are intrinsically connected to the mind via the media of majjā dhātu and mano vaha srotas.

There is a dynamic interplay between the mind and the energy points, and understanding this relationship is essential for healing. In a healthy system, marmāni are sites of vitality where consciousness flourishes and flowers. Pure awareness flows gracefully through the doorways of marmāni and, as all rivers finally merge into the ocean, all pranic energy that courses through the marmāni finally merges in the ocean of awareness.

However, when the mind becomes stagnant or clogged, the flow of prāna is similarly obstructed, like a river that is stagnant or polluted, and the marmāni mirror this. Blockage at a marma is the obstructed flow of awareness. If the mind is overactive, the marmāni reflect this too, becoming painful, sensitive or tender. Likewise, disturbance at the level of a marma is reflected in the mind—revealing the inherent mind/body connection. This is why, for rapid spiritual evolution, a comprehensive mind-body program is so helpful;[2] a program that integrates meditation and breathing with purification procedures for the body and nervous system.

---

2. As explained in chapter 18, "Yoga Therapy and Marmāni."

Chakra System

The nature of the mind-body model can also be analyzed and understood in terms of the chakra system. "Chakra" means a vortex of energy. The chakra system comprises seven principal energy centers aligned along the spinal column, from the crown of the head to the tip of the tailbone. Chakras are non-physical in nature, but correspond to major nerve plexuses that relate to the endocrine centers. The chakra system is one of the pathways of mano vaha srotas in Āyurveda. Thus, each chakra is deeply connected to the mind and reflects a specific quality or level of consciousness. For example, survival is associated with the root chakra and enlightenment with the crown chakra. Table 48 on page 258 in appendix A outlines the properties of each chakra and table 49 on page 259 elucidates various subtle therapies based on the chakras.

A brief description of each chakra and its relationship to the elements and koshas follows.

Mūlādhāra. This is the root chakra of survival and groundedness. Related to the earth element, it is where matter meets with matter, environmental matter with bodily matter. Mūlādhāra is connected to the annamaya kosha, the physical or "food body" and is governed by apāna vāyu.

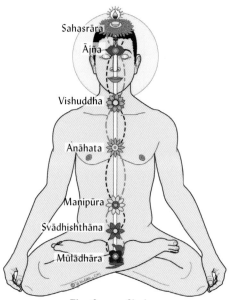

The Seven Chakras

Kundalinī shakti is the divine neuro-electrical energy that, until it is awakened, lies dormant at Mūlādhāra chakra at the base of the spine. Sanskrit texts describe spiritual development and the growth of higher states of consciousness in terms of the ascent of the kundalini energy up the spine through its channel (called sushumnā) from the root or base chakra to the crown chakra. Kundalini is the vehicle for transforming lower consciousness into higher consciousness and unfolding spiritual joy and bliss.

Kundalinī may be awakened in several ways, including deep meditation, prānāyāma or directly by a guru (an enlightened spiritual master), through a transmission of subtle energy known as shaktipat. The Vedic tradition describes four ways shaktipat may be conferred: darshana, the master's look of love; sparshana, the touch of compassion, often carried out when the master presses a thumb on the "third eye" of the disciple, site of the Ājñā marma; mantraya, the gentle whispering of a mantra into the right ear of the disciple, which goes directly into the chitakash, the space of awareness of the disciple; and smarana, remembering the holy scripture, the guru or the sweet name of God. Holding in one's mind and heart the loving face of the master, or remembrance of sacred texts or the name of God, stimulate the secretion of molecules in the brain that give rise to the experience of bliss. Smarana or remembrance can occur even if the guru is at a great distance.

Svādhishthāna. The basic survival needs that drive a person dominated by Mūlādhāra chakra are food, shelter and clothing. Once a person has these, he or she thinks about sex and procreation, where the male energy meets the female energy. Svādhishthāna is the chakra of self-esteem, and procreation. This chakra is associated with the water element. Without water, there is no sexual pleasure; dry sex is painful. Both the Cowper's gland in men and the corresponding Bartholin's gland in women secrete a lubricating fluid during sexual intercourse. This gives joy and ecstasy to both partners. Thus, this chakra is the meeting point of male and female energy.

Manipūra. This chakra, literally "the city of gems," is the chakra of power, prestige, and position in society, of ambition, competitiveness and aggressiveness. It is the fire element chakra, and is related to pitta dosha. Once people have food to eat, shelter and a sexual partner, they think about power and politics. Here, leader meets with the led. Like Mūlādhāra and Svādhishthāna, Manipūra belongs to our animal nature. Every animal needs food, shelter, sex and power. Birds have their "pecking order," monkeys have an alpha monkey, a "king," bees have a queen who controls millions of other bees. Most creatures, driven by the need to survive and thrive, vie with each other for dominance in their group.

Humanity today is still operating largely through these lower three chakras. People seek shelter, food and sex; when these needs are satisfied, they turn their attention to power and try to gain authority and control over others. So long as humanity is operating primarily through these lower three chakras, world peace will be very difficult to attain. When people are dominated by these very strong needs and drives, they will pursue them at any cost, even at the expense of other people's lives and the environment.

Between these three lower chakras and the higher chakras is the heart, Anāhata. Until this chakra is awakened, we are not yet truly human; we are just in human form.

Table 3: Chakras, Koshas and Marmāni

Chakras	Related Koshas	Vāyus	Marmāni	Function
Mūlādhāra	Annamaya	Apāna	Trik	Survival, groundedness
Svādhishthāna	Prānamaya	Apāna	Nābhi	Procreation, self-identity, self-esteem
Manipūra	Manomaya	Samāna	Sūrya	Ambition, achievement, power, control
Anāhata	Jñānamaya	Vyāna	Hridayam	Love, immunity
Vishuddhi	Vijñānamaya	Udāna	Jatru	Communication, wisdom
Ājñā	Ānandamaya	Prāna	Ājñā	Intuition
Sahasrāra	Beyond the koshas	Prāna	Mūrdhni	Self realization, bliss

Anāhata. This is the most vital center, standing between the lower three animal chakras and the higher three divine chakras. This is the chakra of human love. The seat of love, compassion and care, it is related to the air element and to prāna vāyu and vyāna vāyu. Anāhata is the meeting point where lover meets with the beloved.

Vishuddhi. Here the inner person meets with the outer. This is the chakra of purity, clarity and communication. Located at the throat, it is the chakra of speech and language. It is governed by udāna vāyu and related to the space (ether) element.

Ājñā. Situated between the eyebrows, the "third eye" is the chakra of insight and intuition. It is the meeting of guru and disciple, the chakra of radical evolution and transformation where alpha meets with omega. This is often said to be the best chakra to have attention on during meditation. As the previous chakras are related to the five elements, Ājñā is related to consciousness.

Sahasrāra. The thousand petalled lotus at the crown of the head is the seat of pure awareness, the meeting point of jīva with Shiva, the lower self with the higher self. It is the chakra of self-realization, bliss and transformation. The primary significance of the chakras for this study is that the marmāni are intimately connected to the chakra system. A marma is a doorway of consciousness, while each chakra is a reservoir of consciousness. Stimulating a marma activates the energy of the corresponding chakra through its pranic energy currents. For example, Trik marma stimulates energy at *Mulādhāra chakra* and Mūrdhni marma stimulates consciousness at *Sahasrāra,* the crown chakra.

Thus, the marmāni help to complete the meeting points, those polarities of male and female, inner and outer, leader and led and so on, and unfold higher spiritual experiences.

Emotions: Origin, Expression and Healing

The goal of Āyurveda, as we will emphasize throughout this book, is perfect health of body, mind and spirit. Much attention will be paid to the use of marma chikitsā (marma treatment or therapy) in healing the body and promoting clarity of thought and perception. In this section, we will consider emotions, investigating their origin and development as well as the buildup, in the unconscious levels of the mind and in the very tissues, channels and fibers of the body, of unresolved negative emotions.

In terms of this chapter's theme—the spiritual dimension—the aim of Āyurveda is enlightenment, full awakening to the Self or Spirit at the root and core of our being. Enlightenment cannot blossom in a body clogged with āma, the toxic by-product of food that is old, stale, spoiled, or poorly digested. Nor can enlightenment—a state of supreme clarity and love—dawn in a mind and heart filled with *mental* or *emotional* āma, generated by negative thoughts and emotions.

Emotions are natural expressions and responses that occur in our daily interaction with the external world. They are the consequence of the outer world meeting with the inner world, particularly the world of memory.

In pure awareness, the mind is still and prāna is motionless. The movement of prāna transforms awareness into perception, perception into feeling, feeling into thought and thought into emotion. When the mind stirs and prāna begins to flow, awareness takes a direction and becomes attention. The moment attention passes through the doors of perception (eyes, ears, nose and so on), it becomes perception. Perception brings sensations, which flow into feelings. Then mind steps in and, based on its stored-up memories, begins to create thoughts, which carry judgment. True perception is the ability to see clearly without any judgment or bias. However, when mind becomes involved, the person feels attraction or aversion, and judges experiences as pleasant or unpleasant. The innocent pure perception is obscured. Emotion is thus a reaction born of memory meeting the present challenge of the outer world.

For example, we all carry around images of the people in our lives, created out of conscious and subconscious emotions. You have an image of your husband or wife, your boyfriend or girlfriend. Whenever you look at your husband or wife, or listen to them, these layers of images filter the information. Therefore, you always receive very little actual information in your relationship. You look through the screen of these images. Whatever you receive is filtered; it is not total perception, but partial. You may sleep with your wife but you may be miles and miles apart from her because she is engrossed in her own image-making machinery and you in your own.

The nature of emotion is to flow within and through us, just as the tide ebbs and flows on the seashore. Emotions should not be repressed, but allowed to mature and flower in awareness.[3] Just as ripened fruit drops from a tree and leaves fall from their branches in the autumn, emotions must be released. The beauty of emotions is to experience them in full bloom and then let them go. This natural rhythm requires first recognizing the emotion, being in touch with it, allowing it to mature and then letting it go. Letting go of emotions is surrender. Surrender is a journey towards the heart. The consistent practice of witnessing emotions rise up, blossom and dissolve in freedom trains the mind to settle into an expansive state of pure meditative awareness and leads to the unfoldment of higher consciousness. The individual lives in increasing harmony with his or her thoughts, feelings, emotions and environment. Ultimately, the goal is unshakable peace and tranquility, a life of freedom and unbounded love, beyond the influence of fluctuating emotions and the vicissitudes of the external world.

Unfortunately, modern society does not provide the necessary tools for adequately processing emotions and

experiences. Every thought, feeling and emotion has an origin and a maturation process that is important to honor. When feelings and emotions rise up, it is important to be with them. But we rarely pay attention to the inner process. Every emotion has something to convey, a story to tell, but we are not ready to listen. Either we are not there, or we control it, suppress it, pack it and store it. As a result, emotions become suppressed, leading to mental toxicity (āma).

Toxicity represents a blockage of the mind on a subtle level, and an eventual obstruction within tissues, organs and channels. Just as physical āma may be produced from eating old, stale or improper food, or from food that is inadequately digested, mental āma is created from unripe, unprocessed raw emotions, thoughts and feelings. Āyurveda describes these toxins as unresolved, "crystallized" emotions that deposit into the deep connective tissue and consequently the marmāni. Sensitivity at a marma diagnostically reflects either physical or mental disturbance. Stimulating marmāni addresses the blockages by enhancing the flow of prāna and bringing subconscious, hidden emotions to the surface. Deep bodywork as part of pañchakarma therapy effectively breaks these crystals of emotion and releases them.

In Āyurveda, all emotions are considered doshic reactions, classified as predominantly vāta, pitta or kapha in nature. An individual has a propensity to experience those emotions that correspond to his or her constitution, especially when that dosha is elevated. For example, a vāta individual with high vāta will have a tendency to be anxious or nervous. When pitta is predominant and the person has high pitta, he/she will tend to become angry or irritable, while a kapha predominant individual with high kapha may tend toward depression or attachment. The classification of emotions is summarized in table 5 on page 32.

According to Āyurveda, emotions are associated with particular organs and marmāni. (see table 4) The liver is a seat of anger, the gall bladder the seat of hatred or jealousy, the kidneys the seat of fear and anxiety. The colon is the seat of nervousness, the spleen the seat of attachment and greed, the lungs the seat of grief and sorrow, and the heart is the seat of hurt and worries. Thus, tenderness felt at a marma may indicate organ dysfunc-

---

3. The key phrase here is "in awareness." We are not in any way advocating outwardly acting out or inflicting on others one's anger, etc. but, rather, an inward process of healing self-awareness.

Flow of Awareness

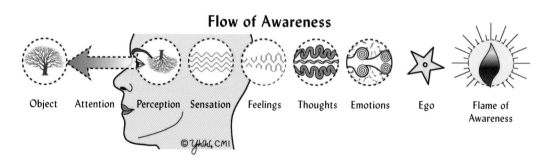

Object   Attention   Perception   Sensation   Feelings   Thoughts   Emotions   Ego   Flame of Awareness

tion, or it may indicate emotional imbalance. For example, Yakrut marma may be tender if unresolved anger lodges in the liver. Vrukka marma may be tender if fear settles in the kidneys. An individual with deep-seated grief and sadness may experience tightness in the chest muscles at Hrid marmāni. Pain in sacral marmāni may be due to a sudden loss of support, or a feeling of instability and ungroundedness.

Marmāni regulate the flow of prāna and consequently influence all perception, sensation, feeling, thought and emotion. With marma chikitsā, perception becomes clearer, thoughts more focused and emotions flow more smoothly. Marmāni are sites where the mind can recognize its limitations and misperceptions, and then allow consciousness to rejuvenate and awareness to flower.

Table 4: Organs and Emotions

Organ	Emotion	Related Marmāni
Lungs	Grief, sadness, melancholy	Apastambha, Agra Patra, Kakshadhara
Kidneys	Fear	Vrukka, Kati
Heart	Worries, hurt	Hridayam, Hrid
Liver	Anger, rage	Yakrut
Gallbladder	Jealousy, envy	Vankri
Spleen	Attachment, greed	Plīhā

Go With the Flow: Marmāni and the Art of Calming the Mind

Mastery of the mind requires discipline and training through techniques such as meditation, prānāyāma (control of the breath) and yoga, which can be creatively integrated with marma chikitsā. The constantly active mind can learn to rest in greater stillness.

An excellent form of meditation is the innocent watching of every thought, feeling and emotion; without judgment, without liking and disliking. In that simple, expansive awareness, there is a letting go. Letting go is another name for surrender, and surrender is a journey towards the heart. In the beginning, there may be many thoughts—bumper to bumper traffic! But if one continues that silent, peaceful watching, thinking eventually slows, and one can clearly perceive a gap between thoughts, memories or emotions; a silence, however momentary. Enter that gap. In time, it will expand into a vast silence that can be experienced during not only

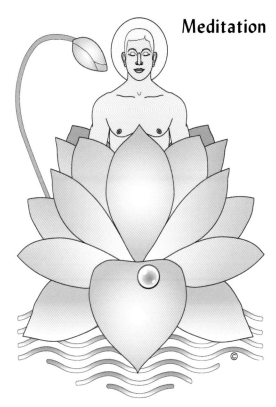

Meditation

meditation periods, but all the time. This silence, this unbounded pure awareness, is your true nature, and to be in this state, awake and aware to whatever is taking place within or in the environment, is meditation.

Placing one's quiet attention at a particular marma point can be considered a form of meditation. It is also a method of marma chikitsā that does not involve physical touch. It enhances awareness and brings the therapeutic qualities of that marma to fruition. Similarly, paying attention to specific marmāni associated with the chakras activates those energy centers according to their unique aspects of consciousness. For example, focusing on marmāni associated with the heart such as Hrid and Hridayam, unfolds the qualities of love, bliss and supreme joy. Refer to chapter 7 for specific meditation techniques.

Prānāyāma is the science of mastering the breath. The breath is intimately connected to the mind. By controlling the breath, the mind is regulated, and vice versa. When the mind is turbulent, the breath will be rapid and shallow. When the mind is still, the flow of breath is smoother and slower. Stimulating the appropriate marmāni, such as Apastambha or the Hrid marmāni (see chapter 11), regulates the breath and calms the mind.

Performing yoga postures (āsana) is another form of self-induced marma chikitsā. Yoga is a complete discipline comprising eight limbs. Meditation and prānāyāma are two branches of the beautiful tree of Yoga, while physical postures are another limb. By aligning the body correctly, and bending and twisting so that pressure is naturally applied to certain marmāni, suppressed emotions crystallized in the tissues are broken up and the flow of energy (prāna) in the body is enhanced, leading to deeper breathing, a calmer mind and overall balanced health. Chapter 17 is devoted entirely to yoga and its relation to marmāni.

In our journey in this chapter through the cells, tissues, fibers and channels of the body and the energy centers through which life energy (prāna) flows, and through the various levels of mind (manas, buddhi, chitta, ahamkāra), we have seen how marmāni can play an influential role in the healing of every level of body and mind as well as opening one's awareness to the pure spiritual dimension of our being. An ancient, mystical Vedic art, marma therapy is both a science of healing and a spiritual science that has the potential to transform life into supreme bliss.

Table 5: Expression of Emotions

Dosha	Imbalanced	Balanced
Vāta	Fear, anxiety, nervousness, insecurity, loneliness, ungroundedness, emptiness, emotional instability, mood swings, restlessness, hysteria, confusion, daydreaming	Clarity, creativity, alertness, perceptiveness, joyousness, excitement, flexibility, readiness to change
Pitta	Anger, rage, irritability, impatience, agitation, frustration, hatred, jealousy, envy, judgment, criticism, aggression, competitiveness, violence, rejection, perfectionism, success-oriented to the point of addiction to success, manipulation	Understanding, comprehension, appreciation, good memory, right recognition (seeing things clearly, as they are), attention, concentration
Kapha	Attachment, greed, possessiveness, longing, craving-for or hungering-after, sense of worthlessness, grief, sadness, depression, gloominess, heaviness, dullness	Love, compassion, care, gentleness, contentment, satisfaction, fulfillment, forgiveness, stability, groundedness

Āyurveda and Traditional Chinese Medicine

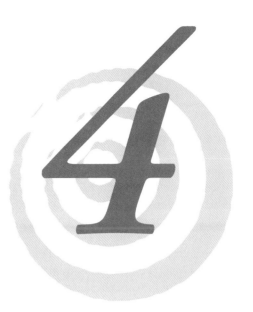

Alongside the Ayurvedic model of marmāni, the most well known system of energy points is found in Traditional Chinese Medicine (TCM), where both pressure and heat (moxibustion) have been effectively used along with acupuncture for thousands of years. Much light can be shed on Ayurvedic marma chikitsā and the role of healing through energy points by examining the great similarities as well as the differences between these two ancient medical systems. Though a comprehensive comparative study is far beyond the scope or intention of this book, we will look in this chapter at their underlying philosophies, concepts of health and disease, and methods for management of pain.

The Creation Model in Traditional Chinese Medicine

• •

Just as Āyurveda is rooted in Sānkhya philosophy, TCM is based upon a Taoist viewpoint that emphasizes tranquility, simplicity and deep attunement to nature and natural law. In this model, all of creation springs forth from the Void (*Wu*), the cosmic, undifferentiated primordial unity also known as the *Tao*, a field of unlimited potential from which all things arise. The *Tao Teh Ching*, a classic Chinese philosophical text dating from at least 2500 BCE, says:

There was something formless yet complete,

That existed before heaven and earth;

Without sound, without substance,

Dependent on nothing, unchanging,

All pervading, unfailing.

One may think of it as the mother of all things under heaven.

Yin and Yang

The unity of the Tao, while remaining eternally unbroken, appears to differentiate into two polar opposites, *yin* and *yang,* which describe the duality inherent within all creation. Yin and yang are considered the "root, fulcrum and backbone" of creation, encompassing the physical, mental and spiritual planes. Present everywhere, they pervade the nature of all phenomena and are expressed in endless forms, levels and degrees of manifestation.

The familiar dark/light symbol for yin and yang is known as *Tai Ji,* the "Supreme Ultimate." This primeval unity, Tao, is oneness that chooses to manifest as duality. From the movement of unity into duality, *qi* (pronounced chi) is generated. Directly parallel to prāna in Āyurveda, qi is the vital life force or energy that is present in all things. In living beings, it differentiates into several types:

* *Yuan qi* (ancestral or inherited energy)
* *Qing qi* (energy of air)
* *Gu qi* (energy of food)
* *Ying qi* (nutritive energy)
* *Zong qi* (energy of the chest)
* *Zang fu qi* (energy of each organ)
* *Jing luo* or *zhi qi* (energy of each meridian or channel in which energy flows)
* *Wei qi* (protective energy, immunity)
* *Xie qi* (pathogenic energy)

Within the human body, qi is related to various organs and meridians. For example, acupuncturists will refer to Stomach Qi or Liver Qi as the energy present within those organs and their corresponding meridians. From qi spring forth the five elements, termed *Wu Xing*: Fire, Earth, Metal, Water and Wood. Yin/yang, qi and the five elements form the pillars of Traditional Chinese Medicine.

The Five Principles of Yin and Yang
Five fundamental principles define the relationship between yin and yang:

1. They are **complementary opposites**; the increase of either one leads to a decrease of the other. This principle allows yin and yang to control and check each other. For example, as the light gradually increases at dawn, the darkness recedes, while the opposite is true at the juncture of dusk.
2. Yin and Yang are **interdependent**; neither can exist without the other because their duality is part of one cohesive whole. Thus, despite terms that appear to create distinctions (dark/light, hot/cold, top/bottom, etc.) yin and yang cannot be correctly viewed as isolated phenomena. In the human body, the superior, anterior and exterior parts are considered to be yang. Yin manifests as the inferior, posterior and interior parts.
3. They are **inter-consuming** due to their dynamic, ever-changing nature. Contraction and expansion, two qualities that describe yin and yang respectively, reflect this relationship of constant flux.
4. They are **inter-transforming**. An extreme of either yin or yang changes to its opposite. When extreme heat consumes the body during a fever, at a critical point, the person begins to experience chills and extreme cold.
5. Both yin and yang are **infinitely divisible**. Even a substance that is very yin has a yang component, and that yang component can be broken down even further into yin and yang. For example, the earth is predominantly yin in nature, but it has a molten core of fire (yang). At the center of the fire is absolute stillness (yin). At times, water is yin because it appears cool, deep, still and tranquil. But it can also be forceful, turbulent and raging, all qualities of yang. Thus, the ability to perceive and classify the ever-transforming, infinitely textured interrelationship of yin and yang within all of nature is endless.

Tai Ji, the symbol of yin and yang, reflects all five basic principles. The white part represents light and corresponds to yang; the black part is yin and signifies darkness. The curved line displays both their opposition and their interdependence. The two halves within the all-encompassing circle illustrate that their duality is part of one whole. The dots demonstrate in the most simple way that each contains the seed of the other, and reveals the potential for inter-transformation. The total symbol

reflects movement and constant flux, depicting yin/yang as dynamic.

Yin is viewed as the material basis for yang and yang as the functional manifestation of yin. Yin functions to cool, nourish and provide rest, while yang has the opposite functions to warm, move, transform, protect and hold. The polarity of yin and yang is reflected in not only the philosophical theory, but also the physical and organic structure of the body, the nature of the organs and meridians, and all physiological functions. In addi-

TCM Creation
Void = Wu or the Tao
Supreme Ultimate, Tai Ji
Feminine Passive — Yin / Yang — Masculine Active
Qi (Chi)
FIRE EARTH METAL WATER WOOD

34

tion, as we shall explore below, the yin/yang framework is used to describe the nature of pathogens, clinical manifestation of symptoms, terms for diagnosis and the principles of medical treatment.

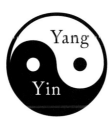

Health and vitality, indeed life itself, come from the balanced interconnectedness of yin and yang. All disease is due to disharmony between them. Thus, treatment in TCM focuses on restoring balance between these two principles.

The energetics of specific organs and meridians are traditionally considered to be predominantly yin or yang. The yin organs include the Heart, Pericardium, Lung, Liver, Spleen and Kidney. They store the five vital substances: qi (energy), *xue* (blood), *jing* (essence), *shen* (spirit) and *jin ye* (body fluids). Yang organs are hollow and responsible for transforming food and drink into their essence and excreting waste products. They include the Large Intestine, Small Intestine, Stomach, Bladder, Gallbladder and San Jiao (see table 6). Yang organs receive, move, transform, digest and excrete substances. Yin organs correspond more to structure, while their paired yang organs govern function. Thus, their energetics should be understood in relation to one another. The

organs are coupled not only because of proximity in some cases, but also similar physiology.

Table 6: The Twelve Primary Organs

Yin Organ	Yang Organ	Corresponding Element
Heart	Small Intestine	Fire
Pericardium	San Jiao	Fire/ Water
Spleen	Stomach	Earth
Lung	Large Intestine	Metal
Kidney	Bladder	Water
Liver	Gallbladder	Wood

The pairing of the Pericardium and San Jiao is a functional organization unique to TCM. The Pericardium is a protective structure for the heart and shares similar energetics with it. The principal difference is their meridian energetics and the Pericardium's greater susceptibility to pathogenic influence. The Pericardium is coupled with the San Jiao, also known as the Triple Burner or Triple Heater. The San Jiao is not a physical organ, but the energetics of various organs working syn-

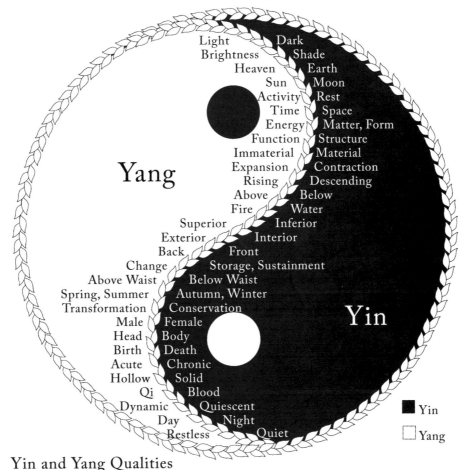

Yin and Yang Qualities

chronistically to regulate water, like a magnificent irrigation system. The three jiaos (areas of water regulation) comprise the upper chest, the area between the diaphragm and umbilicus, and the lower abdomen.

TCM's primary focus on the subtle energetics of the body allows it to view the twelve primary organs as sufficient representations of the entire body's function. The functions of other organs, such as the pancreas and thyroid, are subsumed under the twelve primary organs' energetics.

Table 7: Functions of Organs[a]

Heart	Regulates blood and vessels, houses the mind, spirit, consciousness, memory, mental functions, and regulates sleep
Small Intestine	Receives partially digested food and separates the pure from the impure
Pericardium	Protects the heart, governs emotions and relationships
San Jiao	Regulates water metabolism
Spleen	Transforms and transports food into qi and blood, regulates blood
Stomach	Receives food
Lung	Regulates qi and respiration, regulates water passages and bodily fluids, promotes wei qi (immunity)
Large Intestine	Receives waste material from small intestine, absorbs fluids, excretes feces
Kidneys	Stores jing (essence), dominates reproduction, growth, and development, connected to bones, brain, and marrow, receives qi and aids lungs with respiration, regulates water metabolism
Bladder	Stores and excretes urine
Liver	Stores blood, nourishes eyes, regulates menstrual flow, harmonizes emotions
Gallbladder	Stores and excretes bile

a. (Thyme 1997)

The Five Elements in TCM

Alongside the yin/yang model of describing nature, the Chinese developed what is often called the "five element" model (Wu Xing). However, a better translation of Wu Xing than "five elements" would be "five movements" or "five principles of transformation," which express a more dynamic interpretation, more true to the spirit of Taoism, of the elements as non-static entities as well as the materials necessary for life. For example, Fire and Water are the basis for all food, and Metal and Wood for all production. The model also explains the interaction of the twelve primary organs and meridians that express the energetic of a particular element. The five movements have two primary relationships: a nurturing relationship where each element promotes the growth and development of the element that follows it in the cycle, and a controlling relationship that checks or restrains an element that is out of balance.

The five-element model categorizes all observable phenomena such as the seasons, climate, movement and emotions. In terms of the human body, the elements correlate to the senses and sense organs, substances, tissues and bodily secretions. Table 52 on page 263 in appendix B summarizes these interrelationships.

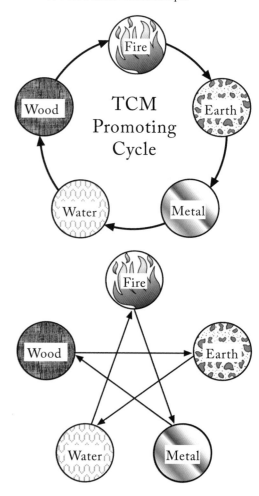

TCM Controlling Cycle

Comparing the Philosophies of TCM and Sānkhya

Unity

A comparison of TCM and Sānkhya philosophy reveals many inherent similarities. The deep wisdom within both venerable traditions not only appears to spring from the same profound source, but also is being increasingly corroborated by the forward march of Western science. In both traditions, as well as in modern science, similar principles have emerged through the process of intuitive insight, observation of nature, developing hypotheses, and testing the validity and usefulness of these hypotheses in practical life.

As we have seen, at the heart of both traditions is a sense of cosmic unity as the source from which all of creation arises. This is termed Wu or Tao in TCM, and is comparable to two concepts in Sānkhya philosophy: Avyakta (the unmanifest) and Purusha, the conscious principle that springs forth from Avyakta. These are eternal, unbounded in space and time, and are the essence of oneness. They are without attributes and beyond name, form and differentiation.

Duality

In both TCM and Sānkhya, the first step of manifestation of the fundamental wholeness or unity is duality. In the Chinese model, the unity expresses itself as yin and yang, which arise together and are eternally and co-equally paired in every aspect of creation. Together, they are the Supreme Ultimate, Tai Ji. Yin and yang co-exist; one cannot exist without the other. Together they constitute a dynamic whole that is inter-transforming and inter-consuming.

The Sānkhya model is significantly different. While the fundamental wholeness, the unmanifest Avyakta, appears to differentiate as Purusha and Prakruti, Purusha is primary, in that Prakruti cannot exist without Purusha, while Purusha can exist without Prakruti. Another subtle difference is that, like yin in TCM, Prakruti is considered feminine, while yang and Purusha are masculine: but yin is viewed as essentially passive, while Prakruti is active. Like yin and yang, Purusha and Prakruti are dynamic entities, but they are not inter-transforming; that is, they do not convert into one another.

Qualities

In contrast to the dualistic model of yin/yang, Prakruti first expresses itself as *three*: the three gunas or qualities of sattva, rajas and tamas. All of creation is imbued with these qualities, which can be compared with the qualities and characteristics of yin/yang. Rajas, for

Sānkhya Creation

Avyākta (the unmanifest)

Purusha
(the conscious principle)
passive

Prakruti
active, creative will

Sattva
passive

Rajas   active

Tamas
passive

Prāna

Pañcha Maha Bhūtani
(the five elements)

ETHER   AIR   FIRE   WATER   EARTH

1. VĀTA   2. PITTA   3. KAPHA

3 Doshas

example, has the active nature of yang, while sattva and tamas possess the passive qualities of yin. Sattva and rajas are yang in terms of being light while tamas is yin because it is darkness. Rajas is the bridge or meeting point between sattva and tamas, but yin and yang do not have a third entity that mediates between them.

While sattva, rajas and tamas are considered to be the *maha gunas* or "great qualities", Āyurveda also recognizes twenty gunas (ten pairs of opposites) that provide a detailed qualitative view of reality and describe

20 Gunas and Their Relationship with Yin/Yang

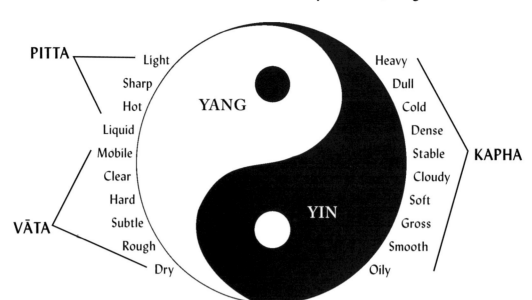

virtually all phenomena. These qualities are directly parallel to the commonly accepted qualities of yin and yang in TCM, as shown in the illustration above.

As the illustration shows, Vāta dosha is cold, light, mobile, clear, subtle, rough and dry. Pitta dosha is hot, sharp, light, liquid, oily and spreading. Kapha dosha can be described as heavy, dull, cold, dense and stable. It is also cloudy, soft, gross, smooth and oily. Thus, vāta and pitta are predominantly yang in nature, while kapha is yin. These characteristics of the doshas suggest the way that qualitative disturbances (such as excessive heat, cold, dryness, roughness, heaviness, etc.) may influence the body by affecting the doshic (or yin/yang) equilibrium and result in disease.

Qi and Prāna

Qi and prāna are virtually equivalent. Both represent energy, the vital life force responsible for the animation of every organism and the life of everything in the universe. Without them, life cannot exist and death is inevitable. Qi is generated from the movement of unity into duality. Prāna, similarly, is the energy that flows through creation from Prakruti to Mahad to buddhi to ahamkāra and lastly into the three gunas and their differentiations into the organic and inorganic universe. Within the body, both flow through the subtle energy pathways, termed meridians in TCM and nādīs in Āyurveda.

Qi and prāna diverge in that prāna is perceived to be not just energy, but the flow of intelligence and awareness. Prāna also exists in conjunction with ojas and tejas, forming a trinity within the microcosm of the body and the macrocosm of the universe. In the body, prāna is cellular awareness, tejas is cellular digestion and intelligence, and ojas is equated with cellular immunity.

Remarkably, the trinity of ojas, tejas and prāna does have an equivalent in TCM. Qi (energy) corresponds to prāna, Shen (spirit) with tejas, and Jing (essence) with ojas. Qi, Shen and Jing are known as the three treasures. Although these concepts do not fully coincide, they provide sufficient grounds for meaningful comparison.

TCM also emphasizes the functional relationship of qi and blood. Qi is yang in nature and blood is yin. Blood is viewed as the mother of qi because of its nourishing nature. Qi is called the commander of blood, because it is thought to lead blood through the channels. In Āyurveda, blood is called *rakta,* and it is intimately associated with prāna in a manner similar to qi and blood, traditionally expressed as *prāno raktānu dhavati,* prāna moves with the blood.

The Five Elements

Essential to both TCM and Sānkhya are the five elements or organizing principles that support life when in balance and create disease when imbalanced. Though expressing it in different language, these traditions share the common perception of a profound harmony between the individual and the cosmos, linking microcosm and macrocosm. The human body is seen to be a microcosm that mirrors the natural world and the universe. Hence, the five elements that are vital, energetic building blocks of the natural world are reflected within the individual.

The five elements do not overlap precisely. Fire, Water and Earth are common to both systems, while the remaining two elements differ. The Sānkhya system includes Space and Air, while TCM has Wood and Metal. But these divergences are not as great as they may initially seem, as metal has many attributes similar to Air and vāta dosha, and Wood shares common attributes with Fire and pitta dosha, because it carries the hidden potential of Fire within it. Space, from the Sānkhya system, does not have a direct correspondence in the TCM model, but it is implied there as the space within which the other elements exist and interact.

In TCM, the elements nourish and regulate each other in a cyclical manner. In contrast, the Ayurvedic five elements arise from a linear, hierarchical progression where one element generates the next in a natural order that mimics the evolution of creation from the soul to the conscious spirit to space and the other elements.

Perhaps the greatest difference is the role the five elements play in each system. In TCM, the structural progression from Tao or Wu through yin and yang stops with the five elements, which form the basis of what the Taoists call "the 10,000 things." In Sānkhya and Āyurveda, the five elements are not the end point in the creation scheme. From their combination emerge the three doshas, the cornerstone of the Ayurvedic lexicon and the heart of its conceptual framework. Thus, the Ayurvedic five elements are not given the same emphasis as the elements in TCM because the doshas play a more prominent role.

Space and Air unite to form vāta dosha, Fire and Water form pitta dosha, and Water and Earth constitute kapha dosha. These three doshas are the governing factors for diagnosis and treatment. Just as the TCM five elements have a "controlling cycle" that maintains self-regulating balance, the three doshas continuously adjust and re-adjust to maintain equilibrium. In both systems, when an element or dosha becomes excessive or deficient, balance is disrupted, leading to specific symptomatology and pathology.

Individual Constitution

De is the Chinese term for an individual's unique nature, which is typically expressed in terms of the five elements. He or she may be predominantly Fire, manifesting as energetic, robust and hot-tempered. Someone endowed with more Metal is organized, meticulous and may be emotionally cold and detached. A person imbued with a preponderance of Earth is good-natured, jovial, grounded, stable and possibly stubborn. An individual influenced by Water may be emotional, sensitive, contemplative and imaginative. Someone controlled by Wood is creative, intuitive, energetic, active and decisive. These constitutional types are discussed in modern interpretations of TCM (most notably in the five element school of thought), but are not mentioned in the ancient texts. However, this typology does provide an interesting ground for comparison with Āyurveda.

In Āyurveda, an individual's constitution (prakruti) is predominantly vāta, pitta, kapha or a combination of these doshas. The science of prakruti provides each indi-

Comparison of the Five Elements

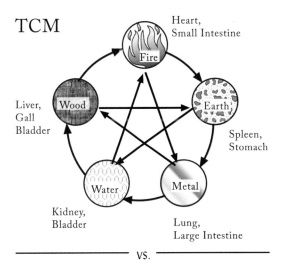

TCM

Heart, Small Intestine — Fire
Liver, Gall Bladder — Wood
Spleen, Stomach — Earth
Kidney, Bladder — Water
Lung, Large Intestine — Metal

— VS. —

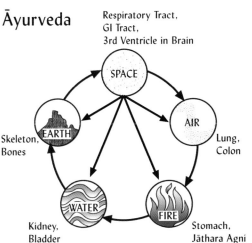

Āyurveda

Respiratory Tract, GI Tract, 3rd Ventricle in Brain — SPACE
Skeleton, Bones — EARTH
Lung, Colon — AIR
Kidney, Bladder — WATER
Stomach, Jāthara Agni — FIRE

vidual with knowledge of his or her psychological and physiological strengths and weaknesses. Knowing the constitution, one can easily discover the best diet and lifestyle habits to maintain vibrant health, as well as predict potential illnesses and imbalances and take precautions to prevent them from arising. In Āyurveda the prakruti is considered to have, in addition to the basic physical, doshic combination, a karmic and genetic component and a mental component. In addition, the present altered state of the doshas, *vikruti,* is also vital to understand. The Ayurvedic practitioner carefully notes the individual's unique constitution and life history, as well as the particular circumstances of his or her life at the moment. This sophisticated analysis and insight is the foundation of all Ayurvedic diagnosis and treatment.[1]

---

1. For a deeper and more extensive exploration of Ayurvedic constitution and its practical applications for life and health, please see chapter 1, "Introduction to Āyurveda," *The Textbook of Āyurveda,* volume 1, chapters 2 and 3, or *The Complete Book of Ayurvedic Home Remedies,* chapter 2.

Health and Disease in Āyurveda and TCM

· ·

The philosophies that shape the foundation of these two great medical traditions each provide a specific outlook with which to view the body and mind and their relationships to health and disease. Understanding these concepts is vital if we are to truly comprehend the perspective these traditions have to offer.

In TCM, health in its simplest definition is the balance of yin and yang in the body. From an energetic viewpoint, health is an abundance of qi that flows smoothly throughout the network of meridians and related organs. Reflecting the intricate relation of microcosm and macrocosm, health is also viewed as harmony between the inner and outer worlds, and between the individual and nature. Disease is the disruption of the balance between yin, yang and qi.

Balance and harmony are also central to the Ayurvedic view of health and disease. Life lived in harmony with the laws of nature governing individual life and the interaction of the individual with others and with the daily and seasonal cycles of nature, is seen as essential to good health, as are a balanced state of body and mind. The Ayurvedic conception of a healthy person is spelled out with great specificity in this verse from Sushruta Samhita (Sūtrasthanam 15.38).

समदोषाः समाग्निश्च समधातुमलक्रियाः।
प्रसन्नात्मेन्द्रियमनाः स्वस्थ इत्यभिधीयते ॥ ३८ ॥

सु.सू. १५

Sama doṣāḥ samāgniś ca sama dhātu mala kriyāḥ
Prasannātmendriya manāḥ svastha ityaghidhīyate

Su. Sū. 15

The one who is established in Self, who has balanced doshas, balanced agni, properly formed dhātus, proper elimination of malas, properly functioning bodily processes, and whose mind, soul, and senses are full of bliss, is called a healthy person.

Or, to paraphrase and expand a bit, "One who is established in the Self, who has balanced doshas (the governing principles of physiology), balanced agni (healthy appetite and digestion), properly formed dhātus (tissues), proper elimination of malas (wastes), proper functioning *kriyā* (bodily processes), and whose manas (mind), ātman (soul), and *indriya* (senses) are full of clarity and bliss, is known as a healthy person."

When doshas, dhātus, and malas are in proper functional relationship, along with a balance on the cellular

level of ojas, tejas and prāna, there is a perfect balance of body, senses, mind and consciousness, resulting in clarity, happiness, joy, peace and love. Disease, or at least less-than-perfect health, arises when this balance is not maintained.

It is highly significant that in its fundamental definition of health, Āyurveda includes, along with proper functioning of the organs and bodily processes, not only profound happiness but "being established in the Self," the pure divine consciousness that is our true nature.

Etiology and Pathogenesis in Āyurveda

The concepts of health and disease shape the language in which pathology is described. In Āyurveda, the pathogenesis of disease is termed *samprāpti*. The six stages summarized in the table below depict a dosha's journey from balance to imbalance. Imbalance arises from three etiological categories: internal factors, external factors and the mind. These concepts are discussed in detail in chapter 6, "Pathogenesis and Disturbance of Marmāni."[2]

Table 8: Stages of Samprāpti

Stages	Description of Pathogenesis
1. Sañchaya	Accumulation of dosha in home site: vāta in the colon, pitta in the small intestine, and kapha in the stomach
2. Prakopa	Provocation or aggravation of doshas in their home site
3. Prasara	Spreading of doshas leaving their home site and moving to other areas of the body through circulation of rasa and rakta dhātu
4. Sthāna Samshraya	Deposition of doshas into khavaigunya (defective space) in dhātu, organ, or system
5. Vyakti	Manifestation of pathology, symptomatology
6. Bheda	Differentiation of disease, complications

TCM Etiology

In TCM, disease arises from three categories as well: external, internal and miscellaneous factors. The six external pathogens, known as the pernicious influences, are wind, dryness, summer-heat, fire, cold and damp. Wind and dryness can be correlated to aggravation of vāta dosha, summer-heat and fire to an imbalance

---

2. See also *The Textbook of Ayurveda*, vol. II, chapter 2, Lad.

of pitta, and cold and damp to an accumulation of kapha. These invade the body from the exterior: the skin, mouth, respiratory system and sense organs. The first four pathogens are yang in nature, while the last two are yin in nature. Each pathogen has its own symptomatology and is more prone to aggravation in a specific season. The body's immune response depends on the quantity and quality of qi, which varies from individual to individual.

The seven emotions are internal factors that affect the mind: joy, grief, shock, fear, anger, worry and pensiveness. They are normal responses that lead to disease only when excessive. Each emotion affects the circulation and quantity of qi and blood. In response to the emotions, qi may ascend, descend, scatter, stagnate, slow down or become depleted. These emotions also affect the corresponding organs. Each of the five yin organs has a principal emotion associated with it. It is interesting to note that both TCM and Āyurveda have the same correspondences between the organs and the emotions: the heart is connected to joy, the lungs to grief, the kidneys to fear, the liver to anger and the spleen to worry. Each emotion encompasses a broad range. For example, joy represents excessive excitement, ungroundedness, instability and restlessness, all vāta traits. Anger can be associated with rage, irritability, resentment and frustration, all pitta imbalances. Thus, the seven emotions can be seen as doorways into the entire scope of human emotion.

Disease etiology in TCM also includes miscellaneous pathogenic factors in addition to the six pathogens and seven emotions. They include dietary factors, activity levels and environmental influences. All etiological factors cause disease by spreading through the meridian pathways and organ networks.

In contrast, Āyurveda views disease as spreading through multiple avenues (doshas, dhātus, srotāmsi, etc.), not just through a network of channels. Ultimately, most etiology is ascribed to low agni that creates poor digestion and a build-up of āma, a toxic morbid substance. This āma clogs the channels, adversely affects nutrition, reduces resistance and initiates the disease process, which therefore is sometimes called *āmaya* in Āyurveda, meaning that which is born of āma.

TCM Pathology and Diagnosis

Once pathology has occurred, TCM has several methods for examining signs and symptoms, of which the most important are the "eight principles." These categorize all disease phenomena and are differentiated into pairs of opposites: interior and exterior, deficiency and excess, hot and cold, and yin and yang. Interior and exterior describe the location of pathogenesis, whether it is superficial or deep. Excess and deficiency represent the

quantity of qi. Hot and cold represent a set of qualities or symptoms in relation to yin and yang. Heat pathology is due to excess yang or depletion of yin, whereas cold pathology is attributed to excess of yin or a depletion of yang energy. These present themselves in an individual's diagnosis as a complex amalgam of signs and symptoms. The eight principles constitute the foundation for diagnosis and treatment in TCM.

By understanding the nature of the etiological factors and the methods used to observe and classify them, greater insight is shed on how these pathologies manifest. Qi can become stagnant, rebellious (counter-flow), deficient, or collapsed (extreme deficiency). Blood can likewise be described as deficient, stagnant or heated. Yin and yang can become excessive or depleted. The pathologies of wind, cold, heat, damp, dry, fire and phlegm are excesses that manifest in all of the various organ systems. Some organs have a propensity for certain types of pathogenic imbalance. For example, the Heart is more prone to heat pathology, while the Bladder is more prone to damp pathology. In treatment, acupoints are chosen to regulate the flow of qi and blood, dispel stagnation, and harmonize yin and yang.

Diagnosis in Āyurveda

Clinical diagnosis in Āyurveda is a subtle and sophisticated science. Volume II of Dr. Lad's *Textbook of Āyurveda,* subtitled, "A Complete Guide to Clinical Assessment," offers the student of Āyurveda a thorough and detailed store of practical knowledge. This brief section summarizes only a tiny fraction of that material.

In the process of determining the constitution (prakruti) of the patient, investigating the causes of a disease (etiology), and attempting to discover precisely its stage of development in the disease process (samprāpti) in order to devise an appropriate healing regimen, the clinician undertakes a thorough examination. In Āyurveda, this includes three main categories, known as *darshanam* (visual examination), *sparshanam* (palpation), and *prashanam* (questioning). In carrying out the examination, the practitioner employs the traditional Ashtavidhā Parīkshā—the eight methods of clinical examination. They are:

* *Nāḍī Parīkshā* – Pulse
* *Mūtra Parīkshā* – Urine
* *Purīsha or Mala Parīkshā* – Feces
* *Jihva Parīkshā* – Tongue
* *Shabda Parīkshā* – Speech
* *Sparsha Parīkshā* – Touch or Palpation
* *Drig or Netra Parīkshā* – Eyes
* *Ākruti Parīkshā* – Physical Appearance

Āyurveda Picture of Tongue

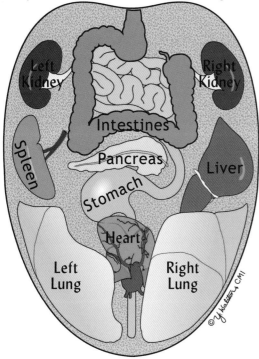

TCM Picture of Tongue

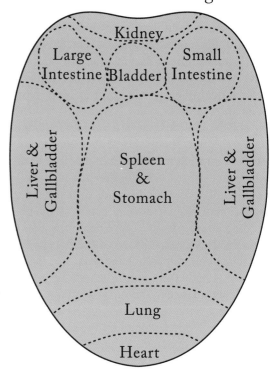

Diagnosis in Āyurveda and TCM

Tongue and pulse diagnosis are common methods in both TCM and Āyurveda to detect and understand pathology and provide a foundation for treatment. However, in Āyurveda, pulse diagnosis[3] includes more than the organ pulses used in TCM. In addition, more organs are included in Āyurvedic tongue diagnosis than in TCM. The tongue diagrams illustrated here contrast the diagnostic systems in the two traditions. On the whole, examination in Āyurveda is more elaborate, utilizing more avenues of investigation, and is thus a highly accurate diagnostic tool.

The similar and sometimes identical perspectives in both traditions provide insight into the ancient way of thinking. Both divide the origin of disease into interior and exterior factors, and recognize the role of the mind and emotions in disease and health. In both, disease is thought to be largely preventable by living in harmony with nature, for example by paying heed to the juncture between seasons, when people are most susceptible to developing imbalance and falling ill. Āyurveda and TCM similarly view the individual as possessing a unique constitution that plays a role in health and disease, although this concept is significantly more developed in Āyurveda.

Models of Pain

• • • • • • • • • • • • • • • • • •

Pain is a universal symptom from which many people desperately seek relief. Yet it is also pain that often brings the patient to the doctor, opening the door to diagnosis and healing. Āyurveda views pain as the body's method of prompting self-awareness, by communicating that something is wrong and needs attending to. It is the language of the body, speaking out about unseen inner doshic pathology.

Acupuncture has become well respected in the West for its dramatic results in modulating pain. Like Acupuncture, marma chikitsā is an effective means not only to alleviate the pain, but also to simultaneously address the underlying condition by promoting balance and healing. Though sometimes relief from painful symptoms is absolutely necessary, the approach of both Āyurveda and TCM is not to treat the patient merely symptomatically, but more importantly, to eradicate the deeper pathological process. Signs and symptoms are like leaves and branches; by merely cutting the leaves and branches, you cannot uproot the tree of the disease.

Pain in TCM

In TCM, pain is primarily due to a stagnation of qi or blood in the meridians. It is termed "Bi syndrome" which is classically defined as blockage or pain. It results from either a pathogenic influence or a weak con-

---

3. Appendix A, page 256–257, has illustrations showing the two methods of the pulse diagnosis.

stitution due to depletion of energy, overexertion, excess sexual activity and/or low immunity. There are four basic differentiations of pain that vary according to the affected body region, the particular organs and meridians involved, the strength of the pathogen and the strength of the patient. (see table 9 on page 44)

These types of Bi can be roughly correlated to disturbance of the doshas. Wandering Bi is vāta, fixed Bi is kapha and heat Bi is pitta. Pain can be alleviated by three primary methods in TCM. The first method is to select acupoints in the region of the body affected (especially those that are painful on pressure), including distal acupoints on the same meridian that traverses the affected area. The second method is to select points according to the principles of relieving pain. These acupoints promote the flow of qi and blood and unblock stagnation. The last method is to choose points relevant to the TCM diagnosis. For example, if pain is due to wind, acupoints that expel wind from the body are chosen even though they may be far away from the area of pain.

Pain in Āyurveda

Pain is termed *duhkha* in Sanskrit, sometimes translated as suffering. Pain in Āyurveda is primarily differentiated according to doshic factors and toxins, summarized in table 10 on page 44. All pain is due to disturbed vāta dosha that governs movement and circulation. There is no pain without vāta imbalance. Pain is attributed to a deficiency of prāna in an area, or stagnant prāna, which is similar to obstructed qi or blood. Prāna can be blocked by pitta, kapha and āma (toxins), leading to various manifestations of pain. Pain is a blockage of energy, similar to TCM, but it may also be due to a physical blockage due to toxins clogging the channels. Doshic pain may also trigger specific emotional factors affiliated with an imbalance of the dosha. For example, vāta type pain may be accompanied by vāta emotions such as anxiety, fear, nervousness and insecurity. The same holds true for pitta and kapha.

Pain can also be viewed in terms of its relationship with the dhātus (tissues). Any disturbance of a dhātu translates into specific types of pain.

- ✳ Rasa dhātu: generalized body ache (excess kapha)

- ✳ Rakta dhātu: burning, inflammatory pain, bleeding (excess pitta)

- ✳ Māmsa and meda dhātu: muscular pain (excess kapha)

- ✳ Asthi dhātu: pain in the joints, arthritis, traumatic injury, may arise from āma (toxins) or excess vāta

- ✳ Majjā dhātu: neurological pain, psychosomatic pain, mental or emotional trauma

- ✳ Shukra and ārtava dhātu: pain in reproductive organs (vāta, pitta, or kapha)

There are several factors to consider when selecting marmāni for pain relief. First, marmāni are chosen according to the affected body area, similar to the TCM method. Second, they are selected by their potential to pacify the dosha in question. Third, points are chosen according to affected tissues, such as muscular pain (muscles) or neurological pain (nerves). Other factors influencing the therapist's choice include the organs and channel system affected, stage of samprāpti, and directional movement (*gati*) of the dosha.

In conclusion, Āyurveda and Traditional Chinese Medicine show striking similarities in philosophy, inclusion of a five-element model, and related concepts of both health and disease. Both reflect a holistic approach involving mind, body, and spirit. Despite their differences, each system presents an integral philosophical and medical model clearly demonstrating the connection between health and living in balance, in harmony with nature. Most notably for this present study, both traditions utilize the energy points as doorways to maintain health and harmony.

Table 9: TCM Types of Pain

Type of Bi	Etiology	Pain Symptoms	Relieved By
1. Xing Bi (Wandering Bi)	Due to wind	Migrating, radiating, unfixed, aggravated by wind	Steady pressure, moxibustion (heat)
2. Tong Bi (Painful Bi)	Due to cold	Severe, stabbing, aggravated by cold	Warmth, pressure, moxibustion, (ginger) compresses
3. Zhuo Bi (Fixed Bi)	Due to damp	Soreness, swelling, numbness, heaviness, fixed painful areas, aggravated by cloudy and rainy days	Movement, moxibustion, dry pressure without oil
4. Re Bi (Heat Bi)	Due to wind-damp transforming into heat	Hot to touch, reddish, swollen, sudden onset, aggravated by touch	Cold, cooling compresses, ice pack

Table 10: Āyurvedic Types of Pain

Doshic Factor	Etiology	Nature of Pain	Relieved By
Vāta (wandering)	Cold, wind, dryness, trauma	Fluctuating, mobile, radiating, shifting, spasmodic, gripping, tearing, throbbing, pricking, shooting, vague, non-localized, non-inflammatory, aggravated with movement	Heat, steady pressure (e.g., with bandage), rest, heating food and drink, basti (medicated enema), oil massage
Pitta (burning)	Heat, spicy food, exposure to sunlight	Sharp, burning, irritating, excruciating, pulling, throbbing, flaring, spreading, sucking, swollen, inflammatory, painful on pressure, possibly accompanied by nausea and vomiting	Cold compress, khus, camphor, sandalwood paste, avoiding exposure to sun and heat, cooling food and drink, virechana (purgation)
Kapha (congesting)	Cold, dampness, eating fatty, fried food, lack of exercise and movement	Deep, dull, mild, heavy, constant, achy, slow manifestation, localized	Application of dry heat, dry massage, movement, stretching, deep pressure massage, inducing vomiting
Āma (clogging)	Low agni, incompatible food combinations, metabolic wastes	Greater near sunrise and sunset and on cloudy days, moves from joint to joint, autoimmune inflammatory changes	Kindling agni, ginger tea, steady pressure, dry massage without oil, heat, movement, stretching, steam, application of ginger paste

Channels, Energy Points and Measurements in Āyurveda and Traditional Chinese Medicine

Here we continue our exploration of the parallels and divergences between Āyurveda and Traditional Chinese Medicine. Here we will focus on the subtle energy channels that run through the body, and the specific points where that energy can be most effectively accessed and influenced to relieve pain, heal disease and promote health and vitality.

The chapter is divided into three principal sections that describe the concept of channels, the classification of energy points, and the measurements that have evolved to help practitioners locate the points. These topics are explored in the language and framework developed within each tradition.

Channels

One of the most striking similarities is that the model of channel systems arose in both traditions several thousand years ago, and has remained at the center of their understanding of how the body works and how to treat its ailments effectively. Both traditions hold that this knowledge came to humanity because the great ancient rishis and sages, through their inner wisdom and meditation, intuitively perceived the elegant organization and intricate flow of energy within the living body. They considered this knowledge sacred, offering a deep insight into the life force. They described how energy flow in the microcosm of the body reflected the macrocosm of nature. The movement of qi or prāna was compared to natural phenomena like the movement of water, which flows effortlessly and gracefully along a river or stream.

Energy in the body flows through an elaborate network of pathways, termed *meridians* in TCM and *srotāmsi* or *nādīs* in Āyurveda. Energy collects in these channels, builds up and ultimately animates the organism. In the literature of both systems of natural medicine, the channels are referred to as vessels, tubes, pipes, ducts, canals, pathways and so on. These structures facilitate movement, such as the transporting of nutrients, fluids or other bodily substances. Equally important, they serve as an immense communication network, conveying information and subtle energy from one place in the body to another.

Both systems utilize the concept of channels to elucidate our place in the cosmos. In TCM, as in Chinese philosophy in general, human beings are viewed not only as an integrated mind-body unity that is part of and intimately connected to nature, but also as a bridge between heaven and earth; as living conduits of cosmic energy. The goal of individual life is to become a "sage," aligned with natural law, the cosmic will. To accomplish this attunement, individuals must become empty vessels, freed from racing thoughts, turbulent emotions, ceaseless desires and inflated egos. Numerous practices are advocated, such as Tai Qi, Qigong, meditation and so on, which serve to quiet the mind and keep the qi (energy) in the meridians of the body flowing in harmony and balance.

In Āyurveda, the subtle channels that connect the individual with cosmic energy are called nādīs. Like individual and universal qi, the prāna that flows through the nādīs in the body is related to the cosmic prāna that animates the universe. And just like with TCM and Chinese philosophy, Āyurveda and the vast Vedic tradition of which it is a part provide almost countless systems and methods, such as Yoga and meditation, to generate higher spiritual awareness and help individuals live enlightened lives in attunement with natural law.

Of course, the notion of channels is not exclusive to Eastern thought; it is also prominent within modern Western medicine's conception of the body and its various systems. This includes the nasal passageways and bronchial tree of the respiratory system, the tubes and ducts of the intestinal network, and the circulation of blood through the complex network of arteries and veins.

Channels encompass the cranial and spinal nerves of the peripheral nervous system as well as the spinal cord itself. All these anatomical structures reflect the principle of channels on a gross physical plane, and correlate to the Ayurvedic system of srotāmsi.

Meridians and nādīs, however, are subtle energy pathways, not solid, visible structures. This has made acceptance of their reality a bit of a stretch for those brought up in the world view dominated by Western science. However, through their training and practice, a great many medical practitioners, body workers and hands-on healers have refined their clinical skills to the point where they can readily sense the channels and points. These gifted individuals can therefore know immediately when a channel or point is open and harmoniously flowing, or when it is blocked and the energy is stagnant, too hot or cold, etc., and needs to be treated. Many patients receiving marma therapy or acupuncture report the ability to feel the flow of energy in the body, and the changes in that flow as a result of treatment.

Channels in TCM

In TCM, the classification of meridians according to their functions and locations and with their often poetic names dates back to antiquity and has been recorded in a host of classical Chinese texts. Perhaps equally ancient, *Qigong*, the practice of cultivating energy, allows one to sense the flow of qi through the meridians and to transmit this energy to others. The meridians' multitude of functions highlights their paramount place in TCM. They regulate deficiency and excess, and harmonize yin and yang. Their management of healthy qi and their role in healing disease is central to TCM and forms the basis of its principles. The functions of the meridians include:

Transport Qi and Blood. They are principally vessels of transportation regulating and directing the flow of qi and blood, as well as providing nourishment to every part of the body.

Regulate Yin and Yang. Meridians inherently balance and regulate all aspects of yin and yang, including right and left, upper and lower, and interior and exterior components.

Protect the Body. The channels are a protective mechanism to prevent pathogens such as wind, cold, damp, dryness, heat and fire from penetrating deeper. When these pathogens are located in the superficial channels, disease is easier to treat. As the pathogens lodge into the deeper channels, the prognosis of disease will be more severe.

Regulate the Flow of Qi. Regulating and stimulating the flow of qi (sometimes called "propagation of qi sensation") in the meridians is essential for therapeutic results and transmitting energy to a diseased area. This can be achieved through needling, pressure, massage, heat and cupping.

Respond to Dysfunction. Channels reflect signs and symptoms of pathology when they respond to dysfunction. They may also express local pathology of stagnation or deficient qi or blood that manifests as pain, tenderness, weakness, distention or numbness and tingling along their pathway. Points along a meridian can become tender or sensitive, rendering them useful diagnostic tools for detecting organ or meridian imbalance.

Integration of Intelligence. The channels facilitate a ceaseless communication or flow of intelligence between the skin, flesh, muscles, tendons, bones, limbs, other tissues and sense organs of the body. They help to maintain the relationships between all aspects of the body, mind and consciousness and the functional integrity of the whole.

Although meridians originate deep within the body, the twelve principal meridians emerge at the surface, linking the interior and exterior. Of these, the six yin meridians run on the medial aspect of the body, while the six yang meridians are situated on the lateral aspect. Most channels run vertically, linking above and below, as well as bilaterally, maintaining the symmetry of the body.

Pathogens enter the body via the skin and are transported through the meridians to the twelve internal organs. The organs are considered the root; the twelve principal meridians, the stems; and the tissues and sense organs, the flowers. Pathology of the organ can affect its corresponding meridian and vice versa. When out of balance, each meridian has its own pathology, which can vary from organ pathology. Meridian disorders can in turn affect corresponding organs or spread disease to a paired organ.

Jingluo, the Chinese term for meridians and collaterals, is often illustrated by an image of a tree with a solid trunk and many branches sprouting from it. Jing is the trunk that comprises the meridians, while luo are the branches comprising the collaterals. Jing includes the twelve primary channels, eight extraordinary vessels and twelve divergent channels that run deeper in the body. Luo are the collaterals that include the Luo channels, minute collaterals that are too numerous to count, twelve sinew channels and twelve cutaneous regions located superficially. These channels are distributed at various levels of the body from the most superficial to the deepest. A brief description of them is listed in table 11.

The twelve primary channels are differentiated into six yin and six yang channels that correspond to the twelve organs. Each has an external pathway that runs superficially and along which the acupoints are located as well as internal pathways that connect to certain organs and regions. Specific indications of the acupoints

Jingluo Meridians and Collaterals

Heart
Pericardium
Lung
Large Intestine
Small Intestine
San Jiao
Spleen
Liver
Kidney
Stomach
Gallbladder
Bladder

3 Yin   3 Yang   3 Yin   3 Yang

Hand   Foot

Correspond to 12 Primary meridians
Ren & Du
Grand Luo of Spleen

Du
Ren
Yin Qiao
Chong
Yang Qiao
Dai
Yin Wei
Yang Wei
8 Extraordinary Vessels

12 Primary Meridians

Luo Connecting Channels

12 Sinew Regions

12 Cutaneous Regions

12 Divergent Channels

* Minute channels
are not shown

* 12 Divergent, Luo, Sinew,
& Cutaneous Regions
correspond to the
12 Primary meridians

can be correlated to the internal pathways. The twelve primary meridians are listed in table 12; illustrations are provided at the end of this chapter.

Energy flows through the twelve channels cyclically, circulating from one organ to the next in the order listed in table 12. There is a rhythm established in this flow from yin to yang, from one element to another, beginning with the Lung channel all the way to the Liver, until the cycle repeats itself. The flow corresponds to various times of the day when the qi of that particular organ or meridian is most dominant. The illustrations on

page 49 show the "organ clock" representing the flow of energy through the organs at regular times throughout the 24 hour cycle for each system.

Energy flow links specific regions of the body. For example, the Lung meridian originates in the chest and terminates at the hands. Its paired meridian, the Large Intestine, originates where the Lung meridian terminates at the hands and flows to the face. This results in the distribution of qi through three yin and three yang channels primarily on the arms and three yin and three yang channels on the legs.

Chapter 5 ~ Channels, Energy Points and Measurements

Table 11: TCM Channels

Channels[a]	Description
Cutaneous regions (12)	Similar in function to the sinew channels, broader region to address pain and meridian pathology
Minute collaterals	Branch off other meridians and transport qi and blood to every area of the body
Sinew channels (12)	Superficially located on the periphery, broadly follow course of associated primary channel, treat muscular pain and limited range of motion
Luo (connecting channels) (15)	Branch out from the primary channels and extraordinary vessels, superficially distributed over the four limbs, strengthen link between paired organs and channels, drain excess and tonify deficiency
Primary channels (12)	Correspond to the twelve organs, contain majority of acupoints, various functions related to energetics of the organ
Divergent channels (12)	Branch off primary channels, distribute qi and blood deeper, strengthen relation between paired organs and channels
Extraordinary channels (8)	Reservoirs of qi and blood, branch off primary channels and interlink them, promote immunity by circulating wei qi, protect against pathogens
Deep pathways of primary and divergent channels	Link areas of the body, transport qi and blood deeper

a. From superficial to deep channels.

Table 12: The Twelve Primary Meridians

Organ (Abbreviation)	Yin or Yang	Element	Chinese Name
Lung (LU)	Yin	Metal	Hand Taiyin
Large Intestine (LI)	Yang	Metal	Hand Yangming
Stomach (ST)	Yang	Earth	Foot Yangming
Spleen (SP)	Yin	Earth	Foot Taiyin
Heart (HT)	Yin	Fire	Hand Shaoyin
Small Intestine (SI)	Yang	Fire	Hand Taiyang
Bladder (BL)	Yang	Water	Foot Taiyang
Kidney (KD)	Yin	Water	Foot Shaoyin
Pericardium (PC)	Yin	Fire	Hand Jueyin
San Jiao (SJ)	Yang	Water	Hand Shaoyang
Gallbladder (GB)	Yang	Wood	Foot Shaoyang
Liver (LR)	Yin	Wood	Foot Jueyin

Table 13: Directions of Meridian Flow

Origination → Distribution	Meridians	Yin/Yang
Chest → descends down arms	Lung, Heart, Pericardium	Yin
Hand → ascends up arms	Large Intestine, Small Intestine, San Jiao	Yang
Face → descends down legs	Stomach, Bladder, Gallbladder	Yang
Foot → ascends up legs	Spleen, Kidney, Liver	Yin

TCM and Āyurveda Organ Times

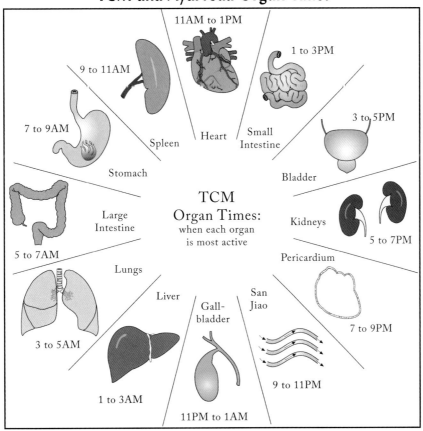

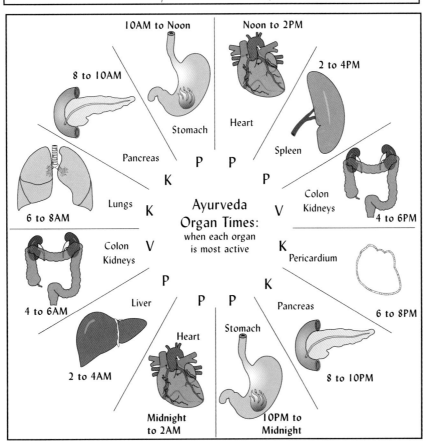

Channels in Āyurveda: Srotāmsi and Nādī

In contrast to TCM's multi-layered system of meridians, the Ayurvedic classification of channels contains two distinct levels, subtle and gross. Like meridians, nādīs are subtle energetic pathways. Srotāmsi, on the other hand, are larger and comparatively more gross structures created from various tissue components (dhātus) that facilitate the movement of fluids and other bodily substances. They are part of the body's anatomy and physiology. One srotas may carry several nādīs. A key difference between them is that srotāmsi govern functional activity, while nādīs govern energy (pranic) activity. Like the soul within the body, the nādīs control or animate the srotāmsi. Without nādīs, srotāmsi cannot operate.

Another way to understand the difference between nādīs and srotāmsi is that srotāmsi are anatomical structures with physiological functions, while nādīs are subtle energy channels that have primarily psychological functions; they carry thoughts, feelings and emotions. For example, prāna vaha srotas are the channels of the respiratory system, including the trachea, bronchi and bronchioles. *Prāna vahini nādīs* are similar, but they are more refined, non-physical energy pathways.

Nādīs

Nādīs are also referred to as prāna vahini nādīs, meaning channels that propagate the pranic current throughout the body. This gives a hint of their extremely refined nature. The term nādī may be translated as tube, duct, cord or vessel. It also represents a channel, stream, river, pulse or flow of time. The Sanskrit root *nād* means sound vibration and movement. All of these various meanings have the same connotation of flow, whether it is the flow of a river, the flow of time or the flow of energy.

There are 72,000 nādīs that branch off the seven chakras and pervade the body. The *īdā, pingalā* and *sushumnā* are the three principal nādīs. Sushumnā is the central nādī that originates in the mūlādhāra chakra at the base of the spine, ascends along the spinal cord, and enters the brain and crown chakra, terminating at Mūrdhni marma. An anterior branch travels to Brahmarandhra marma and a posterior branch to Shivarandhra marma. All other nādīs are connected to this central nādī. Kundalinī energy ascends through the sushumnā for higher spiritual awakening to occur. The sushumnā contains within it the fiery Vajra nādī and the cooling Chitra nādī that balance each other. Each of these channels has its own energetics, which are beyond the scope of this book.

The īdā and pingalā, two channels that ascend the spine parallel to the sushumnā, regulate the breath and

play an important role in awakening spiritual energy. The īdā opens into the left nostril and the pingalā the right nostril. About every ninety minutes, the pattern of the breath changes, dominance (stronger, easier flow) in one nostril giving way to dominance of the other. The īdā channel on the left is feminine, lunar energy and primarily yin. Directing the breath through this channel during the practice of prānāyāma or breath control increases relaxation and sattvic energy. The pingalā channel is masculine, solar energy and primarily yang. It is responsible for stimulating energy, vigor and stamina. The right breath cycle controls the activity of the left brain and vice versa. Mastery of the breath is linked with mastery of the mind.

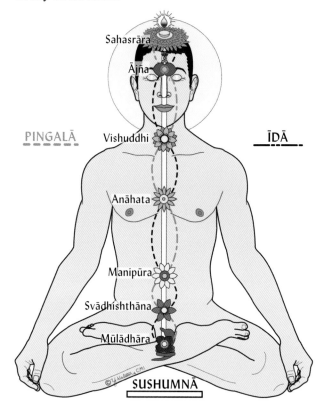

Īdā, Pingalā and Sushumnā Nādīs and the Seven Chakras

These three vital channels (īdā, pingalā and sushumnā) are joined at their root in the mūlādhāra chakra. This meeting is known as *yukta triveni,* or the meeting of three streams. As all three ascend the spinal cord, the īdā and pingalā criss cross at each chakra, alternating their flow until they meet again at Ājñā marma (third eye) and Ājñā chakra. This second meeting is termed *mukta triveni,* translated as "liberated three streams." Yogis strive to master these three streams of consciousness. Kundalinī may be awakened by a guru or master stimulating Ājñā marma, or through deep meditation, yoga postures or prānāyāma. It may even appear to awaken spontaneously in a person who has purified and refined the body-mind through prayer, fasting, devotional practices and so on. When the channel is activated, kundalinī shakti awakens, leading to expanded consciousness, bliss and internal harmony.

The *Shiva Svarodaya,* an ancient dialogue between Lord Shiva and his consort, Pārvatī, outlines the ten principal nādīs and their connection with the ten bodily gates, as listed in table 14. Even though these channels are located in the interior of the body, they link to the exterior via the sense organs. The channels that carry the objects of perception—sight, sound, taste, smell and tactile sensation—are known as *tanmātrā nāḍī.*

Each of the ten principal nādīs and the srotāmsi flower into a sensory "gate." This is reminiscent of the Chinese description of sense organs that flower off the stems or meridians. In TCM, the Lung meridian opens into the nose, Liver meridian opens into the eyes, Kidney meridian opens into the ears, Spleen meridian opens into the mouth and Heart meridian opens into the tongue. Thus, the sensory organs can be equated with both the nādīs and srotāmsi, and with the meridians.

Srotas

Srotas is the singular form and srotāmsi the plural of the Sanskrit word for channel. Compared to nādīs, srotāmsi represent a mostly visible physiological network of channels that are comprised of the dhātus (tissues). Ayurvedic anatomy has a rich vocabulary to describe various types of srotāmsi; for example, arteries are called *dhamanī,* while veins are known as *sirā. Mārga* means any large passage. These channels are subsidiaries of the srotāmsi system and correspond to anatomical structures. Examples of srotāmsi are anna vaha srotas, the food-carrying channel or gastrointestinal tract, prāna vaha srotas, the respiratory tract and mūtra vaha srotas, the urinary tract. Āyurveda highlights fourteen major srotāmsi: three receiving channels, three eliminating channels, seven corresponding to the tissues, and mano vaha srotas, the channel for the mind.

The subtlest srotāmsi are *anu srotas* and *atyanu srotas,* existing at the cellular level. Anu is translated as cell, the most basic functional unit of the body; anu srotas is a channel that receives and conveys the nutrition of the cell. Atyanu srotas operates at the nuclear level. It is present in the genes and transmits genetic information to neighboring cells.

The principal functions of both channel systems—nādīs and srotāmsi—are summarized below. For more about the channels, please see chapter 16, where we discuss disturbances of the channels and their healing and balancing using marmāni.[1]

Table 14: Āyurvedic Channels

10 Principal Nādīs	10 Bodily Gates	Related Organs	Srotāmsi
Sushumnā	Fontanel	Brain	Parashabdha vaha srotas; Ākāshīya srotas
Īdā	Left Nostril	Left testicle and ovary, left kidney, lung, and thyroid, spleen and right brain hemisphere	Prāna vaha srotas (cooling)
Pingalā	Right Nostril	Right testicle and ovary, right kidney, lung and thyroid, liver, right chambers of the heart, left brain hemisphere	Prāna vaha srotas (heating)
Gandhari	Left Ear	Left Ear	Shabda vaha srotas
Hastajihva	Right Ear	Right Ear	Shabda vaha srotas
Chakshusha	Left Eye	Left Optic Pathway	Rūpa vaha srotas (cooling)
Alambusha	Right Eye	Right Optic Pathway	Rūpa vaha srotas (heating)
Sarasvati	Tongue (Speech)	Mouth and oral cavity	Rasa vaha srotas (gustatory, as in the perception of the six tastes)
Kuhu	Guda (excretory organs)	Rectum	Purīsha vaha srotas
Shankhini	Genitals	Prostate and cervix	Shukra vaha srotas; Ārtava vaha srotas

Functions of Srotāmsi and Nādīs

* *Prīnana:* nutrition, immunity

* *Jīvana:* life function, oxygenation, regulation of flow of prāna

* *Lepana:* plastering, covering, protection, movement, strength

* *Dhārana:* support, structure

* *Snehana:* lubrication, insulation, beauty

* *Pūrana:* communication, learning, memory

* *Prajanana:* procreation

Comparison

Some interesting and important distinctions can be made between the channels in TCM and those in Āyurveda. As explained above, both nādīs and meridians are subtle, refined pathways of intelligence and energy, while the srotāmsi are more physical and functional entities. Nādīs and meridians form an interconnected network; srotāmsi do not. Meridians are classified according to location and function, while the nādīs are not. Meridians are accessible on the exterior surface of the body, while nādīs and srotāmsi are internal pathways that do not surface, though they can be influenced from the surface by such means as marma massage or the application of heat. Unlike meridians, nādīs and srotāmsi cannot be mapped on the exterior surface of the body.

Interestingly, both systems recognize fourteen major channels. Each of the fourteen principal meridians in TCM is delineated by acupoints that trace the flow of energy in a continuum from the first point on the meridian to the last. From the terminal point, energy flows to the first point on the meridian that follows it in sequence, such as from the Lung meridian to the Large Intestine. In contrast, the related points of a srotas are not traditionally seen as associated with each other on a continuum. However, the srotāmsi do have internal connections to specific related organs. Meridians in TCM are closely linked to their associated organs, while srotāmsi are more closely related to tissues and functions. Despite these differences, all the channel systems and energy networks facilitate communication, transportation, intelligence and vitality and promote optimal functioning of the body.

Energy Points

Energy points are referred to as acupoints in TCM and marmāni in Āyurveda. Although both acupoints and marmāni are located and "worked" on the surface of the body, one striking difference between the two medical systems is that a majority of acupoints have been "mapped" onto meridians on the exterior surface of the body, while marmāni have not been mapped with reference to either the nādīs or srotāmsi, which are both internal pathways. However, marmāni can be associated with nādīs or srotāmsi that travel from one region of the body to another. Shankha marma, for example, located at the temple, is an effective marma for treating nausea and vomiting. Why? It is situated where a prāna nādī connects to the stomach. Marmāni are also related to the fourteen srotāmsi in terms of regulating their functions and treating their disturbance.

The marmāni of Āyurveda have not been systematized in a great network like the Chinese meridian system. However, they are far from isolated energy points. All marmāni have not only local effects at the point or region of their position, but also, like Shankha marma mentioned above, may stimulate, pacify or balance aspects of mind and body both near and far away.

Classification of Acupuncture Points

In TCM, acupoints are locations at which qi is infused and surfaces on the body. The Chinese term for acupoint can be translated literally as hole or aperture, signifying an opening for qi and a place where the energy of the respective meridian and organ can be modified. They serve as focal points both for diagnosis and for treatment, for responding to disease and strengthening qi and bodily resistance. The therapeutic potential of each point is unique, depending on its location, the meridian it is situated on and the abundance of qi at that point.

The names of acupuncture points are both elegant and profound, capturing imagery of nature such as the mountains, sky and water. Many incorporate the Chinese term for gate, window, palace or opening, conveying a place where qi is stored and through which it moves. Thus, the movement and flow of qi so central to TCM is implied through acupoints as well as meridians. Names can also describe anatomical locations, such as elbow, wrist, bone or thigh. Some names reflect the point's therapeutic properties; for example, the "Sea of Blood" or "Sea of Qi", where these substances are abundant.

Much of acupuncture imagery is based on the management of water as it flows through irrigation canals, ditches, reservoirs, rivers and so forth. Just as the water in an irrigation network can be directed and channeled, certain acupoints govern the ebb and flow of qi in the body. These influential points, five on each of the twelve primary channels, are known as *shu* points. They originate at the extremities and terminate near the elbows or

---

1. See also *The Textbook of Ayurveda,* volume I, Srotamsi chapter.

knees. Each has specific indications for treatment, based on the flow of qi at these foci. They include:

1. *Jing-Well* point: where meridian qi starts to "bubble"
2. *Ying-Spring* point: where meridian qi starts to "gush"
3. *Shu-Stream* point: where meridian qi "flourishes"
4. *Jing-River* point: where meridian qi "pours abundantly"
5. *He-Sea* point: where meridian qi "flows generously"

The classification of acupuncture points can be summarized briefly as follows:

✳ Regular points, 361 in number, located on the fourteen principal meridians and most commonly used in clinical practice.

✳ Extra points that have specific names and locations, but are usually not located on the fourteen meridians.

✳ *Ashi* points, unfixed tender spots with no specific names or locations, are principally used for the treatment of pain syndromes. The *Ling Shu,* one of the most revered Chinese medical texts, says "Where there is pain, there is an acupoint." (Cheng 1987) Thus, there is no place on the body that is not potentially an acupoint.

Additional classifications for the acupoints of the twelve primary channels are summarized in table 16 on page 55.

Classification of Marmāni

Like their counterparts in TCM, Ayurvedic marmāni have also been described according to various classifications that illuminate their myriad roles, including their function, location, relationship to the five elements, association with doshas and subtypes, corresponding organs and srotāmsi, and degrees of vitality. The whole of chapter 2 is devoted to marmāni classifications.

Measurements

• •

Both traditions developed precise measurements to map the locations of energy points on the surface of the body. These measurements are standardized not according to an unvarying absolute standard, such as an inch or a millimeter, but according to the proportions of each individual's body. These basic units of measurement are known as *cun* in TCM and *angula* (plural *anguli*) in Āyurveda. In part 2, chapters 9 through 14, the location for each individual marma is given in terms of anguli. The corresponding acupoints are discussed in terms of cun measurements. It is very important to note that

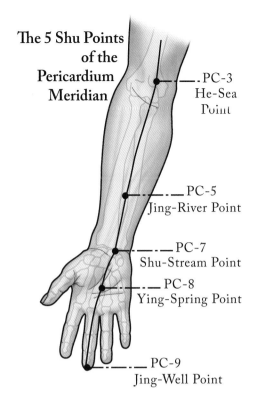

The 5 Shu Points of the Pericardium Meridian

PC-3 He-Sea Point
PC-5 Jing-River Point
PC-7 Shu-Stream Point
PC-8 Ying-Spring Point
PC-9 Jing-Well Point

measurements are taken according to the patient's proportions and anatomical landmarks and not the practitioner's. Therefore, each person's unique body size will result in different sized cun or anguli.

In TCM, one cun is most commonly taken to be the width of the thumb. The breadth of the fingers placed side by side is also used for a number of measurements. The combined width of the index and middle finger is equivalent to 1.5 cun. The width of all four fingers taken across the fingers is three cun, but four cun if measuring from the knuckles. These are depicted in the illustrations below. TCM practitioners also standardized cun measurements for specific regions of the body used for reference in locating acupoints. For example, from the occiput to the anterior midline of the hairline is a distance of 12 cun.

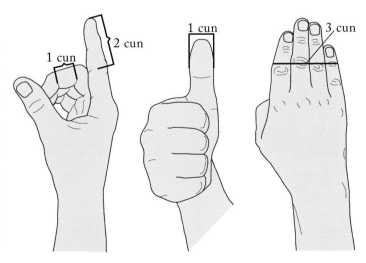

1 cun
2 cun
1 cun
3 cun

In Āyurveda, Sushruta described the unit of measurement, the angula, as the width of the middle finger measured across the medial interphalangeal joint. The entire width of the hand when all the fingers are outstretched is one *tada* or 12 anguli. Seven tadas correspond to the maximum length (height) of the human body, as well as the maximum arm span, measured from the middle fingertips. Seven tadas are equivalent to a total of 84 anguli.

An important differentiation is that one cun is calculated by the width of the thumb and one angula by the width of the middle finger. Thus, one cun is slightly larger in size than one angula. They can be converted by following the simple equation that one angula is equivalent to .8 cun or one cun is equivalent to 1.25 anguli. Table 15 will facilitate quick conversion.

Table 15: Conversion Table

Anguli to Cun	Cun to Anguli
.5 anguli = .4 cun	.5 cun = .625 anguli
1 angula = .8 cun	1 cun = 1.25 anguli
1.5 anguli = 1.2 cun	1.5 cun = 1.875 anguli
2 anguli = 1.6 cun	2 cun = 2.5 anguli
3 anguli = 2.4 cun	3 cun = 3.75 anguli
4 anguli = 3.2 cun	4 cun = 5 anguli
5 anguli = 4 cun	5 cun = 6.25 anguli
6 anguli = 4.8 cun	6 cun = 7.5 anguli
10 anguli = 8 cun	8 cun = 10 anguli

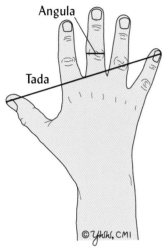

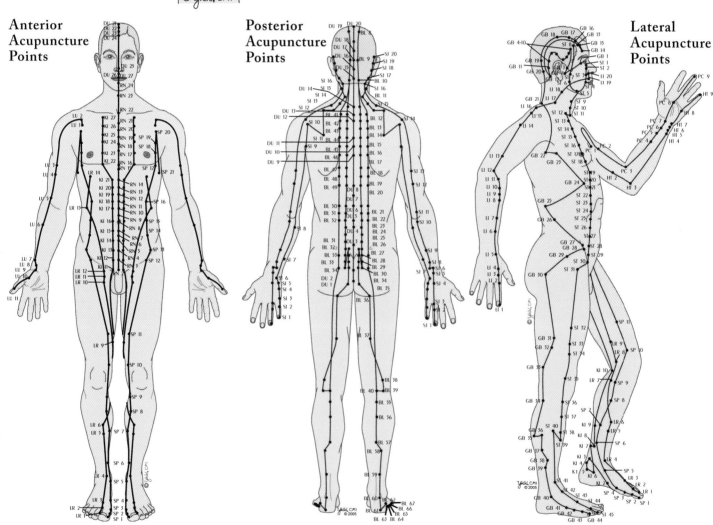

Anterior Acupuncture Points

Posterior Acupuncture Points

Lateral Acupuncture Points

Table 16: Additional Classifications of Acupoints

Acupoints on 12 Meridians	Description of Point Categories
Source points	Copious amounts of qi, located on the limbs
Luo points	Link coupled meridians, treat disorders transmitted between related meridians
Xi (cleft) points	Treat acute disorders, where qi and blood of meridian is deeply converged
Jing-well points	Clear heat, restore consciousness, treat fullness and stagnation in the chest
Ying-spring points	Clear heat in the organ, treat diseases of yin organs and yang channels
Shu-stream points	Treat heaviness of the body, pain in the joints, intermittent diseases
Jing-river points	Treat cough, shortness of breath, chills and fever, diseases of the sinews and bones
He-sea points	Treat digestive disturbances, disorders of yang organs
Front mu points	Diagnostic for organ disturbance, on surface of chest and abdomen
Back shu points	Diagnostic for organ disturbance, run parallel to the spine
Crossing points	Located at intersection of two or more meridians, 90 total
Confluent points	Where regular meridians communicate with extraordinary vessels, located on the limbs, 8 total

Samprāpti: Pathogenesis and Disturbance of Marmāni

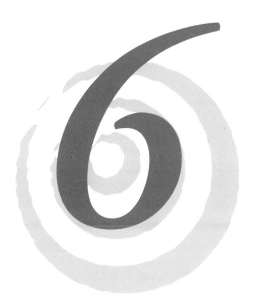

Disease does not appear from nowhere. Behind every illness or dysfunction is a causal chain of events and influences that lead step by step to the condition that finally presents on the surface as a full-blown disease. The underlying causes are like a seed that contains the potential illness, sprouts and begins to grow invisibly underground, eventually breaking into view. In the case of illness—as opposed to gardening—the wise and expedient action is to nip it in the bud, that is, to detect the incipient problem and reverse the process at an early stage, before it grows and becomes difficult to treat.

One of the great contributions of Āyurveda to medical knowledge is a detailed, in-depth explanation of precisely what stages occur, and what occurs at every stage, as a minor imbalance or dysfunction develops into a serious disease. Along with this, Āyurvedic physicians have cultivated the companion art of diagnosis to such a degree of refinement and precision that a skilled practitioner can perceive the very earliest stages of the disease process, and prescribe means to reverse course and regain health and balance. Indeed, any individual with sufficient motivation and a little knowledge and training, can learn to observe the fluctuations within his or her own body, through pulse diagnosis and other subtle diagnostic tools, and self-treat most imbalances while they are still in their early stages, before professional help is required.

In this chapter we will explore the disease process (pathogenesis or, in Sanskrit, *samprāpti*) with reference to the causative factors that disturb doshic balance, the stages of disease development and the pathways of disease propagation in the body. Then we will look at how imbalance and illness affect the marmāni, with an eye toward understanding how these vital energy points can be used not only to restore health when illness has arisen, but also, to maintain good health and prevent future problems from cropping up.

Etiological Factors

In considering health and illness, Āyurveda always looks at the big picture. This means not only the "whole person," mind, body, and soul or spirit, but also, the person's relationships to other people and to the environment, both social and natural. Nothing that touches on one's life can be set aside as irrelevant. Thus, the Ayurvedic physician takes into consideration the individual's constitution, diet, typical kind of exercise or lack of it, lifestyle habits and daily routines, relationships, the climate, air quality, season, age, profession, stress level and so on. All these, and more, influence both health and disease. These factors can be grouped into three broad categories: mental, physical and environmental.

The mind can be a cause of imbalance and illness due to such factors as psychological trauma, worry, extreme stress, repressed or excessive emotions, and *prājñāparādha*. Prājñāparādha, literally "crimes against wisdom," results from not listening to the body's innate intelligence, or failing to act on one's knowledge and understanding. This requires no further elaboration than to say that every one of us sometimes does something we know we shouldn't, whether it is eating wrong food, staying up too late, being a workaholic, etc. The body is brilliantly self-regulating and self-righting, and most minor infractions against natural law or the wisdom of experience cause little or no harm, but in the long run actions do have their consequences, and we reap what we sow.

External factors that may contribute to the early stages of doshic imbalance leading to disease formation include environmental components such as seasonal influences, extreme climatic conditions, high noise levels, exposure to pollen, air and water pollution, and numerous similar factors. Difficult relationships, workplace stress, excessive travel, rush hour traffic and other potentially stressful interactions with the environment

Samprāpti, the Process of Disease

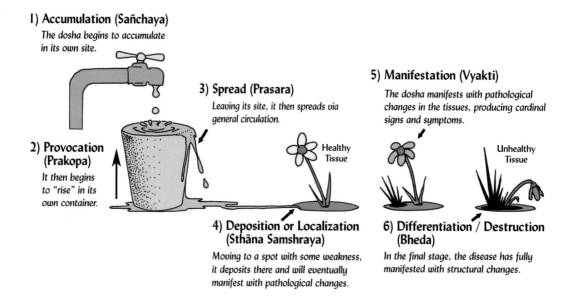

1) Accumulation (Sañchaya)
The dosha begins to accumulate in its own site.

3) Spread (Prasara)
Leaving its site, it then spreads via general circulation.

5) Manifestation (Vyakti)
The dosha manifests with pathological changes in the tissues, producing cardinal signs and symptoms.

2) Provocation (Prakopa)
It then begins to "rise" in its own container.

Healthy Tissue

Unhealthy Tissue

4) Deposition or Localization (Sthāna Samshraya)
Moving to a spot with some weakness, it deposits there and will eventually manifest with pathological changes.

6) Differentiation / Destruction (Bheda)
In the final stage, the disease has fully manifested with structural changes.

can also lead to doshic imbalance and plant the seeds of future disease.

Many physical factors also play a role. Physical injury and trauma, over-exertion and under or over-exercise, dietary indiscretions and sleep deprivation are just a few. Inattention to what will best serve the body's fundamental constitution, and thus making choices that will throw off the balance of the system, is a major cause of disease. There are also genetic predispositions, congenital weaknesses and areas of disease proneness that may lead to health concerns. Āyurveda also holds that it is unhealthy to suppress natural urges such as the need to sneeze, cough, yawn, belch, vomit, urinate, defecate and eject flatus. One is advised to eat when hungry, drink when thirsty, sleep when tired and cry when miserable.

Improper dietary choices are considered in Āyurveda to be one of the leading causes of disease. Consuming leftovers or food that is not fresh, and eating incompatible food combinations can all disturb the doshas. Fast foods, foods that have been frozen or are extremely cold, hot, excessively spicy, microwaved, fermented, heavy or oily impair digestion. Indulging in any of the six tastes (sweet, sour, salty, pungent, bitter or astringent) in undue proportion can disturb doshic balance. Overeating, undereating, prolonged fasting, eating late at night or eating in a hurry are lifestyle choices likely to cause health problems.

All these etiological factors have the potential to trigger the beginning of the disease process.

Samprāpti (Pathogenesis)

Samprāpti, the Sanskrit term for pathogenesis, means "the process of birth and manifestation of disease." An understanding of the disease process is vital for every health practitioner, in order to correctly diagnosis the nature and stage of the disease that the client or patient presents, and to accordingly prescribe treatments that will be maximally efficacious.

Āyurveda has distinguished six distinct stages in the development of disease, each with its own symptomatology specific to the aggravated dosha. Each stage describes the journey of the dosha from its home site in the gastrointestinal tract to the rest of the body. These six stages are:

* *sañchaya* (accumulation)
* *prakopa* (provocation)
* *prasara* (spreading)
* *sthāna samshraya* (deposition)
* *vyakti* (manifestation)
* *bheda* (differentiation or complications)

The first three stages describe the development of disease at a subtle, as yet unmanifested, level. Ayurvedic clinicians can detect which of these stages are involved from pulse diagnosis and other subtle signs. The second three stages are less subtle and involve the manifestation of disease into observable signs and symptoms.

Āyurveda differentiates symptomatology into two classifications. Prodromal symptoms are known as *pūrva rūpa,* meaning before form or manifestation—these are "warning bell" symptoms. Cardinal symptoms, termed *rūpa,* reflect the spectrum of symptomatology that is widely recognized by patients and medical practitioners. Pūrva rūpa manifests at the junction between the third and fourth stage of pathogenesis, when the dosha enters the dhātu, while rūpa is revealed in the fifth stage of manifestation. Some symptoms may occur in more than one stage, but they reflect increasing levels of severity as they progress through each stage. The Ayurvedic clinician aims to detect disturbances at the beginning stages of samprāpti when they are significantly easier to treat.

Sañchaya (accumulation). In the first stage of pathogenesis, etiological factors trigger the dosha to accumulate in its home site within the gastrointestinal (GI) tract. Vāta accumulates in the colon, pitta in the small intestine and kapha in the stomach. Symptoms at this stage are relatively mild. Excess vāta may create gaseous bloating and abdominal distention; over-abundant pitta leads to hyperacidity, acid indigestion, and intestinal discomfort; high kapha results in fullness and heaviness in the epigastric area, low appetite, slow digestion, and sleepiness after food.

Prakopa (provocation). When the level of a dosha rises in its own site to a critical point, it can become provoked. Vāta in the prakopa stage rises into the hepatic and splenic flexure, causing generalized abdominal distention (bloating) and discomfort, constipation, even difficulty breathing. Provoked pitta is experienced as nausea, periumbilical pain, belching, heartburn or acid reflux. Aggravated kapha creates salivary belching, excess salivation, fullness of the stomach, thick mucus salivary secretions and drooling.

Prasara (spreading). In the third stage, excess doshas leave the GI tract and spread into the general circulation through the medium of rasa and rakta dhātus (plasma and blood). Each dosha primarily gravitates towards regions in the body for which it has an affinity, known as secondary sites of the dosha, but can also circulate to any other area of the body. Vāta goes under the skin, creating poor circulation, goose bumps, cold hands and feet, and twitching sensations in subcutaneous tissue. The same principle holds true for pitta and kapha. Pitta has an affinity for the skin and can produce hives, rash, urticaria and acne; heartburn and burning eyes may also appear. Kapha, via rakta and rasa dhātu, moves from its seat in the stomach to the lungs, head, sinuses and elsewhere, creating cold, clammy skin, profuse mucus secretion, sinus and lymphatic congestion, water retention, heavy breasts and catarrh.

Sthāna samshraya (deposition). After circulating in rasa and rakta dhātus, the doshas are as if seeking a place to lodge, and will enter a site or space that is weak or vul-

Table 17: Doshas and the Six Stages of Disease

Six Stages	Vāta	Pitta	Kapha
Sañchaya (accumulation)	Bloating, abdominal distention	Hyperacidity, intestinal discomfort	Fullness in stomach, heaviness, drowsiness
Prakopa (provocation)	Constipation, bloating, difficulty breathing	Nausea, vomiting, belching, heartburn, acid indigestion	Lack of appetite, congestion and excess mucus, cough
Prasara (spreading)	Dry skin, cold hands and feet, heart palpitations, tinnitus, insomnia, anxiety, nervousness	Intense heartburn, hives, rash, urticaria, burning eyes, irritability, anger	Sinus congestion, lymphatic obstruction, tightness in chest, heavy feeling, water retention
Sthāna samshraya (deposition)	Cold, dryness, dry cough, sneezing	Irritation, infection, inflammation, ulceration	Congestion, edema, consolidation, mucus formation
Vyakti (manifestation)	Radiating pain, weakness, fatigue, emaciation, tremors, tics, spasms, stiffness and muscle wasting	Inflammation, infection, excruciating and throbbing pain	Metabolic changes, weight gain, dull pain, kidney or gallbladder stones
Bheda (differentiation)	Loss of function, osteoporosis, degenerative changes, paralysis, deformity	Perforation, ulceration, abscess formation, gangrene, hemorrhage	Profuse edema, stagnation, tumor formation, obstruction, occlusion of arteries

nerable due to genetic predisposition, trauma, accumulated stress, repressed emotions, or other factors. (These weak spots are called *khavaigunya,* a defective space.) Signs and symptoms of sthana samshraya will vary according to the site of deposition. In general, during this stage vāta will create dry, rough, stiff and abnormal movement at the site of deposition. The person may feel weakness in that organ. For example, if vāta deposits in the lungs, it will produce dry cough, sneezing, wheezing and difficulty breathing, accompanied by chest pain. Pitta will produce local inflammation, irritation and infection, which can give rise to fever. If pitta goes into the lungs, it will create bronchitis, with a cough accompanied by greenish-yellowish mucus, indicative of infection. Due to this infection, there may be fever. Kapha will follow a similar track. It will percolate into an organ, creating congestion, swelling, mucus secretion, and thickening of the tissue, leading to consolidation. If kapha goes into the lungs, it will produce profuse bronchial secretions, leading to cough and expectoration. The aggravated kapha may create lung edema, thickening of lung tissue, and pneumonia.

Vyakti (manifestation). In the fifth stage, the disease process manifests with intensifying levels of severity. Vāta vyakti creates radiating or fluctuating pain, weakness, fatigue and emaciation. It also manifests as tremors, tics, spasms, stiffness and tissue wasting. Pitta dosha expresses itself through inflammation, irritation and infection with burning pain. Kapha at this stage will create more congestion, obstruction, consolidation and lead to solidification and fibrotic changes within the organ of deposition. In the lungs, this may express as lobar pneumonia, and as gallbladder or kidney stones in their respective organs.

Bheda (differentiation, complications). The final stage in the development of disease, bheda, brings serious complications, systemic involvement, and deformity in the organs. Western medicine's forté is addressing this level of pathogenesis, where symptoms are the most severe and can be potentially life threatening. Āyurveda's strength is recognizing imbalance at the beginning stages of pathogenesis and preventing it from progressing further. Vāta dosha in bheda may lead to loss of function, osteoporosis, degenerative changes, paralysis, deformity or neuromuscular dystrophy. The bheda stage of pitta includes ulceration, perforation and abscess formation, leading to hyperpyrexia with febrile convulsions and hemorrhage. Obstruction, severe edema, neoplasm (tumor formation) and occlusion of the

arteries are typical kapha manifestations. table 17 on page 59 summarizes the six stages and provides examples of doshic disturbances in each stage.

Vyadhi Mārga, the Three Pathways of Disease

In addition to recognizing the stages of pathogenesis, a clinician must carefully observe the pathways in which disease occurs, termed *vyadhi mārga. Mārga* is translated as passage or pathway and *vyadhi* as disease. In the beginning of our biological life, the body is created from three vital layers of the embryo, the ectoderm, mesoderm and endoderm, the outer, middle and innermost layer respectively. These same layers that are responsible for the origin of the body later become pathways for the creation and progression of disease. In the process of pathogenesis, disease may flourish in one of the three pathways, *bāhya mārga* (outermost pathway), *madhyama mārga* (middle pathway) and *abhyantara mārga* (innermost pathway).

In the first two stages of samprāpti, doshas undergo accumulation and provocation in their own sites in the GI tract, which is the abhyantara mārga. If balance has not been restored and the doshas spread to rasa and rakta dhātu and begin to circulate through the body, they enter the bāhya mārga where they affect the extremities, capil-

Vyadhi Mārga

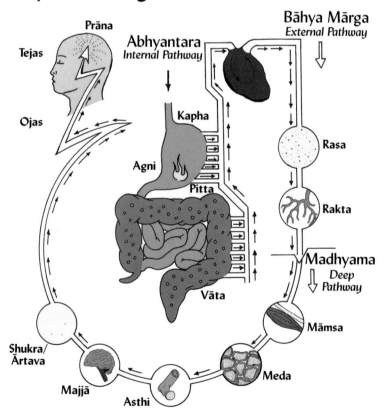

laries and skin, causing skin diseases such as eczema, dermatitis and psoriasis. If the disease is allowed to progress further without being checked, the doshas enter madhyama mārga where, during the fourth stage, they deposit into the deep tissues (māmsa, meda, asthi, majjā and shukra/ārtava) and in the fifth and sixth stages penetrate deeper, and affect the vital organs such as the heart, liver and kidneys. Diseases beyond stage four are complicated and become difficult to cure. That is why Āyurveda so strongly emphasizes healthy lifestyle practices in order to prevent the development of disease, and why Āyurvedic practitioners are so thoroughly trained in the subtle arts of diagnosis, in order to detect incipient health problems long before they manifest as overt symptoms.

Effective management of any condition depends upon understanding and applying this valuable knowledge. These pathways are summarized in table 18.

Vikruti, the Present Imbalance

Doshic disturbance, whether generated by external, internal or psychological factors, results in changes in the individual's doshic balance. External influences include diet, lifestyle and environment, such as weather conditions. Internal physical factors include the condition of one's agni or digestive fire; āhāra rasa, the quality of chyle, the end-product of digestion; the production of āma, toxic morbid metabolic waste; dhātu kshaya, degenerative change or depletion of tissue; and mārgavarodha, blocking of the srotāmsi. Psychological factors include anger, fear or attachment. This imbalance is termed *vikruti*. Vikruti always exists in relation to *prakruti*, the individual constitution, and can be detected by clinical observation such as symptomatology, pulse and tongue diagnosis, and by systemic examination through darshanam (observation), sparshanam (palpation) and prashnam (questioning). Vikruti may constantly fluctuate in response to internal and external factors, but prakruti remains constant. Thus, each person's state of imbalance depends on his or her constitution.

For example, a vāta constitution is more prone to vāta vikruti (imbalance) in dry, windy environments; pitta types to pitta imbalance in hot, humid weather, and kapha individuals to kapha imbalance in cold, damp climates. Thus, prakruti has specific vikruti proneness within it, and vice versa: within the disorder of vikruti lies the potential for restoration of order, prakruti.[1]

Role of Marmāni in Relation to Samprāpti and Pathways of Disease

Marmāni are a component of the connective tissue and more specifically the majjā dhātu (nervous tissue). Both are part of the madhyama mārga, the pathway of disease that is affected during the third and fourth stage of spreading and deposition. Marma samprāpti (pathogenesis) is the spreading of the doshas from the GI tract (abhyantara mārga) to the skin (bāhya mārga) and then penetrating to the level of the marmāni (madhyama mārga).

Vāta dosha has an affinity towards vāta marmāni, such as sandhi (joints) and asthi (bones) marmāni. This includes Kūrpara (elbow), Jānu (knee), Trik (coccyx), and Bhaga (pubic bone), to name a few. Pitta spreads towards pitta-type marmāni such as Yakrut (liver), Plīha (spleen), Hrid (heart) and points related to heat, such as Sūrya (stomach) and Nābhi (umbilicus). Lastly, kapha penetrates to snāyu (fat) and māmsa (muscle) marmāni such as Kaksha (armpit) and Sphij (gluteal fold). It also gravitates towards Jatru (manubrium sterni), Kantha (throat) and Apastambha (upper chest), where mucus tends to accumulate.

Marma vikruti is doshic imbalance that exists at the level of a marma. It results from āma lodging into the space of the marma and blocking its functions. Vikruti and āma can be differentiated as vāta, pitta or kapha in

---

1. Even though each prakruti (vāta, pitta, kapha) has a proneness toward imbalance of its own doshic type (vāta prone to vāta imbalance, etc.), when the etiological factors are strong, vāta prakruti can develop pitta or kapha vikruti, and so on.

Table 18: Pathways of Disease and Prognosis

Vyadhi Mārga (Pathway)	Embryological Layer	Constituent	Stage of Pathogenesis	Prognosis
Abhyantara mārga (Internal)	Endoderm	Gastrointestinal tract within the boundaries of the mucous membrane	Stages 1, 2	Good
Bāhya mārga (External)	Ectoderm	Skin, extremities, peripheral capillaries	Stages 3, 4	Fair to Poor
Madhyama mārga (Middle)	Mesoderm	Deep connective tissue, seven dhātus, vital organs: brain, heart, liver, kidneys and all vital marmāni	Stages 4, 5, 6	Bad

nature. Vikruti also has various levels of severity. Sadyah pranahara marmāni possess the most vitality and thus disturbance at these sites is the most severe. (see page 23) Vitality is greatest when ojas, tejas and prāna are most abundant at the site of a marma. At other marmāni with less vitality, vikruti may be mild or moderate. Thus, prognosis depends on the dosha involved, type of marmāni affected and severity of symptoms. By understanding the three doshas in terms of their qualities and the regions of the body for which they have an affinity, it is possible to predict which marma sites the excessive doshas might seek to lodge within.

Disease affects ojas, tejas and prāna, the vital essences, via the marmāni, at the level of connective tissue. Hence, marmāni are the perfect vehicle to re-establish balance of the doshas. That is, we can address doshic imbalance anywhere in the body by enlivening or triggering ojas, tejas and prāna at the level of marmāni.

Marmāni as Khavaigunya

Doshas penetrate into a marma when it is *khavaigunya,* a defective space or weakened site. This concept is unique to Āyurveda. It can be defined as any vulnerable area of the body that invites disease because of genetic predisposition, improper functioning, repressed emotions or a lack of cellular intelligence. The defective space can be an organ, srotas or nādī (channel), dhātu (tissue), upadhātu (by-product), sensory opening or marma. The space can be in either the physical body or the mind. When the dosha leaves its home site in the GI tract, it seeks a place to lodge and infiltrates that space (khavaigunya). Several factors may contribute to both the creation of a defective space and disease etiology. These factors include:

* Genetic predisposition
* Congenital defect
* Fingerprints of previous disease or trauma
* Low immunity
* Unresolved repressed emotions
* Poor diet and lifestyle
* Build-up of toxins (āma)
* Low dhātu agni and pīlu-pithara agni
* Unfinished past life karma

A marma may be a defective space or "black hole" for any of the above reasons.

Genetic predisposition is described as cellular memory in Āyurveda. We carry the cellular memory of our parents' and grandparents' illnesses; our genes possess the fingerprints of their previous diseases.

One of the fundamental causes that trigger marma involvement is the association of marmāni with organs and channels. For example, if high vāta lodges in the heart and affects cardiac functions, it may directly penetrate to marmāni related to the heart. The same principle holds true for any organ disturbance. This explains why marmāni are such excellent diagnostic tools for disturbance in any area of the body, and also why they are so therapeutically effective: Stimulating marmāni enlivens intelligence at the site of the khavaigunya and helps to restore health. In this way, the weakened or defective sites become the space or doorways for healing. Thus, marmāni are not just anatomical sites, but centers for either health or disease to flourish.

Marmāni in Relation to Āma and Agni

Āma, the Sanskrit term for toxins, is a central concept in Āyurveda, though it is discussed only briefly here. Āma accrues—toxins build up—whenever agni is low, enabling various etiological factors to aggravate the doshas. Agni is the fire principle of digestion or metabolism that exists in every tissue, organ, channel and cell. There is no aspect of the body in which agni is not present. *Jāthara agni* is the central fire present in the stomach, *bhūta agni* exists in the liver, *kloma agni* in the pancreas, and so on. *Dhātu agni* is the fire component of the tissues and *sroto agni* is the fire component of the channels. Similarly, there is agni present at the level of the marmāni, known as *marma agni.* Ideally, all types of agni function together harmoniously.

Āyurvedic internal medicine is sometimes called *Kāya Chikitsā,* the therapy of agni. All Āyurvedic treatment is geared towards awakening agni to ensure optimal body function. Balanced agni creates functional integrity between the doshas, dhātus (tissue) and malas (waste product), and plays a crucial role in health. When agni is disturbed, pathogenesis ensues. Likewise, it is only when marma agni is negatively affected that imbalance occurs at the level of the marma.

The basic qualities of agni are *ushna* (hot), *tīkshna* (sharp), *laghu* (light), *sukshma* (subtle), and *rūksha* (dry). The very existence of āma is dependent on diminished agni and doshic imbalance. *Doshic āma* is formed by the qualities of the dosha that counteract agni's characteristics. For example, kapha is gross, dull, cold, heavy and oily, qualities that inhibit the subtle, sharp, hot, light and dry qualities of agni. If pitta increases in its liquid and oily qualities, it becomes like hot water, i.e., if you pour it on fire, the fire goes out. In this way, pitta can suppress agni, creating pitta-type āma. Vāta opposes agni by its cold and mobile qualities. Drinking cold water increases vāta and suppresses agni. And as a gusty wind will blow out a candle, excess vāta dosha diminishes the fires of agni.

Āma is not always formed in the GI tract by aggravation of doshas. Invasion of virus, bacteria and para-

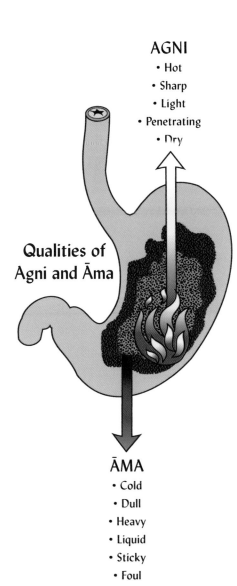

AGNI
- Hot
- Sharp
- Light
- Penetrating
- Dry

Qualities of
Agni and Āma

ĀMA
- Cold
- Dull
- Heavy
- Liquid
- Sticky
- Foul

sites can also disturb localized dhātu agni and produce āma. When the agni of a particular tissue, organ or channel is low, āma accumulates in those respective structures. The general symptoms of āma are:

* *Sroto rodha* (clogging of channels)
* *Bala bhramsha* (fatigue)
* *Gaurava* (sense of heaviness)
* *Anila mūdhata* (retrograde vāta)
* *Ālasya* (lethargy, malaise)
* *Apakti* (indigestion)
* *Sanga* (stagnation or congestion)
* *Aruchi* (loss of taste, perverted taste, lack of interest in everything, depression)
* *Klama* (sexual debility)
* *Sāma jihvā* (tongue coating)
* *Roma rujā* (roots of hair ache)
* *Sarvanga sāda* (generalized body ache)

* *Moha* (mental confusion)

As a result of āma, these toxins may enter into related marmāni, known as *marma gata āma*, which makes the marmāni tender and sensitive to the touch. When vāta dosha is aggravated, it will tend to affect māmsa, asthi, majjā, shukra and ārtava marmāni. Pitta dosha primarily influences rakta marmāni and kapha dosha the rasa and meda marmāni. Table 19 summarizes symptomatology of tissue disturbance.

Table 19: Marmāni Tissue Disturbances

Dhātu	Symptoms
Rasa marmāni	Lymphatic congestion, lymphatic swelling, enlargement of the lymph nodes, generalized lymphadenopathy, edema, pallor
Rakta marmāni	Hives, rash, urticaria, irritation, Inflammation, bleeding disorders, itching, burning, hemorrhage, skin disorders, hot flashes
Māmsa marmāni	Muscle twitching, muscle spasms, muscular pain, muscle fatigue, muscle tumor, fibrocystic growth (fibroid tumor)
Meda marmāni	Multiple lipoma (fatty tumors), obesity, uneven distribution of fat, undue perspiration, lipofibroma
Asthi marmāni	Joint pain, cracking, popping, aching of the joints, calcaneal spur, dislocation of joints, arthritis, osteoporosis
Majjā marmāni	Lack of sensation, tingling, numbness, hypertonia, hypotonia, lack of coordination, neuralgia, mental or emotional disorders
Shukra marmāni	Premature ejaculation, low libido
Ārtava marmāni	Painful coitus, depletion of ojas

Toxins may also travel from the marma to the tissue, to the channel and ultimately to the organ. General symptoms of channel disturbance include overflow (*ati pravrutti*) such as diarrhea or vomiting; stagnation (*sanga*) such as lymphatic congestion or constipation; swelling or tumors (*sirā granthi*); and entry into the wrong channel (*vimārga gamanam*) which can result in many forms of bleeding or perforations. Classifying these according to doshic involvement:

* Vāta: hyperactivity, overflow and entry into the wrong channel

✳ Pitta: inflammation, ulceration, irritation and perforation

✳ Kapha: congestion, swelling, stagnation, tumors and clots

The space of any bodily structure, whether marma, tissue, organ or channel, becomes stagnant due to toxins, accumulated doshas or unresolved emotions. The function of the mind, too, is affected adversely when one's mental space becomes clouded by emotions such as anxiety or confusion. Because of toxicity, communication is impeded, cellular intelligence disrupted and disease eventually ensues.

The identical principle is true in the subtlest of spaces. Marmāni are the doors of perception. They require functional clarity, integrity and synchronization with each other. When āma builds up and they become clouded by toxicity, their crucial role of facilitating communication between organs and body regions, and between the individual and the external world is interrupted and impaired.

With this understanding of pathogenesis from the Ayurvedic perspective, it is logical to turn our attention to the many modes of Ayurvedic treatment, and particularly the application of marma therapy (*marma chikitsā*) in the prevention and healing of disease. This will be our theme for the following two chapters, and then we will begin our point-by-point examination of each of the 117 marmāni of Āyurveda.

Introduction to Chikitsā, Āyurvedic Therapy

याभिः क्रियाभिर्जायन्ते शरीरे धातवः समाः ।

सा चिकित्सा विकाराणां कर्म तद्विषजां स्मृतम् ॥३४॥

च. सू. अ. १६ सू. ३४

yābhiḥ kriyābhir jāyante śarīre dhātavaḥ samāḥ
sā cikitsā vikārānāṃ karma tadbhiṣajāṃ smṛtam

Charaka Saṃhitā Sūtrasthāna, ch. 16, vs. 34

Translation: The measures by which the bodily dhātus are brought back to equilibrium constitute the therapeutics (treatment of disorders). This is the function of the physician.

"By any method, by any means, by any technique or system, if it creates balance between dosha, dhātu, mala and agni, between prakruti and vikruti, between ojas, tejas and prāna, and re-establishes harmony between body, mind and consciousness, that is called chikitsā."

~ *Commentary by Vasant Lad, M.A.Sc.*

Chikitsā means therapy, treatment or management. It comes into play after thorough investigation and diagnosis of the condition of the patient. Āyurvedic chikitsā is a broad umbrella that encompasses many branches and methods of treatment. Among them, marma chikitsā is the understanding and therapeutic use of marmāni—energy points—to balance body, mind and spirit. Marma chikitsā is a complete and highly sophisticated science that has been refined over many centuries. Yet like all Āyurvedic therapies, it is rarely used alone, but rather in conjunction with others. This chapter explores the role of energy points in various types of Āyurvedic treatment, and within Āyurveda as a whole.

Types of Chikitsā and the Role of Marmāni

Marma chikitsā is utilized as an integral part of numerous Āyurvedic healing and rejuvenative modalities, including *shodhana* (cleansing), *shamana* (palliation), *rasāyana* (rejuvenation), *apunarbhava chikitsā* (preventative measures) and *sadyah phaladai chikitsā* (first aid therapy). *Tanmātrā chikitsā* involves each of the five sensory pathways of perception as an avenue for treatment. For example, sound therapy uses mantras (sound vibrations), touch therapy uses marma chikitsā and massage, visual therapy utilizes colors in chromotherapy, and olfactory therapy utilizes essential oils in aromatherapy. Each therapeutic modality has a role and place within Āyurvedic treatment. Although these therapies are vast topics in themselves, they are presented briefly here according to their relevant context within marma chikitsā.

Shodhana, Cleansing through Marmāni

Shodhana is cleansing and detoxification. Pañchakarma (*pañch* = five, *karma* = action) is one widely utilized branch or sub-classification of shodhana that incorporates *basti* (medicated enemas), *virechana* (therapeutic purging), *vamana* (therapeutic vomiting), *nasya* (nasal administration of medicated oils and herbal powders) and *rakta moksha* (blood-letting). To prepare the body for pañchakarma, snehana (oleation) and svedana (sudation) are performed first. Then, through the five cleansing actions, accumulated doshas that are present in the marmāni, tissues, organs, channels or other khavaigunyas (defective spaces) are removed from the body. Herbal remedies, fasting and exercise also cleanse the body and are a form of shodhana.[1]

---

1. Pañchakarma is explained in detail in *The Textbook of Āyurveda*, vol. 3.

Marmāni are avenues of cleansing and detoxification for their related doshas, tissues, organs and channels. For example, marmāni that relate to specific organs such as Yakrut (liver), Plīhā (spleen), Vrukka (kidney) or Hrid (heart) are direct avenues for cleansing those organ systems. Nasal marmāni clear the nasal passages, relieve congestion, enhance respiration and the flow of prāna, and thereby cleanse prāna vaha srotas (respiratory channels).

Marmāni facilitate the cleansing of vāta dosha and help to re-establish its normal directional flows. All sub-types of vāta (vāyus) have their own *gati* (vector). When a vāyu moves in an improper direction, imbalance can arise. These flows can be corrected by stimulating the marmāni corresponding to each vāyu. For example, udāna vāyu rises upwards, as in coughing. Marmāni in the throat region pacify udāna vāyu, relieve cough and cleanse the bronchi. When apāna vāyu fails to move downwards, there is retention of urine. If pressure is applied to Bhaga or Basti marmāni, strengthening and cleansing of mūtra vaha srotas (urinary channels) and ambu vaha srotas (channel of fluids) is enhanced. Thus, the aggravated doshas, toxins, unwanted accumulations and impurities are eliminated from the system.

Table 20: Gati (Vectors) of Vāta

Prāna vāyu flows inwards
Udāna vāyu rises upwards
Apāna vāyu pushes downwards
Samāna vāyu moves horizontally
Vyāna vāyu circulates throughout the body

Shamana, Palliation of Doshas via Marmāni

Shamana or palliation therapy pacifies aggravated doshas by enkindling agni, but does not eliminate the excess doshas from the body. Shamana involves techniques such as fasting, exercise, prānāyāma (breath control) and sun or moon bathing. Other methods include oil massage, application of herbal pastes, and shirodhāra (pouring a gentle stream of warm oil on the forehead and "third eye" area). Marmāni can also be used to kindle agni and pacify the doshas. For example, stimulating Nābhi marmāni pacifies pāchaka pitta, enkindles samāna vāyu and jāthara agni, and addresses vāta-type intestinal pain. Stimulation of Jatru marma pacifies udāna vāyu, stimulates lung agni and immediately calms wheezing. For palliation, essential oils such as nutmeg and mustard are used for treating vāta marmāni, sandalwood and khus for pitta, and vacha or camphor oils for kapha.

Shamana is a milder therapy than shodhana, recommended when the body is too weak to undergo pañchakarma. The primary difference between them is the state of the doshas. In shodhana, the doshas should be "ripe" or mature (*utklishta*) and ready to be eliminated out of the body, so stronger measures are required. In shamana, the doshas are aggravated but not ripe enough to be expelled. Shamana is the phase of burning āma and neutralizing excess doshas locally. The same marma may be used for shodhana or shamana, depending on the state of the doshas. For example, pressure on Yakrut marma cleanses and detoxifies the liver, moving stagnant doshas into the GI tract during shodhana. Stimulating Yakrut during shamana enkindles the agnis of the liver, known as bhūta agni, and pacifies the local doshas.

Rasāyana, Rejuvenation via Marmāni

Rasāyana is a unique aspect of Āyurvedic therapy. When the doshas have been pacified, the organs and channels cleansed, and any disease eradicated, the mind and body still require a deeper rejuvenation. Rasāyana unfolds *rasa,* the juice of life, by restoring the body's innate intelligence and maintaining optimal function. A supportive therapy that nourishes and rejuvenates the tissues at the cellular level, rasāyana uses herbal and lifestyle regimens.

Marmāni also aid in rejuvenation by balancing ojas, tejas and prāna. These three vital essences of life are present at the site of each marma. Rejuvenation can occur by stimulating the vital sadyah prānahara marmāni, where ojas, tejas and prāna are most abundant. Treatment using marmāni that correspond to various organs or channels rejuvenates those structures. For example, massaging marmāni on the chest clears the bronchi and rejuvenates the lungs. Energy points that belong to prāna vaha srotas rejuvenate prāna and allow it to flow smoothly through its channels.

Apunarbhava Chikitsā, Preventive Therapy through Marmāni

Perhaps the greatest strength and contribution of Āyurveda is *apunarbhava,* the preventive approach that emphasizes living with awareness, in harmony with nature and natural law. Apunarbhava Chikitsā incorporates a personalized daily routine (*dīnāchārya*) adjusted according to a person's prakruti (constitution) and vikruti (present imbalance) as well as to the time of year. The preventive approach to health care involves a healthy diet, suitable exercise, yoga, meditation and prānāyāma (breath control).

The dīnāchārya typically includes a brief daily self oil massage, which stimulates a great many marmāni, thereby communicating with corresponding tissues, organs and channels and promoting healthy functioning of those structures. Self-massage also releases stagnant emotions, pacifies the doshas and helps to prevent illness. Performance of yogāsanas also stimulates numerous marmāni (see chapter 18, "Yoga Therapy and Marmāni"). Thus, even without learning about specific marmāni, marma chikitsā can play a major role in an Āyurvedic prevention program.[2]

Sadyah Phaladai Chikitsā, Marmāni as First Aid Therapy

Sadyah phaladai means that which instantly bears fruit or gives immediate results. Most herbal regimens achieve this, but marma therapy may also be used as a first line of treatment. Certain marmāni can instantaneously relieve acute pain and discomfort. For example, Skandadhara[3] marma relieves intense shoulder pain, Apānga and Kanīnaka marmāni alleviate periorbital pain, and Nābhi marmāni soothe acute abdominal pain. It is important to note that ***these energy points are not a substitute for medical treatment or acute emergency care.*** Chapter 17, which is devoted to the role of marmāni in the management of specific illnesses and conditions, begins with a long section on Āyurvedic first aid, listing marmāni that are helpful in healing or relieving dozens of painful symptoms.

Tanmātrā, Five Element Chikitsā

The tanmātrā (subtle elements) are the objects of the senses—sound, touch, vision, taste and smell. These are the major pathways of our inner pharmacy, which unfold subtle healing. They are connected to the five gross elements and the senses by hearing, feeling, seeing, tasting and smelling. Tanmātrā chikitsā are therapies that involve the five sensory perceptions and the five cognitive sense organs responsible for these perceptions. The table below summarizes the connection between the sensory organs, sensory perception, subtle elements and associated therapies. Refer also to the illustration in chapter 1, page 10, "The Five Elements and Their Manifestation in the Body." Each therapy in tanmātrā chikitsā is briefly discussed below in reference to marma

2. For a thorough description and guidelines for dīnācharya, please see *The Complete Book of Ayurvedic Home Remedies*, chapter 5.
3. Also called Kakshadhara.

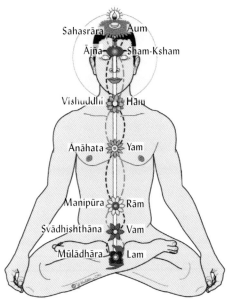

Bīja Mantras for the Seven Chakras

chikitsā, except for dietary therapy (taste), which is explained in the book *Ayurvedic Cooking for Self-Healing* by Usha Lad and Dr. Vasant Lad.

Shabda (Sound)

Mantra chikitsā is the origin of all sound therapy. A mantra is a sacred syllable or string of syllables from the Sanskrit alphabet. Space is intrinsically related to sound because it gives sound the freedom to travel, expand and communicate. *Sukha,* or health, is translated as contented space. *Duhkha,* illness or pain, means unhealthy space that may be distorted, congested, inflamed or clogged with toxins. The principle of mantra chikitsā is that the vibration of sound—the particular sound of the appropriate mantra—can create balance in the cellular space and thus restore health. Each of the seven chakras has a corresponding bīja (seed) sound as well.

Sound has an affinity for space; it also permeates the space of the marma. Marmāni occupy space within the nervous tissue and on the surface of the body. They are the doorways for sound to penetrate to the space of a tis-

Table 21: Tanmātrā and Chikitsā

Tanmātrā	Related Element	Cognitive Organ	Sensory Perception	Associated Therapy	Effect
Shabda (Sound)	Space	Ears	Hearing	Mantra chikitsā	Balances space element of cell
Sparsha (Touch)	Air	Skin	Feeling	Marma chikitsā	Improves cellular communication
Rūpa (Form or Color)	Fire	Eyes	Seeing	Chromotherapy	Enhances pīlu agni and pithara agni and balances cellular metabolism
Rasa (Taste)	Water	Tongue	Tasting	Dietary Therapy	Improves cellular nutrition
Gandha (Odor or Smell)	Earth	Nose	Smelling	Aromatherapy	Creates mineral balance at cellular level

sue, organ, or channel, or to deeper cellular and synaptic spaces of the central nervous system. Every organ has an affinity to a particular sound and an associated marma, as shown in table 23 on page 70. For greater effectiveness, the marmāni that correspond to the organ may be massaged while the healing sound is recited, either aloud or silently.

Sparsha (Touch)

Of the five tanmātrā, sparsha or touch is the one through which marma chikitsā primarily operates, and we devote an entire chapter (chapter 8) to exploring in depth the array of techniques utilized in touch therapies. The following remarks are but a brief introduction.

While touch can convey a variety of feelings, emotions and qualities, from anger, fear, hatred, temptation or lust to tenderness, compassion, love and healing, sparsha chikitsā utilizes pressure, massage and other techniques of touch for the purpose of healing. The therapeutic effect is connected predominantly to vāta dosha and specifically to prāna vāyu. Touch may be direct physical contact or an intangible transmission of prānic energy. A *prānachārya*, a master of prāna, can direct pranic energy within his/her own body or a patient's body for healing purposes. Similarly, in TCM, *Qigong* is the practice of cultivating qi and transmitting energy through what in Āyurveda is known as Tala Hrida, the marma located at the heart of the palm. A Qigong master is able to "touch" the patient at a deep level to facilitate healing.

Rūpa (Vision)

Rūpa is form, shape or color, which is perceived only through the sense of sight. Certain marmāni in close proximity to the eyes are related to ālochaka pitta, the subdosha that governs sight. These include Apānga, Kanīnaka, Vartma and Ashrū marmāni. Specific marmāni distinguish color vibrations and their unique healing effect. This is commonly known as chromotherapy. In pañchakarma detoxification treatment, light may be emitted along the midline of the body directly above each of the seven chakras, affecting corresponding marmāni in those regions, e.g., Ājñā, Jatru, Hridayam, Agrapatra, Sūrya, Nābhi and Bhaga. Table 50 on page 260 in appendix A outlines therapeutic properties for each color. Red, orange and yellow are hot, sharp and penetrating colors that stimulate pitta dosha. Green, blue and violet are cold, calming and soothing colors that stimulate vata and kapha dosha and pacify pitta dosha.

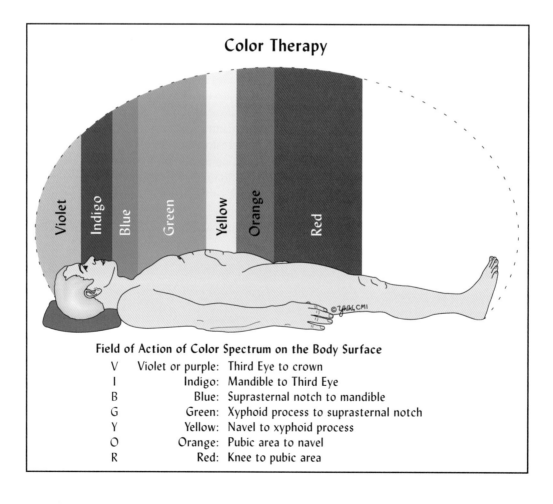

Color Therapy

Field of Action of Color Spectrum on the Body Surface

V	Violet or purple:	Third Eye to crown
I	Indigo:	Mandible to Third Eye
B	Blue:	Suprasternal notch to mandible
G	Green:	Xyphoid process to suprasternal notch
Y	Yellow:	Navel to xyphoid process
O	Orange:	Pubic area to navel
R	Red:	Knee to pubic area

Colors and Their Healing Effects on the Doshas

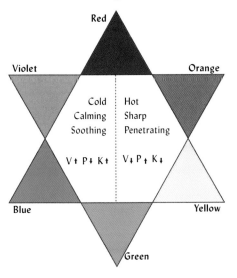

Rasa (Taste)

The moment we put a substance on the tongue, the first experience is the taste. Taste, according to Āyurvedic teachings, has a great therapeutic value. Sweet taste, for example, pacifies vāta and pitta but may increase kapha. Taste also affects the emotions as shown in the table below. In Āyurveda, herbal and dietary therapies each consider the effects of taste in the consumption of any substance. These modalities are beyond the scope of this book, but you can find a thorough discussion of the six tastes (sweet, sour, salty, pungent, astringent, bitter), their relationship to the five elements and the bodily organs, and their psychological and pharmacological actions in *The Textbook of Āyurveda,* volume I, Digestion chapter, as well as *The Complete Book of Āyurvedic Home Remedies,* chapter 8.

Gandha (Smell)

Aromatherapy, an important aspect of Āyurveda Chikitsā, relies on *gandha,* the sense of smell. Essential oils, attars, and incense trigger the olfactory pathways and influence body, mind and spirit. Chapter 15 discusses the art of aromatherapy and the therapeutic healing abilities of essential oils.

Context of Marma Chikitsā within Āyurvedic Therapy

• •

Āyurveda is a complete, integrated program of healing. It includes education and individualized recommendations for the patient about diet, useful herbal remedies, lifestyle factors and daily routine, meditation, yoga, exercise, rejuvenative therapies and many other factors, including marma chikitsā or marma therapy. The well-trained and experienced Āyurvedic practitioner has a vast array of therapies available to offer the patient, each with its own healing power.

As mentioned at the beginning of this chapter, marma chikitsā is rarely used as an isolated or self-contained method of healing, but rather is put to use within the context of Āyurveda as a whole. It can be used to cleanse, detoxify, energize, pacify and rejuvenate the body. Treating marmāni can restore balance or prevent imbalance. It can be almost instantaneously effective for certain conditions when used as first aid. When combined with other Āyurvedic treatments, it is a marvelous tool for healing through the sense of touch.

Every patient is a living book. To read that book, and to create a healing story with a happy outcome, is as much an art as it is a science. The Āyurvedic clinician who wants to master both the art and science of healing should study with a master and build a solid foundation in anatomy, physiology and clinical insight. In treating a patient, he or she must ascertain the patient's constitution, current state of imbalance, which doshas, dhātus and srotāmsi are involved, the stage of pathogenesis, and the severity of symptoms. It takes great sensitivity to read the pulse, eyes, skin, tongue and other aspects of the patient that deliver clues and insights into his or her condition. Further, the practitioner must carefully gauge the strength of the patient and the patient's agnis, and the strength of the disease. Many other factors, such as the person's relationships and work stresses, and the season of the year, also come into play in understanding the patient's condition and determining the course of treatment. There is enormous wisdom accumulated in the millennia-old tradition of Āyurveda, which incorporates so many facets of experience, knowledge and practical skill.

In the next chapter we will begin the truly practical phase of this book, by looking at specific techniques of marma chikitsā, and then proceed to the chapters detailing the 117 marma points of Āyurveda.

Table 22: Effects of the Six Tastes

Taste	Positive Effect	Detrimental Effect
Sweet	Love	Attachment
Sour	Determination, discrimination	Judgment
Salty	Enthusiasm	Agitation
Bitter	Withdrawal, introspection	Harshness, austerity
Pungent	Comprehension, digestion of experience	Anger
Astringent	Compactness, binding, holding together, integrity	Repression, 'stuck' emotions

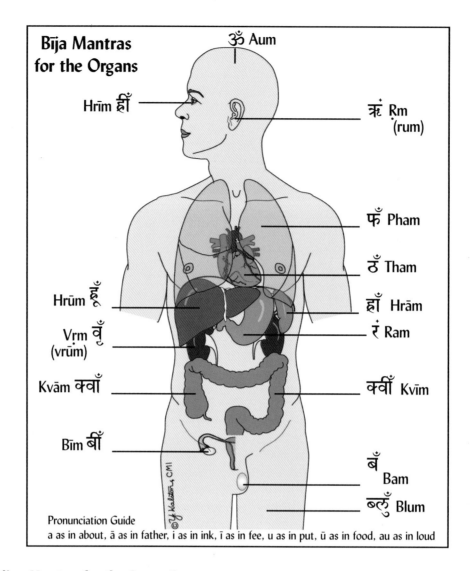

Bīja Mantras for the Organs

ॐ Aum

Hrīm ह्रीँ

ऋं Rm (rum)

फँ Pham

ठँ Tham

ह्राँ Hrām

रं Ram

Hrūm ह्रूँ

Vrm वृँ (vrūm)

Kvām क्वाँ

क्वीँ Kvīm

Bīm बीँ

बँ Bam

ब्लूँ Blum

Pronunciation Guide
a as in about, ā as in father, i as in ink, ī as in fee, u as in put, ū as in food, au as in loud

Table 23: Healing Mantras for the Organ Systems

Marma Name/Location	Organ System or Tissue	Bīja Sound
Mūrdhni, Brahmarandhra	Cerebral cortex	Aum
Apānga, Kanīnaka	Lacrimal glands	Hrīm
Karnamūla, Karnapālī	Ear, Parotid gland	Rum
Hrid 1, 2, 3, Agra Patra	Heart, pericardium, thymus	Thum
Kakshadhara, Apastambha	Lungs, bronchus, bronchioles	Phum
Yakrut	Liver, gall bladder	Hrūm
Sūrya (Solar Plexus)	Stomach, cardiac valve, pylorus	Ram
Plīhā	Spleen, tail of pancreas	Hrām
Vrukka	Kidneys, adrenals	Vrūm
Nābhi 3 (Unduka)	Ascending colon, cecum, ileocecal valve	Kvām
Nābhi 4 (Malāshaya)	Descending colon, sigmoid colon, rectum	Kvīm
Vankshana, Yoni Oshtha	Ovaries, fallopian tubes, bulbourethral glands (Bartholin's gland)	Bīm
Vrushana (in males)	Testicles, bulbourethral gland (Cowper's gland)	Bum
Ūrū	Femoral triangle, femoral artery and nerve, cremaster muscle	Blum[a]

a. Ūrū marma is a very delicate point. In females, it may stimulate Bartholin gland secretions. In males, it is the location of the cremasteric reflex, a testicular retraction. In both sexes, it may increase sexual energy. Blum is the Bīja mantra for ojas.

Techniques of Marma Stimulation – Guidelines for the Practitioner

Chapter 7 placed Marma Chikitsā within the broad context of Āyurveda and its multiple therapeutic modalities. Now it is time for a few final but critical considerations before moving into the central portion of the book, where we look at each marma point, its precise location and its uses. In this chapter, we will set out the various techniques employed by generations of Ayurvedic physicians for stimulating the marmāni, and offer guidelines for the practitioner to follow during treatment in order to be most effective in maintaining and restoring the health and vitality of the patient.

Techniques of Marma Chikitsā – 10 Methods of Stimulating Marma Points

Sparsha chikitsā (literally "touch therapy") provides an array of techniques to stimulate marmāni. Touching the skin activates the subdoshas of bhrājaka pitta (the skin), prāna vāyu (conveyor of the sensation of touch), vyāna vāyu (circulation and distribution of touch sensation) and rañjaka pitta (the blood). The skilled practitioner must determine which technique or combination of techniques is most appropriate for the specific condition of the individual. These techniques should be practiced only with proper training and guidance from a skilled teacher. They include:

* *Snehana* (oleation, application of oil to the skin)
* *Svedana* (sudation, sweat or steam therapy)
* *Mardana* (deep, connective tissue dry massage)
* *Pīdana* (deep pressure without oil)
* *Veshtana (*binding)
* *Lepana* (application of paste)
* *Trasana* (deep stimulation)

* *Agni karma* (application of local heat)
* *Sūchi bharana* (puncturing with a needle)
* *Rakta moksha* (bloodletting)

With the exception of snehana and svedana, all these techniques are also practiced in traditional Chinese medicine (TCM), some even more so than in Āyurveda. Sūchi bharana is equivalent to the Chinese art of acupuncture, agni karma is similar to moxibustion and trasana to *plum blossoming*. (see page 74) Rakta moksha, the therapeutic art of bloodletting, and lepana, the application of medicated pastes to various regions of the body are also common practices in TCM. The practitioner of *tui na,* or TCM therapeutic massage, utilizes various amounts of pressure, comparable to the Ayurvedic massage techniques of mardana, pīdana and veshtana.

Snehana (Oleation)

Snehana literally translates as love, and as oiliness. Massaging the body with medicated oils brings many benefits. It promotes psychological well-being by calming the mind and inducing a deep sense of relaxation and inner tranquility. Gentle massage and pressure also soothe the nervous system as the oil penetrates the fascia into the nerve endings, permeates to the level of all seven dhatus and rejuvenates the tissues. This releases muscle tension and strain and improves arterial, venous and lymphatic circulation. This strong action influences neural reflexes and corrects autonomic dysfunction. Oleation pacifies all three doshas, because it opposes and balances the dry quality of vāta, the hard quality of kapha and sharp quality of pitta. It especially calms vāta dosha and acts on prāna and vyāna vāyu. Oleation softens the skin, promotes flexibility and enhances immunity.

Oil may be applied to the hands or fingertips to stimulate marmāni. The site of the marma has the potential to be a defective space where disease may flourish. Localized oleation encourages stagnant, excessive doshas and impurities in the form of mental and physical toxins to soften. The liquefied toxins are released from the marmāni into the general circulation of rasa and rakta dhātu (lymph and blood). From there, they return to the gastrointestinal tract and are more readily eliminated from the body.

Snehana is an important technique used in preparation for pañchakarma (detoxification). During pañchakarma, the whole body is massaged with oil with special attention given to the marmāni specific to the individual's healing needs. This oleation facilitates cleansing of the marmāni and subsequently detoxifies the corresponding tissues, organs and channels of the body and helps free the mind of negative thoughts and emotions.

Oils are selected for both the individual's constitution (prakruti) and present imbalance (vikruti). Sesame oil can be beneficial for all three doshas, but because it is hot, sharp and penetrating, some pitta people cannot tolerate it. It is the best choice for vāta individuals, along with castor oil. Sunflower, safflower and coconut oils are cooling and gentle, and optimal for pitta pacification. For kapha dosha, mustard, corn and olive oils are the most appropriate invigorating oils. Mahānārāyana oil, made from a mixture of many potent herbs, is a strong analgesic and muscle relaxant. It can be used topically to relieve any type of doshic pain or pain in virtually any region of the body.

Svedana (Sudation)

Svedana is the therapeutic use of heat, in the form of a steam bath, sweat box or direct local application of steam. The medicated steam from herbs or essential oils used in svedana calms the doshas, liquefies āma (toxins) and promotes their elimination through perspiration. The heat of svedana kindles agni, dilates the srotas and brings the doshas back to the GI tract for further elimination. It also improves blood flow and cleanses the skin. Steam can be directed through a small tube to a specific area of the body, such as the joints, for localized relief. In general, steam from nirgundi oil is recommended for vāta disorders, sandalwood oil for pitta disorders, and eucalyptus oil for kapha disorders. Svedana is performed after oleation, but both techniques are contraindicated when there is high toxicity (āma) in the body. An experienced clinician can determine whether this is the case and suggest herbal remedies that can be used first to enkindle agni and eliminate āma. Important: snehana and svedana, as deep cleansing procedures, are contraindicated for women during menstruation and pregnancy.

Mardana (Deep Connective Tissue Massage)

Mardana, deep connective tissue work, helps to break up accumulated crystals of unresolved emotion. Mardana means crushing or grinding, an apt description of the strong nature of this type of massage. It is a dry massage without the use of any oils. Mardana is recommended for kapha individuals, obese patients and athletic individuals with well-developed muscles. These patients require deep stimulation, not gentle massage. In general, deep connective tissue massage is indicated for areas with large muscles, such as the gluteal area, thighs, calves, low back and arms. Many patients enjoy the somewhat "rough" feeling of mardana, however, it is not recommended for delicate areas near the heart, kidneys or thyroid. Practitioners should be aware that as long-held toxins, stresses and painful cellular memories are released, the patient may experience some physical pain as well as some therapeutic emotional release, often in the form of crying. But within a few treatments, a desirable release of muscle tension, enhanced flexibility and deep relaxation are generally achieved.

Pīdana (Deep, Dry Pressure)

Pīdana is the application of localized deep, dry pressure (without oil) that is relatively less forceful than mardana. It is indicated for the same types of individuals, conditions and regions of the body as mardana. Pressure is increased steadily, based on the patient's pain tolerance. A small, blunt rod, called a *shalākā*, is sometimes used to emit steady, deep pressure. (It can also be used to transmit heat; see below under agni karma.) The shalākā may be a rounded rod, probe, thin bar or small stick. It is usually made of wood, but other materials may be used that are suited to each dosha: copper for reducing kapha, gold for reducing vāta and silver for reducing pitta. The concept of shalākā also exists in TCM, which may employ various objects to maximize pressure and stimulation of the energy points.

Veshtana (Binding or Holding)

Veshtana involves applying firm steady pressure for a few minutes by grabbing or holding a painful area. The binding action is antagonistic to the mobile quality of vāta dosha that is responsible for creating cramps, spasms, tremors and intense pain. This stabilizing force calms vāta dosha that is lodged in māmsa dhātu (muscle tissue) and facilitates relaxation and muscle release.

Lepana (Application of Paste)

Lepana is the application of pulp or paste from freshly ground herbs, leaves, roots and barks. TCM also applies paste over certain regions of the body and specific energy points. The qualities of these substances penetrate through the skin into the superficial and then deep fascia and thus to the nerve endings. Through the marma, each herb's properties, such as rasa (taste), *vīrya* (heating or cooling energy) and *vipāka* (post-digestive effect), are carried to the nervous system. For example, ginger paste applied to the skin promotes heat because the rasa of ginger is pungent. The vīrya of ginger is also heating to the skin and improves circulation upon application of the paste. The vipāka of ginger paste made from powdered ginger is pungent, hence it burns āma (toxins) and relieves pain.

Āyurveda has long employed numerous *lepa* (pastes) and catalogued their therapeutic properties. For example, nutmeg paste induces tranquility and sound sleep. Punarnava paste reduces edema and swelling by stimulating the diuretic action of the kidneys. The clinician must combine understanding of doshic involvement with the region of the body affected and apply paste to the appropriate marmāni. An example is shringa shunthi lepa (a paste of deer horn ash and ginger) applied to the Hrid (heart) marmāni for cardiac pain. Ginger paste can be applied to Shankha, Ājñā and Ganda marmāni to relieve sinus headaches. The table below lists a number of lepa and conditions that they can address.

Table 23: Lepa (pastes) and Their Uses

Lepa (paste)	Related Condition
Camphor	Pitta type pain
Dashamūla	Vāta type pain
Garlic	Vāta headache, vāta type pain
Ginger	Sinus headache, kapha congestion
Guggulu	Arthritis
Haridra (turmeric)	Infection or inflammation
Hina	Vāta type pain
Hing (asafoetida)	Muscle spasms
Khus	Pitta headache
Musta	Muscle ache, pitta inflammation
Nutmeg	Insomnia, migraine, agitation
Punarnava	Edema
Red sandalwood	Inflammation, sprain
Sandalwood	Pitta headache, inflammation, burning
Shringa shunthi	Cardiac pain, angina

Agni Karma (Application of Heat)

Agni karma, the application of local heat, is comparable to moxibustion in TCM. It allows heat to spread throughout the body, from the marma to the tissues, organs and channels. With its sharp penetrating action, it can sometimes be more effective than deep, connective tissue massage or puncturing with needles. Agni karma acts instantaneously to improve circulation, unblock stagnation, calm vāta dosha and facilitate all vāta subdoshas to move in the proper direction. In addition, it improves digestion by enkindling agni (*agni dīpana*) and digesting toxins (*āma pachana*).

Moxibustion involves burning the herb *artemisia vulgaris,* also known as mugwort, close to or directly on the skin, so the properties of the herb penetrate into the energy points and meridians. Agni karma is a similar procedure. It may be performed using a piece of dried turmeric root heated until it is red-hot, held close to the skin by tongs or forceps. Or a shalākā, the blunt rod described above, may be used to radiate heat above the point. In ancient times, gold, silver, copper and brass rods were used for the royal family, while clay chalk-like rods were for common people. Gold is best suited for treating vāta individuals, silver for treating pitta and copper for kapha. Agni karma is effective for people with raw ojas (unprocessed ojas), high kapha or excessive fat, and is commonly used for arthritic pain and calcaneal spurs. It is contraindicated for diabetics, for a number of reasons. Diabetics generally have low resistance and poor circulation, and are prone to infections; even a minor burn or blister due to the heat may become infected and cause a great deal of trouble, even leading to gangrene.

Sūchi Bharana (Puncturing with Needles)

Sūchi bharana means to puncture with a needle. In ancient times, needles were created from bamboo shoots or the thorns of the babul bush and sterilized with antiseptics such as neem oil. Very fine, sharp needles were inserted gently into the subcutaneous tissue at tender spots, stimulating the nervous system. However, the art of acupuncture never became popular in the subcontinent of India. A likely reason is that, due to the centrality of the principle of *ahimsā* (non-violence) in both Hinduism and Buddhism, the insertion of needles came to be considered too invasive, a form of violence to the body. Thus, acupuncture did not continue to develop in Āyurveda compared to other methods of marma chikitsā.

Trasana (Irritation)

Trasana means to trouble, torture or irritate. *Gharshana* is a synonym meaning to rub the skin surface roughly and agitate it. Trasana is a dry massage, in which a rough surface, such as that of a brush or stone, is rubbed against the skin, creating a friction like fine-grained sandpaper. Intense rubbing stimulates the skin and marmāni. Trasana enhances local circulation of vyāna vāyu, which releases stagnant prāna and activates rañjaka pitta (blood) and bhrājaka pitta (the pigmentation layer of the skin).

In TCM, plum blossoming is a technique that accomplishes a similar action. It uses an instrument with a flexible shaft and multiple small needles at the head. The technique's name derives from the image of a plum blossom with its red color, as the skin surface reddens when it undergoes irritation. The technique is effective for conditions such as extreme muscle tightness.

Cupping is another method used in TCM that works by virtue of irritation. During cupping the practitioner places heated glass cups on the skin, creating a vacuum of negative pressure. This technique successfully draws toxins to the skin surface, relieves pain and increases local circulation.

Rakta Moksha (Bloodletting)

Rakta moksha, therapeutic bloodletting, is a technique that improves local circulation. It can be used in pañchakarma for treatment of clots, thrombosis, excess pitta, and locally stagnant prāna. In India, Ayurvedic clinicians have traditionally used leeches for this purpose. The leech injects saliva into the capillaries and sucks approximately 100cc of blood, preventing the blood from clotting. The leech's saliva contains hirudin, which is a heparin-like, anticoagulant substance. Needles or venipuncture can also accomplish localized rakta moksha.

Blood-letting is also commonly used in TCM for reducing excess heat or stagnation in the meridians. The jing-well acupoints adjacent to the finger and toe nails (see chapter 5, pages 53 and 55), are pricked with a needle to release a couple of drops of blood. These points correspond to the beginning or end of the twelve principal meridians and have a clearing action on the entire pathway of the meridian.

> Marma chikitsā is a powerful, divine science that can potentially activate both good and bad energies. That is why, while doing marma therapy, the therapist should meditate, to make the mind calm and the heart full of compassion and love. While doing marma chikitsā, he or she should feel that God is watching, so that his or her energy will not go in a wrong direction.

Guidelines for Practitioners of Marma Chikitsā

Marma therapy, as we have seen, utilizes numerous techniques to stimulate marmāni for healing purposes. Ultimately, however, it is the practitioner's skill, knowledge, attention and awareness, on a solid platform of love and compassion, that are crucial for attaining effective thera-

peutic results. This section includes practitioner guidelines regarding clinical knowledge, fundamentals of touch during treatment and methods such as meditation that calm the mind and increase self-awareness and focus.

Clinical Knowledge

Marma chikitsā is a great yoga, requiring skill in action. It is similar to archery. An unskilled archer launches several arrows, hoping one will reach the target, while an expert archer requires only one arrow to hit the target efficiently and effortlessly. The identical principle is reflected in acupuncture, where one needle may be all that is necessary to achieve the desired therapeutic effect. This ability stems from mastery of clinical knowledge that results in precision in selecting the most appropriate therapeutic approach or, in marma chikitsā, the correct marma or marmāni.

The patient's prakruti (constitution) and vikruti (present imbalance) must be considered so marmāni do not aggravate the doshas. The clinician will also consider the subdoshas, tissues, organs and channels that are affected by the condition, or that he or she wishes to influence for healing. For pain management, marmāni may be chosen according to the region of the body affected.

Important considerations to keep in mind when selecting marmāni:

* The patient's perception of pain or tenderness at the affected site is important. Pay attention to the patient's reactions and let them guide your treatment – how hard or how long to press, and so on.

* The degree of tenderness at a marma does not necessarily correlate with severity of dysfunction.

* Sensitivity at a marma is not reliably indicative of a specific stage of pathogenesis.

* Points have their own "sphere of influence;" some are more powerful than others. Thus, two or more points may address the same disturbance, but with varying levels of efficacy.

* The therapeutic effect of any marma will vary in different situations, conditions and individuals.

Meditation and Breath Awareness

The practitioner's skill is cultivated through experience and meditative awareness. Stillness of the mind is the fruit of meditation and may be cultivated in many ways, such as through awareness of the breath. A quiet mind allows a practitioner to be creative, intuitive and focused. So'Hum and Empty Bowl meditation are two processes to achieve stillness.

In **Empty Bowl Meditation**, the natural movement of the breath is observed as it flows gently in and out, with awareness of the lungs expanding and contracting. The meditator's attention follows as the breath enters through the nose, travels through the respiratory pathways to the lungs and diaphragm and then deep into the abdomen, behind the navel. Careful, quiet observation reveals a natural stop before the exhalation begins. Staying with the process, one's attention follows the breath back up as it exits the body, moving outward to about nine inches away from the nostrils, to a second natural stop that occurs before the next inhalation.

When you practice empty bowl meditation, stay in each stop, even though it may be for just a moment at first. In those brief stops of the breath, time stops, because time is a movement of breath; when there is no breath, there is no time. We exist, without breath, without time. And in that stop there is no mind, because mind, too, is the movement of breath. Mind and breath are intimately connected. Breathing is the physiological component, and thinking the psychological component of the same phenomenon.

So in that stop during meditation, breath stops, mind stops, time stops, and you enter into silence. You become completely like an empty bowl. The moment you become an empty bowl, divine lips will touch you, God will come to you to pour out his love.

In the beginning, the stop rarely lasts more than a few seconds. But if you practice this meditation for ten minutes in the morning and in the evening, and for ten minutes on your bed before you go to sleep, just quietly watching the breath and the stop, slowly the stop will increase, up to 30 seconds, 40 seconds, one and a half minutes. With time, resting in these two natural pauses becomes more natural, and the feeling of inner peace and contentment is more easily sustained.

So'Hum meditation[1] has existed in India throughout the ages. It synchronizes the movement of the breath with the mantra that fits naturally into the inhalation (So) and exhalation (Hum). *So* is felt and said *mentally* during the whole phase of inhalation and *Hum* during the exhalation. The literal translation of So'Hum is "I am that," while the deeper meaning is "I am that pure awareness." This mantra calms the mind, yet simultaneously focuses and sharpens it. When the Ayurvedic physician or marma therapist utilizes this technique, a sense of tranquility and clarity pervades the patient-practitioner interaction, enhancing communication and receptivity.

So'Hum Meditation

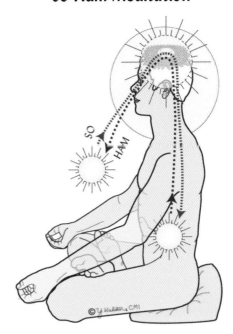

Inhale from 9 inches away from the nostrils and mentally say 'so…ooo' as you inhale. Bring your awareness to the 'so' as that 'so' goes inward, into the center of the brain, and stops. Stay there for a fraction of a second, then exhale as you feel and say 'hammmm' throughout the phase of exhalation. You exhale out of the body and ham dissolves into the outer space.

Within these two stops, so and ham, within that gap, there is a canvas of pure awareness. On that canvas, your whole life is painted. Be with that canvas and then you will feel the pure essence of your being. Your being is god, your being is reality, your being is the love divine. Just stay there. With this practice, so'ham will unfold inner beauty, inner joy, and inner truth.

Guidelines for Touch and Pressure

Part 2 of this book, which follows immediately after this section, contains specific and detailed guidelines for treating over 100 marmāni. The following are general guidelines for every practitioner regarding breath, posture, application of pressure on the marmāni and selection of the correct points for treatment.

Whenever possible, maintain a stable and comfortable posture, with the spine held straight. Proper posture enables the breath to flow freely and the suitable amount of pressure to be exerted.

You will find it helpful if you settle your breath by the meditation techniques described above and then synchronize your breath with your patient's breath. During the course of treatment, the patient's breathing will naturally become smoother and slower, or he or she may let out a sigh or begin to cry. These are indications of relaxation, relief and release and are good signs. Some temporary faster or heavier breathing may also signal a release.

---

1. So'Hum is actually spelled So'Ham but for ease of pronunciation, in the text we spell it as it sounds.

Apply steady pressure to each marma for approximately one to two minutes. Unless gentle pressure is specifically called for, begin with medium pressure and gradually increase it when the patient exhales, if you feel it is necessary or would be helpful. Maintain pressure at a deep level, according to the patient's tolerance. Pressure may be applied for a slightly longer duration if there is significant pain relief or reduction of tenderness.

When applying pressure to a marma, you can hold your fingers steady at the marma site, rotate them clockwise or counterclockwise, or move in a linear direction from one marma to another. These movements pacify or stimulate the doshas and have other therapeutic effects. Clockwise movement is tonifying and stimulating, pacifying vāta and kapha, but possibly triggering pitta. Counterclockwise movement is calming and pacifying. It soothes pitta dosha but may stimulate vāta and kapha. Linear movement also balances vāta dosha.

The finger a practitioner uses to exert pressure on a marma is also significant. Each finger corresponds to one of the five elements and releases the subtle energy of that element during treatment. The thumb corresponds to the space (ether) element, the index finger to air, the middle finger to fire, the ring finger to water, and the little finger to earth energy. The thumb also signifies vast limitless consciousness. That is why a guru or spiritual master may initiate a disciple by pressing Ājñā marma with the thumb.

During a pañchakarma massage, two practitioners simultaneously massage the body and synchronize their breath with each other and with the patient. They coordinate their movements and their pressure and give equal emphasis to the marmāni on the right and left sides of the body. Marmāni on the right side can be used for treating male patients and those on the left side for female patients. However, they are generally stimulated bilaterally.

Every individual responds uniquely to stimulation, depending on many factors, including his or her constitution, current condition, sensitivity and underlying strength. Also, some individuals are open to change and will readily relax and let go of tension and areas where unexpressed emotions are held, while others may be more resistant.

Prakruti (constitution) is a major influence on an individual's response and sensitivity to touch. Vāta individuals tend to be the most sensitive. They respond to gentle, superficial and delicate touch. Kapha types are relaxed and less sensitive. They require deep and vigorous pressure. Pitta individuals like strong and firm pressure.

Certain marmāni are dosha-sensitive in specific individuals or constitutional types. For example, Yakrut and Plīhā marmāni are often more sensitive in pitta individuals, while Bhaga and Trik marmāni tend to be more sensitive in vāta individuals. Kapha people may be more reactive to Apastambha and Jatru marmāni.

Thus, knowledge of an individual's constitution and current condition determines not only which marmāni are selected, but also the degree of pressure and direction of rotation that will be most effective.

Finally, selecting medicated oils best suited for each individual's constitution and condition adds effectiveness to the treatment. Chapter 15 describes the properties and applications of 27 of the main medicated oils that can be used for marma chikitsā. See also table 26 on page 212 and table 27 on page 215 where the information on oils is summarized for quick reference. Considering all these factors makes marma chikitsā specific to the individual and his or her condition, leading to the desired therapeutic results.

Marma chikitsā can be repeated on a daily basis or periodically until symptoms resolve.

Āyurveda views each and every individual as a unique manifestation of cosmic consciousness. Thus, stimulating the energy points in marma chikitsā (as in acupuncture as well) should always be done with great sensitivity and awareness. When touching the human body, there must be a great deal of clarity, compassion and love in one's heart. The ultimate level of service is to treat the patient with the highest respect and love.

The preceding chapters have offered a wealth of information about Āyurveda, Marmāni and Marma Chikitsā as well as some fascinating and, we hope, useful parallels with Traditional Chinese Medicine. Now it is time to dive into the knowledge of the 117 Ayurvedic marmāni. Part 2 of the book provides detailed descriptions of marma locations, energetics and therapeutic applications for each of the marmāni. Uniquely, this part of the book also presents some delightful stories about many of the marmāni from the Hindu and Vedic tradition, along with insight into the significance and practical value of these energy points for spiritual evolution and growth of consciousness.

Introduction to Part Two

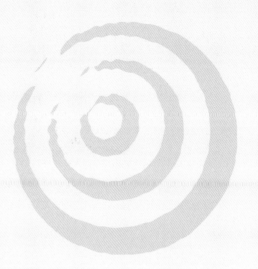

This central part of the book presents the heart of the practical aspect of marma therapy. The material in this section has been organized to systematically elucidate each of the 117 marmāni according to the following categories:

* Sanskrit name
* Anatomical location
* Associated doshic subtypes
* Actions
* Indications
* Commentary
* Treatment
* Corresponding acupoint
* Commentary on the acupoint and comparison with marma
* Anatomical diagram

To preserve authenticity, the authors refer to marmāni by their Sanskrit **Names,** rather than their English translations. Due to the multi-layered richness of the Sanskrit language, each name may have a number of meanings, often replete with medical, poetic and spiritual significance. In the Commentary, several possible interpretations of the name may be mentioned. On occasion, a marma may also be known by two names. To avoid confusion, the marma is referred to by only one name throughout the text. Due to the oral tradition of transmitting information from generation to generation, certain names do not correspond to those used in classical literature, but correlate to modern popularly-used terminology.

The **Locations** of marmāni have been carefully worded to be as anatomically precise as possible. They are also represented in anatomical diagrams. Some of these locations differ slightly from those in the ancient literature because Sushruta believed the marmāni to cover a greater region than a single fixed spot. As a surgeon, his focus was on areas where prāna was concentrated and vitality would be disrupted by an incision. With due respect to Sushrutacharya, the great founder of marma therapy and highly renowned Ayurvedic surgeon, based on the author's four decades of clinical practice with thousands of patients, Sushruta's locations have sometimes been narrowed to specific fixed points that are easier to locate and stimulate.

The **Associated Doshic Subtypes** whose functions are influenced by the marma are listed. Reference can be made to chapter 1 where we outline the specific functions of the subdoshas.

In presenting the basic **Actions** of each marma, great care has been taken to convey technical Ayurvedic terms in equivalent English terms. Sometimes no acceptably precise translation is available, as when an Ayurvedic term encompasses a wider range of functions than a seemingly equivalent term in western medicine. For example, "stimulating prāna" indicates much more than "enhancing respiration". Often a marma may be said to "benefit" a specific organ, body region or function. "Benefit" is loosely synonymous with influence, stimulate, activate or improve function.

The **Indications** for each marma are grouped together in related categories whenever possible. Often a general function such as "relieves pain" will be followed by specific functions, such as "relieves pain—headaches, abdominal pain, liver pain" and so forth. Or a general function, such as "benefits the eyes", will list a variety of eye disorders as specific indications.

The **Treatment** section offers the practitioner valuable guidelines on:

❋ *Essential oils* that may be used to stimulate the marma, often delineated according to doshic constitution or symptoms.

❋ *Specific techniques* for stimulation or massage of the marma, a group of related marmāni or a certain body region.

❋ *Breathing techniques or yoga postures* that can be beneficially used in conjunction with the marma. This topic is explored more fully in chapter 18, "Yoga Therapy and Marmāni."

The **Corresponding Acupoint** with its Chinese name, English translation and commonly used abbreviation are provided. The abbreviations represent the meridian on which the acupoint is located. For example, ST 1 indicates the first point on the Stomach meridian. Refer to table 54 on page 265 in appendix B for the meridian names and abbreviations. Almost 75 of the 117 marmāni correspond exactly to acupoints. Where there is no one-to-one correspondence, major acupoints that are in close proximity are mentioned whenever relevant. References to corresponding acupoints are limited to those located on the fourteen principal channels outlined in table 54 on page 265 in appendix B and certain other important points. This is because the specialized traditions and subsystems within the field of acupuncture, including Chinese, Korean, Japanese and Vietnamese styles, are too numerous to include in this presentation. Acupuncturists, regardless of their individual traditions, agree on the acupoints of the fourteen major meridians.

This section includes comparison of the energetics of the marma and the acupoint. Often, understanding the salient information mentioned for the acupoint facilitates a deeper appreciation of the marma's function. For example, a better grasp of a marma's energetics can be gained by becoming acquainted with its location on a particular meridian. When the functions of both marma and acupoint match, the commentary sheds light on this conjunction within the language of each medical system. To provide a detailed description of the acupoint and its energetics surpasses the scope of this book.

The **Commentary** integrates information from the previous categories to offer greater insight into the marma's energetics. It may include some or all of the following topics: the Sanskrit name with alternate translations and meanings, anatomy, physiology and the correlation of functions and indications to doshic theory. The relevance of the marma for spiritual experience and development may also be considered.

Finally, **Diagrams** of the anatomical sites are provided to facilitate exact location of the acupoint or marma.

These versatile points have a remarkable ability to produce results quickly, relieving pain and other symptoms of distress. They are also highly effective for balancing body, mind and spirit over the long term. A thorough knowledge of these points and their potential applications is a huge addition to the therapeutic armamentarium of any professional dedicated to the healing arts.[1]

---

1. **Disclaimer:** As stated on the copyright page of this book, marma therapy is not a substitute for regular medical treatment or consultation with a qualified medical practitioner. It is intended to be an adjunct to other treatments.

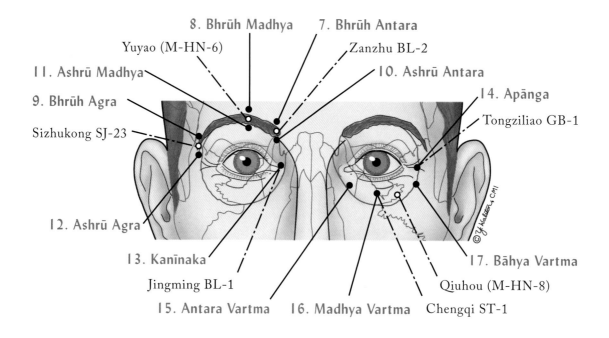

8. Bhrūh Madhya
7. Bhrūh Antara
Yuyao (M-HN-6)
Zanzhu BL-2
11. Ashrū Madhya
10. Ashrū Antara
9. Bhrūh Agra
14. Apānga
Tongziliao GB-1
Sizhukong SJ-23
12. Ashrū Agra
13. Kanīnaka
Jingming BL-1
17. Bāhya Vartma
Qiuhou (M-HN-8)
15. Antara Vartma
16. Madhya Vartma
Chengqi ST-1

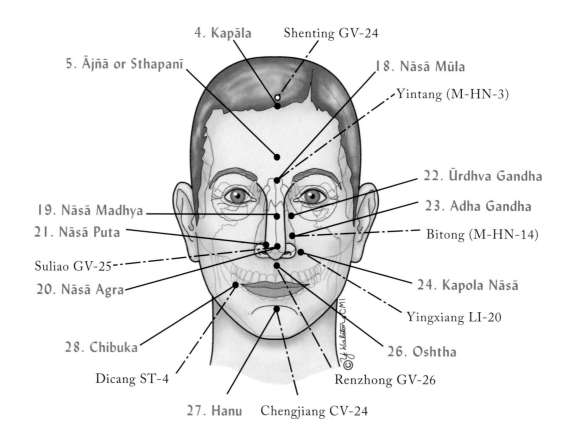

4. Kapāla
Shenting GV-24
5. Ājñā or Sthapanī
18. Nāsā Mūla
Yintang (M-HN-3)
22. Ūrdhva Gandha
23. Adha Gandha
19. Nāsā Madhya
Bitong (M-HN-14)
21. Nāsā Puta
Suliao GV-25
24. Kapola Nāsā
20. Nāsā Agra
Yingxiang LI-20
28. Chibuka
26. Oshtha
Dicang ST-4
Renzhong GV-26
27. Hanu
Chengjiang CV-24

Mukha (Face) and Shiro (Head) Marmāni

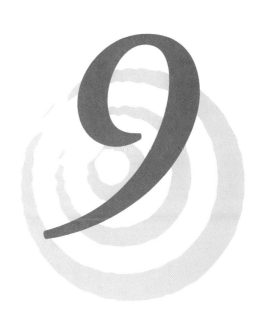

Mukha (Face) and Shiro (Head) Marmāni (28)

#	Marma Points	Page	Acupoint
1	Mūrdhni or Adhipati	82	≈GV 20 ≈GV 21
2	Brahmarandhra	84	GV 22
3	Shivarandhra	86	GV 19
4	Kapāla	88	≈GV 24[a]
5	Ājñā or Sthapanī	89	≈Yintang
6	Shankha	91	≈Taiyang
7	Bhrūh Antara	92	≈BL 2
8	Bhrūh Madhya	92	≈Yuyao
9	Bhrūh Agra	92	≈SJ 23
10	Ashrū Antara	94	≈BL 2
11	Ashrū Madhya	94	≈Yuyao
12	Ashrū Agra	94	≈SJ 23
13	Kanīnaka	95	BL 1
14	Apānga	96	GB 1
15	Antara Vartma	97	≈ST 1, BL 1
16	Madhya Vartma	97	ST 1
17	Bāhya Vartma	97	Qiuhou, ≈GB 1
16	Nāsā Mūla	99	Yintang
19	Nāsā Madhya	100	_____b
20	Nāsā Agra	101	GV 25
21	Nāsā Puta	102	_____
22	Ūrdhva Ganda	103	≈Bitong
23	Adhah Ganda	104	Bitong
24	Kapola Nasa	105	LI 20
25	Kapola Madhya	106	_____
26	Oshtha	107	GV 26
27	Hanu	108	CV 24
28	Chibuka	110	ST 4

a. ≈ means marma is in close proximity to this acupoint.
b. The dashed line means there are no acupoints that correspond to this marma point.

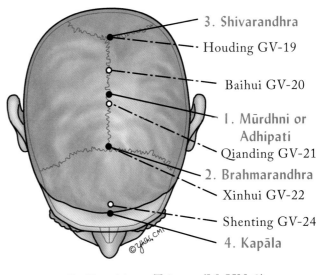

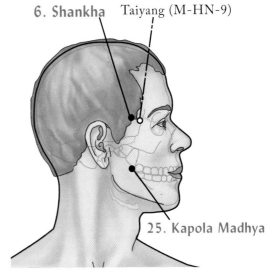

Mūrdhni or Adhipati

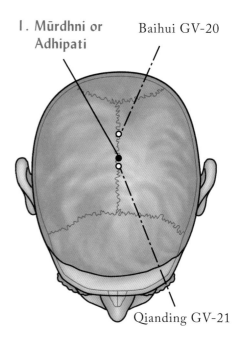

1. Mūrdhni or Adhipati   Baihui GV-20

Qianding GV-21

Location
On the vertex at the midline of the head, 10 anguli above the glabella (midpoint between both eyebrows). Locate by putting the base of the palm on the eyebrows and reach back to where the middle finger touches, or locate by drawing a line from each ear apex meeting at the vertex.

Actions
♦ Regularizes prāna, synchronizes prāna and apāna vāyu
♦ Enhances cerebral circulation and circulation of cerebral spinal fluid (CSF)
♦ Restores consciousness
♦ Treats sensory and motor dysfunction, aids in coordination
♦ Facilitates optimal functioning of pituitary and pineal gland, regulates hormonal secretions
♦ Regulates frontal lobe activity
♦ Stimulates memory, attention and concentration
♦ Relieves headaches
♦ Calms mind, balances emotions

Associated Doshic Subtypes
Directly related to Prāna Vāyu, Sādhaka Pitta, Tarpaka Kapha; indirectly related to Apāna Vāyu, Udāna Vāyu, Vyāna Vāyu.

Indications
♦ Cerebrovascular accident (CVA) or stroke
♦ Muscle spasticity, rigidity, flaccidity
♦ Muscle twitching, spasms
♦ Pituitary dysfunction, hormonal imbalance
♦ Syncope (transient loss of consciousness)
♦ Seizure disorders
♦ Migraines, tension headache, sinus headache, headache in vertex region
♦ Disorientation, confusion, drowsiness, vertigo (dizziness)
♦ Poor memory, poor concentration, attention deficit hyperactive disorder (ADHD), insomnia
♦ Sinus and nasal congestion, nosebleeds, asthma
♦ Nausea, vomiting
♦ Inguinal hernia
♦ Palpitations
♦ All emotional disturbances. Vāta: fear, anxiety, nervousness, insecurity, loneliness, restlessness; pitta: anger, rage, irritability, impatience, frustration, envy, aggression; kapha: sadness, depression, greed, attachment.

Treatment
Brahmī and **jatamāmsī oil** act on majjā dhātu (nervous tissue) and are especially effective for nervousness, anxiety and similar emotional disturbances. **Nutmeg oil** induces tranquility and deep sleep. **Mustard** or **vacha oil** may be helpful to balance the structure and function of the pituitary gland.

Corresponding Acupoint
None

Close to GV 20, Baihui (Hundred Meetings) and GV 21 Qianding (In Front of the Crown)

Mūrdhni is located slightly posterior to GV 21 about 2 anguli anterior to GV 20. GV 21 does benefit the head and eliminate wind, but Mūrdhni is much closer in function energetically to GV 20.

Baihui, translated as "one hundred meetings," parallels the Ayurvedic description of Mūrdhni as the meeting point of a thousand nādīs. This acupoint is said to be capable of treating "the one hundred diseases," reflecting its diversity of function. GV 20 shares many functions and indications with Mūrdhni. It is a principal point to regulate qi, in the same way that Mūrdhni governs prāna.

In the Chinese meridian system, Baihui is the meeting of all yang energy. It balances deficient yang in the form of prolapse, similar to Mūrdhni's regulation of prāna and apāna to counter prolapse. In addition, it addresses excessive yang in the form of migraines, heat, hypertension, hypotension and agitation.

GV 20 also treats Wind disorders, classified in TCM as headache, dizziness and stroke; from an Ayurvedic standpoint, these correlate to disturbances of prāna vāyu.

From this point, the GV meridian descends to the tip of the nose, revealing why it is effective in treating several nasal conditions, such as sinus congestion and sinus headaches. Because the anterior pathway of the GV meridian ascends through the heart, GV 20 can be effectively used to soothe the mind and balance the emotions.

Commentary

Adhi means first or origin and *pati* translates as husband, father or master. *Adhipati* is the first master of all marmāni. This pre-eminent importance is due to its location at the topmost part of the body. Adhi also means before creation, and pati means owner. By concentrating attention on this marma, yogis achieve mastery over their senses and ultimately over the mind. By paying attention to the adhipati marma, a person can gain extrasensory perception (ESP). This mastery is essential for higher spiritual development.

Mūrdhni is known as the meeting point of a thousand nāḍīs and the ultimate opening of kundalinī shakti. (For more on nāḍīs, see pages 45 and 50.) Located at the highest peak of the body, it is the seat of spiritual energy and leads to a profound expansion of consciousness. It stimulates kundalinī energy to rise from mūlādhāra chakra in the pelvic cavity and ascend through *sushumnā*, the central channel of pranic currents in the body. Kundalinī's ultimate destination as she ascends the spinal cord to the crown chakra is Mūrdhni marma. *Sahasrāra* is the crown chakra, which means thousand-petaled lotus. This marma is found at the center of the lotus. Through Mūrdhni, all other chakras can be activated.

Many meditative practices involve focusing the awareness on this marma, to promote the merging of individual consciousness with cosmic consciousness. This merging is yoga, which means *union*. A yogi is not someone who merely performs yogāsanas (postures). Yogis are enlightened beings who are always merged with cosmic consciousness in their daily lives. They live in a state of bliss and choiceless, passive awareness in every moment of life. At the time of death, a yogi's soul departs the body through Mūrdhni marma and is transported to a higher level of consciousness, termed *satyaloka* or the abode of truth. Thus, Mūrdhni is the door to *samādhi* (spiritual absorption) and *moksha* (ultimate liberation).

The name *Mūrdhni* derives from the root *muhu*, which means moment-to-moment and implies movement. Spiritually this name is significant because it implies moment-to-moment awareness. True awareness is never static; it moves gracefully from one moment to the next. All time is rooted in the principle of movement, from the past to the present and to the future. Mūrdhni regulates the movement between one thought and the next, between the birth of a thought and its translation into an action, and between a sensory stimulus and its eventual motor response. Meditation is the witnessing of this movement of time, creating stillness of the mind and cultivating moment-to-moment awareness. The name Mūrdhni also derives from the word *mūrchana*, which means fainting. Hence, it is a point used to restore consciousness during an attack of fainting. This is reflected in Sushruta's classification of the marma as *sadyah prānahara*, meaning an extremely vital center of consciousness. A severe injury to this marma can result in loss of consciousness or coma.

Mūrdhni's relationship to the anatomy of the brain clearly illustrates its influence on the functions of various neural structures and its role in treating their disturbance. It is related functionally to the subarachnoid space that contains cerebrospinal fluid (CSF). Appropriate pressure on the marma regulates the function of CSF and tarpaka kapha to lubricate and nourish the entire nervous system. Furthermore, it is believed to enhance cerebral circulation, especially of the middle cerebral artery. A significant number of strokes occur in the territory supplied by this artery. Mūrdhni is also associated with the mid-cranial fossa where the Broca's area for motor speech and the Wernicke's area for auditory comprehension are located.

Mūrdhni facilitates optimal functioning of the hypothalamus and the pituitary gland, which is often referred to as the master gland of the endocrine system because it regulates the functions of many other glands. Because of its effect on the neuroendocrine axis, Mūrdhni has a profound influence on hormonal balance and pituitary function.

Mūrdhni's association with the pineal gland and psychomotor areas of the brain suggest its importance in treating emotional disorders such as grief, depression and anxiety. The pineal gland was believed by René Descartes to be the "seat of the soul." Although its function is not fully understood by western scientists today, it is thought to regulate the "internal clock" by secreting melatonin. Tenderness at Mūrdhni indicates that the pineal gland is working under stress and there is insufficient prāna. Insufficient or disturbed prāna results in emotional imbalances that are vāta, pitta or kapha in nature. The regular application of pressure here facilitates a state of tranquility, joy and happiness. This may be due to the release of mood-enhancing neurotransmitters such as serotonin. A deficiency of these neurotransmitters can lead to depression and disturbed mental function.

Mūrdhni influences the emotions and well-being of the fetus in the mother's womb. The fetus floats in a sea of amniotic fluid that nourishes and calms the baby through this marma.

As the principal seat of prāna in the body, Mūrdhni promotes communication and sensory perception. Daily massage here increases the flow of prāna. Prāna is the most important governing factor for life and acts as the bridge between body, mind and consciousness. It sustains life through respiration, circulation and many other physiological mechanisms. Children with attention deficit hyperactive disorder (ADHD) have de-stabilized prāna. By stabilizing prāna, calming the emotions and

Face
Head

harmonizing the mind, Mūrdhni produces excellent results in ADHD.

Mūrdhni treats asthma when the flow of prāna is blocked, prolapse of organs when prāna has descended, and vomiting when prāna is moving retrograde. A stroke is a serious disturbance of prāna, in which brain functions become disrupted. Treatment at Mūrdhni can restore the flow of prāna in the brain and enhance recovery from the devastating consequences of stroke.

Mūrdhni principally balances vāta dosha and its sub-dosha, prāna vāyu. It also balances sādhaka pitta and tar-paka kapha, as the functions of these three sub-doshas are intricately linked. They work in harmony with one another, each promoting the functions of the other two. Due to its influence on tarpaka kapha, pressure to this marma relieves sinus and nasal congestion. Tarpaka kapha is also associated with memory, so it is helpful in treating forgetfulness and disorientation. Mūrdhni calms the emotions and promotes increased attention, concentration, perception and understanding, all functions affected by sādhaka pitta.

Brahmarandhra

Location
On the midline of the head, 2 anguli anterior to Mūrdhni and 8 anguli above the glabella (midpoint between the eyebrows).

Actions
♦ Regularizes sādhaka pitta functions
♦ Relieves headaches
♦ Facilitates optimal pituitary gland functions
♦ Regulates frontal lobe activity
♦ Improves cerebral circulation and CSF circulation
♦ Promotes creativity and intelligence, stimulates memory
♦ Calms the mind, transforms feelings and emotions into pure consciousness

Associated Doshic Subtypes
Sādhaka Pitta, Prāna Vāyu, Tarpaka Kapha, Udāna Vāyu

Indications
♦ Migraines, tension headache, sinus headache, headaches in frontal area
♦ Anterior cranial fossa conditions, strokes and space-occupying lesions such as tumors and abscesses
♦ Increased intracranial pressure
♦ Pituitary dysfunction
♦ Syncope (transient loss of consciousness), vertigo, seizure disorder
♦ Insomnia, poor memory, ADHD
♦ Hiccups
♦ All emotional disturbances, whether *vāta*, *pitta* or *kapha* in origin.

Treatment
Brahmarandhra may be gently stimulated with **nutmeg**, **vacha** or **eucalyptus oil**. Brahmī with **jatamāmsī oil** will pacify pitta and treat emotional disturbances. **Mustard** or **vacha oil** may be helpful to balance the structure and function of the pituitary gland.

Corresponding Acupoint
GV 22 Xinhui (Fontanelle Meeting)

GV 22 is located 5 cun anterior to GV 20 and 2 cun posterior to the anterior hairline. The acupoint does not share as many of the mental or emotional indications assigned to Brahmarandhra but it does treat palpitations, somnolence, and fear. In the Chinese medical system, it is specifically used for disorders of Wind that manifest

2. Brahmarandhra Xinhui GV-22

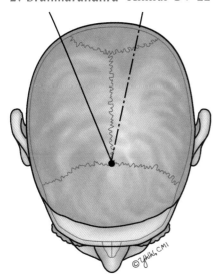

as headaches and dizziness. It also benefits the nose and treats congestion, nosebleeds, and nasal polyps. Since GV 20 is more energetically influential, GV 22 is not as commonly used.

Commentary

Brahmarandhra is translated as the opening to the creator. It has the function of unfolding creative intelligence. *Brahma* means creation or the expansive state of consciousness. Creativity is attributed to the movement of vāta dosha that expresses itself as the dynamic movement of one's mind and thoughts. It is only with this freedom of movement that creativity can flourish.

This marma is functionally related to the anterior cerebral artery, anterior cranial fossa and olfactory bulb. Its association with the pituitary gland explains Brahmarandhra's role in treating hormonal imbalance, similar to Mūrdhni marma. When a baby is born, the two frontal bones of the skull are not yet fused together, allowing sufficient space for the growth of the brain. If a child is born without an anterior fontanel (the space between the bones), the brain lacks this vital space for growth and expansion, which can result in mental retardation. When there is sufficient space, growth occurs and creativity can bloom.

Brahmarandhra is related to the frontal lobe of the brain, which is the seat of emotions. It is also associated with the limbic system, which is connected to emotional behavior. In Āyurveda, emotions are classified by their doshic nature and correspond to distinct segments of the brain. For example, the superior frontal gyrus controls emotions related to vāta dosha, such as anxiety, fear, loneliness, nervousness and insecurity. The middle frontal gyrus regulates pitta type emotions such as anger, irritability and rage. Kapha type emotions such as sadness, grief and depression are connected to the inferior frontal gyrus.

Brahmarandhra transforms feelings and emotions into pure consciousness through sādhaka pitta. Sādhaka pitta processes cognitive functions including perception into knowledge. Brahmarandhra can be stimulated for sādhaka pitta disorders, such as poor memory, impaired judgment and reasoning, and disturbed concentration. This subdosha in the brain is functionally related to the vagus nerve, the tenth cranial nerve, which is directly linked to the cardiac plexus. The brain and heart have an intimate association. Sādhaka pitta in the brain is responsible for processing knowledge into wisdom, while in the heart it processes emotions into compassion. Brahmarandhra can also be stimulated for relief of depression and other emotional disturbances.

Due to its proximity to Mūrdhni, Brahmarandhra shares similar indications, such as fainting, dizziness, cognitive dysfunction, poor memory and emotional disturbance. It ameliorates sinus, tension and migraine headaches because of its strong local action. The marma also treats hiccups that are due to hyperactive udāna vāyu. As udāna rises upwards, it can ascend to and disturb the topmost point at the crown close to this marma.

All the body's anterior nādīs meet at Brahmarandhra. In meditative practice, a yogi directs kundalinī shakti to Brahmarandhra, opening the doors to spiritual liberation. When prostrating before the guru, one touches this point to the guru's feet. This gesture of humility and surrender is symbolic of saying to the guru, "Take away my mind. This is an offering of my ego."

Shivarandhra

Location
On the midline of the head, 2 anguli posterior to Mūrdhni and 12 anguli posterior from the glabella (midpoint between eyebrows).

Actions
♦ Regulates tarpaka kapha
♦ Relieves posterior or occipital headaches
♦ Enhances cerebral circulation and circulation of CSF
♦ Facilitates optimal function of pituitary gland
♦ Relieves meningeal irritation
♦ Stimulates memory
♦ Calms the mind, balances emotions

Associated Doshic Subtypes
Tarpaka Kapha, Sādhaka Pitta, Prāna Vāyu

Indications
♦ Migraines, tension headache, headache in occipital and parietal region
♦ Neck pain
♦ Cervical spondylosis (arthritis of the spine)
♦ Increased intracranial pressure
♦ Posterior cranial fossa conditions: strokes and space-occupying lesions such as tumors and abscesses
♦ Tinnitus (ringing in ears), vertigo
♦ Poor memory, insomnia, ADHD
♦ Emotional disturbance. *Vāta:* fear, anxiety, nervousness, insecurity, loneliness, emotional instability, restlessness.

Treatment
Shivarandhra should be gently stimulated using **nutmeg** or **dashamūla oil**. **Brahmī** or **jatamāmsī oil** helps to calm emotional disturbances.

Corresponding Acupoint
GV 19, Houding (Behind the Crown)

GV 19 is similar to Shivarandhra in that both are used to calm the mind and treat insomnia, headaches and dizziness. It does not share many of the other indications listed for the marma. It is located 1.5 cun posterior to GV 20. Due to its close proximity to an acupoint that is significantly more powerful, GV 19 is less frequently used.

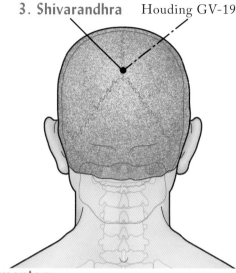

3. Shivarandhra   Houding GV-19

Commentary
Shivarandhra, translated as "opening to Shiva," is located at the top of the sushumnā, along with Mūrdhni and Brahmarandhra. The marma is functionally related to the posterior cerebral artery, posterior fontanel, posterior cranial fossa, cerebellum, posterior pituitary and third ventricle of the brain. It improves circulation in the parietal eminence and occipital lobes. It is no coincidence that the parietal lobe is the seat of memory and Shivarandhra enhances positive memory. Memory is recorded within tarpaka kapha, a subtype of kapha that is located within the cerebral spinal fluid and the white matter of the brain.

Meningitis is a condition in which the covering of the brain and the spinal cord (meninges) become inflamed, usually due to an infection. Treatment to Shivarandhra marma can relieve meningeal irritation by relaxing the tentorium cerebelli or cerebral diaphragm. Shivarandhra also relieves neck rigidity, a complication of meningitis. It subdues occipital and parietal headaches, and relieves migraines.

The five vāyus or sub-doshas of vāta can be ascribed to various regions of the brain according to their sphere of influence. The occipital area is governed by apāna vāyu, the frontal area by prāna vāyu, central area by samāna vāyu, parietal area by udāna vāyu, and lastly the temporal area by vyāna vāyu. Due to these associations, headaches in the parietal region are associated with grief, sadness and the memory of being hurt. This corresponds to udāna vāyu, which is associated with recall of memory.

Due to its proximity to Mūrdhni and Brahmarandhra, Shivarandhra shares similar indications, such as poor memory, insomnia and ADHD. The marma is also associated with emotional disturbances that are primarily classified as vāta imbalances. It can be used to treat anxiety occurring during either the wakeful state or nightmares.

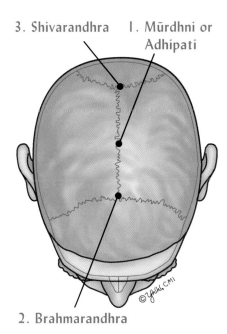

3. Shivarandhra   1. Mūrdhni or Adhipati

2. Brahmarandhra

Spiritual Aspects of Mūrdhni, Brahmarandhra and Shivarandhra

The spiritual aspects of these three marmāni deserve special mention. Brahmā, Vishnu and Shiva are the principal trinity in Hinduism, and are the deities of creation, preservation and destruction, respectively. The trinity correlates with the three *maha* (great) marmāni located at the top of the head, which are considered pre-eminent among all marmāni. Mūrdhni, located at the vertex, is the residence of Lord Vishnu (the preserver). His abode is known as Vishnu loka or Vaikuntha, translated as the place where all desires end. Brahmarandhra, located anterior to Mūrdhni, is the abode of Lord Brahma (the creator) and is known as Brahmā loka. Shivarandhra, located posterior to Mūrdhni, is the residence of Lord Shiva. Lord Shiva is known as the destroyer and his abode is termed Mount Kailas or Shiva loka. The Ganges, holiest of rivers in India, is considered to be of celestial origin. In Ayurvedic tradition, it corresponds to the cerebrospinal fluid in the central nervous system. These three marmāni, it is said, regulate the flow of neuro-electrical impulses in the same manner that the trinity of deities directs the flow of the celestial sacred river Ganges as if flows down from the heavenly realms.

Directing one's attention toward these vital points during meditation awakens the energy of Brahmā, Vishnu or Shiva within one. Similarly, when yogis concentrate their energy at the marmāni at the time of death, they are said to journey to the abode of their chosen deity. These deities are considered heavenly beings of cosmic significance as well as representations of inner experiences. Focusing on Brahmarandhra, Mūrdhni and Shivarandhra, the yogi goes to Brahmā loka, Vishnu loka and Shiva loka, respectively. The profound science explaining the transmigration of the soul after death has been elaborated by many yogis, but is beyond the scope of this commentary.

In the Hindu tradition, all of creation stems from the sacred trinity. Thus, injury to one of these three marmāni disrupts the energy of the trinity that resides in the human body, and a severe injury may result in instantaneous death.

These marmāni unfold the divine qualities of Brahmā, Vishnu and Shiva within us. They manifest our creative forces, preserve our values and overcome those personality attributes that limit our spiritual development. From the Hindu and Ayurvedic standpoints, we embody divinity. The purpose of life is to realize this highest truth. The body is the vehicle for this self-realization. Gentle stimulation of these marmāni has the potential for profound healing and spiritual growth.

Mūrdhni, Brahmarandhra and Shivarandhra are part of the sahasrāra chakra. The ultimate destination of kundalinī shakti is the crown chakra, generally, and these three marmāni, specifically. The yogi's awareness must pass through one of these marmāni to achieve moksha (liberation). There are two ascending pathways of the sushumnā, (the central channel). The anterior path, known as the path of bhakti (devotion), travels through the third eye (ājñā) to Brahmarandhra. The yogic pathway is posterior, moving from the sushumnā to Shivarandhra. It is a mystic pathway for unfolding enlightenment and merging into cosmic consciousness.

Thus, these three vital marmāni are the doorways to clear perception and higher consciousness.

Table 24: The Divine Trinity

	Brahmā	**Vishnu**	**Shiva**
Lord of	Creation	Preservation	Destruction
Abode	Brahmā loka	Vishnu loka (Vaikuntha)	Shiva loka (Mount Kailas)
Associated Marma	Brahmarandhra	Mūrdhni	Shivarandhra
Qualities Unfolded	Creativity, spiritual growth	Sustenance of spirituality	Transformation of jīva into Shiva
Related Subdoshas	Sādhaka pitta	Prāna vāyu	Tarpaka kapha

Kapāla

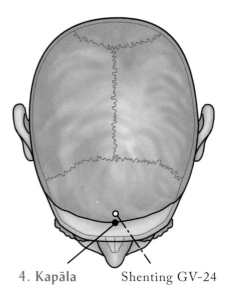

4. Kapāla   Shenting GV-24

Location
At the hairline, 4 anguli superior to the glabella (Nāsā Mūla/Yintang) and on the midline of the forehead.

Actions
♦ Relieves headaches
♦ Facilitates optimal function of pituitary gland
♦ Benefits eyes and nose
♦ Calms mind, balances emotions, relieves stress

Associated Doshic Subtypes
Sādhaka Pitta, Prāna Vāyu, Tarpaka Kapha

Indications
♦ Frontal headaches
♦ Pituitary dysfunction, hormonal imbalance
♦ Irritation of eyes and itching of the nose
♦ Insomnia, mental stress
♦ Emotional disturbance

Treatment
Gentle pressure with cooling oils such as **brahmī, jatamāmsī** or **coconut oil** soothes pitta and treats disturbances of the marma. The entire forehead can be massaged along with Kapāla marma to provide deep relaxation. See Treatment section under Ājñā marma on page 89 for discussion of shirodhara treatment.

Corresponding Acupoint
None

Close to GV 24, Shenting (Courtyard of the Spirit)

GV 24 is located 0.5 cun posterior to the anterior hairline. Kapāla is located directly at the midpoint of the anterior hairline, 0.5 cun anterior to GV 24. The acupoint shares Kapāla's indications, in addition to treating dizziness, mania, and eye and nasal disturbances. GV 24 is the point where the stomach meridian intersects with the GV channel, offering a possible explanation why Kapāla may be useful to treat headaches due to hypoglycemia. Situated on the GV meridian, Kapāla is influenced by its energetics. Hence, Shenting has a crucial role in calming the mind, relieving stress and balancing emotions.

Commentary
The prefix *ka* means time and *pala* means ruler. Thus, *Kapāla* means the ruler of time. Kapāla may also be translated as forehead. This marma is effective for treating people who feel bound by time, who are constantly in a hurry and always seem impatient, anxious or stressed. According to Ayurvedic facial diagnosis, people who are stressed continuously may develop worry lines or creases that run horizontally along the forehead. Kapāla relieves many types of emotional disturbances. It pacifies mental stress and insomnia by calming the thoughts that race through the mind.

Kapāla is functionally related to the anterior cranial fossa, optic chiasma, frontal sinuses and olfactory bulb. It is also associated with the frontal lobe, considered one of the seats of the mind and emotions. It relieves irritation of the eyes and nose and treats frontal headaches. In addition, it pacifies headaches due to hypoglycemia by virtue of its connection to the stomach, pancreas and pitta dosha. Even though this marma is said to promote the functions of the pituitary gland and to treat hormonal imbalance, it does this to a lesser degree than the previous marmāni: Mūrdhni, Brahmarandhra and Shivarandhra.

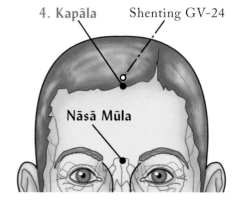

4. Kapāla   Shenting GV-24

Nāsā Mūla

Ājñā or Sthapanī

Location
On the midline of the forehead, one angula above the glabella (Nāsā Mūla/ Yintang).

Actions
♦ Regulates tarpaka kapha and enhances cerebral circulation
♦ Facilitates optimal function of pituitary and pineal gland, regulates hormonal secretions
♦ Relieves headaches
♦ Improves concentration, stimulates memory
♦ Unfolds intuition and insight
♦ Calms mind, balances emotions, relieves stress
♦ Relieves intraocular pressure
♦ Benefits eyes and nose

Associated Doshic Subtypes
Tarpaka Kapha, Sādhaka Pitta, Prāna Vāyu

Indications
♦ Migraine headaches
♦ Pituitary dysfunction, hormonal imbalances
♦ Lack of concentration, poor memory, ADHD
♦ Stress, insomnia
♦ Emotional disturbances
♦ Sinus conditions, nasal obstruction or discharge, nasal polyps, deviated nasal septum
♦ Glaucoma, eye strain

Treatment
Application of **vacha oil** to Ājñā marma may help to relieve intraocular pressure, which is often associated with glaucoma. Vacha oil nasya, which is the medicated oil administered through the nose, effectively treats kapha disorders such as sinus congestion and nasal discharge. This same oil on the third eye is effective for treating growth problems due to kapha imbalance, such as rebalancing the secretion of growth hormones. **Sandalwood oil** can be applied for thyroid problems and pitta type migraines, and to cool the entire body during summertime. **Brahmī** and **jatamāmsī oils** act on majjā dhātu and effectively treat ADHD.

Shirodhāra is one of the treatments used in pañchakarma to balance the three bodily doshas. In shirodhāra, a continuous stream of warm oil is applied to Ājñā and Kapāla marmas. The effect is tremendously calming and tranquilizing, making it highly effective for stress management. **Sesame oil** soothes vāta dosha, **sunflower oil** calms pitta dosha, and **corn oil** pacifies kapha dosha.

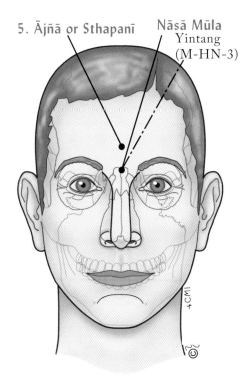

5. Ājñā or Sthapanī — Nāsā Mūla Yintang (M-HN-3)

Corresponding Acupoint
None

Close to Yintang

Although Ājñā does not have a corresponding acupoint, it is located slightly superior to Yintang, which shares many similar functions and indications with Ājñā. It is located on the GV meridian whose energetics calm the mind and emotions, paralleling the acupoint's functions. In addition, the GV meridian descends to the nose, perhaps explaining why Ājñā marma addresses nasal conditions.

Commentary
Ājñā means order. This important marma brings order in the body, mind and consciousness. It steadies the fluctuations of the mind, thoughts and emotions to induce mental tranquility and a profound sense of inner peace. Emotional fluctuations are due to doshic imbalance. Another name for the marma is *Sthapanī*, which is translated as establishment, steadiness or stability. It creates stability of the mind and steadiness in oneself.

Ājñā is functionally related to the hypothalamus, optic chiasma and frontal lobe. It creates a bridge between the pineal and pituitary glands and helps to achieve hormonal balance. Ājñā is indicated for eye disorders, headaches in the frontal region and pitta type migraines that are sharp in nature.

Ājñā effectively relieves stress and insomnia by quieting the mind. Treatment here improves ADHD, lack of concentration and poor memory. In the yogāsana (posture) known as the child's pose, Ājñā marma is naturally stimulated when the forehead touches the ground. This posture induces a deep state of relaxation and is often used to treat insomnia.

Many yoga practitioners focus their energy and attention on Ājñā marma during meditation. It is a principal point in the chakra system, sometimes known as the seat of the guru. A spiritual Master may awaken kundalinī shakti in a disciple by touching this marma point with his or her thumb, a process known as *shaktipat*.

Steady concentration at Ājñā slows the breath and allows one to witness the flame of inner awareness. Kabir, a famous mystic and poet from India, labeled this flame *Atma Jyotis,* the light of the Self.

Flame of Awareness

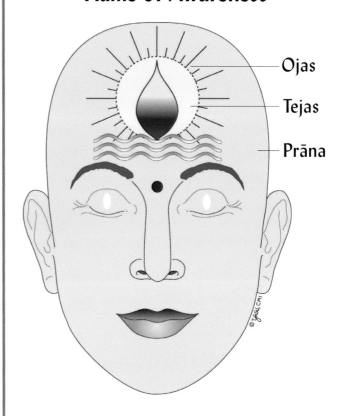

Ojas

Tejas

Prāna

Shankha

Location
At the temple, in a depression 1–2 anguli posterior to the eyebrows.

Actions
♦ Strongly pacifies pitta
♦ Relieves headaches
♦ Relieves stomach pain, decreases acidity
♦ Regulates colon
♦ Benefits ears, eyes, teeth and face
♦ Influences speech
♦ Reduces emotional stress, calms mind

Associated Doshic Subtypes
Sādhaka Pitta, Pāchaka Pitta, Udāna Vāyu, Apāna Vāyu

Indications
♦ Migraines, headaches in temporal region
♦ High acidity, gastritis, peptic ulcer, duodenal ulcer
♦ Gastroesophageal reflux disease (GERD)
♦ Gallstones, colitis, colon dysfunction
♦ Vertigo in Ménière's disease, eye disorders
♦ Otitis media, tinnitus
♦ Temporomandibular joint (TMJ) pain, dental pain, speech disorders
♦ Trigeminal neuralgia, Bell's palsy (facial paralysis)
♦ Emotional disturbance

Treatment
Avoid heavy pressure and irritant substances that may be harmful to the eyes. These include vacha oil, mustard oil, eucalyptus oil and Tiger Balm®. **Brahmī**, **jatamāmsī** or **sandalwood oil** pacify pitta.

Corresponding Acupoint
None

Close to Taiyang

Taiyang, or Supreme Yang, is a frequently used extra point in TCM. It treats many of the same problems as Shankha marma, including dizziness and eye disorders. Taiyang is located in the depression one cun posterior to the midpoint of the outer canthus and lateral end of the eyebrow (Sizhukong SJ 23). It is slightly inferior to Shankha. The acupoint clears heat and decreases swelling, both pitta-pacifying actions. Taiyang is specifically used for unilateral headaches in the tempo-parietal region.

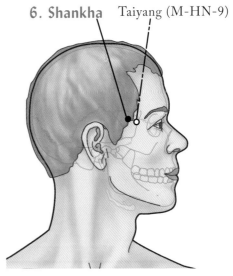

6. Shankha   Taiyang (M-HN-9)

Commentary
Shankha, translated as conch, derives its name from the fact that the temporal bone resembles part of a conch shell. The marma is functionally related to the temporal lobe, superior and mid-temporal gyrus, mid-cranial fossa and temporalis muscle.

The three primary indications of this marma are colon dysfunction, stomach acidity and headaches in the temporal region. Shankha marma on the right corresponds to the stomach and ascending colon. It is sensitive when high acidity results in gastritis or ulcers. On the left side, it is related to the duodenum and descending colon. Sensitivity could indicate gallstones, colitis or a duodenal ulcer. All these conditions reflect high pāchaka pitta. Shankha effectively pacifies pitta and reduces its manifestations as inflammation, infection and heat in the body.

Shankha is the best site for treating migraines and emotional stress. It pacifies all emotions identified with intense pitta. Pressure on Shankha may trigger bitter memories buried deep in the subconscious. Bitter memories are connected to the stomach, liver and gallbladder and can be closely associated with anger and rage. Shankha also treats TMJ pain that may develop from repressed emotions.

Near to the ear and jaw, Shankha treats otitis media, tinnitus, dental pain, trigeminal neuralgia and Bell's palsy. Shankha also addresses Ménière's syndrome, where dizziness is accompanied with tinnitus. Stimulating the marma benefits speech disorders by its association with the Broca's area, the brain's speech producing and language processing center.

Sushruta classified Shankha as an extremely vital marma. It is considered an asthi marma. In ancient martial art traditions, it was also considered a vital spot, having the potential to result in unconsciousness when struck with force.

Face Head

Bhrūh Antara / Bhrūh Madhya / Bhrūh Agra

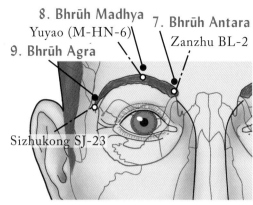

8. Bhrūh Madhya
Yuyao (M-HN-6)
9. Bhrūh Agra
7. Bhrūh Antara
Zanzhu BL-2
Sizhukong SJ-23

Location

These three marmāni are located just above the eyebrows. Bhrūh Antara is immediately superior to the medial border of the eyebrow (closest to the center of the face). Bhrūh Madhya is immediately superior to the midpoint. Bhrūh Agra is immediately superior to the lateral border.

Actions

◆ Benefits eyes, enhances circulation of aqueous and vitreous humor
◆ Relieves headaches
◆ Enhances circulation in frontal lobe of brain
◆ Releases suppressed emotions in the form of tears
◆ Relieves stress, calms the mind

Associated Doshic Subtypes

Ālochaka Pitta, Sādhaka Pitta, Vyāna Vāyu, Tarpaka Kapha

Indications

◆ Ophthalmic migraines, sinus headaches, frontal headaches
◆ Glaucoma, pressure behind the eyes, supraorbital pain
◆ Red itchy eyes, ptosis (drooping of eyelid)
◆ Insomnia, stress, anxiety, suppressed emotions

Treatment

When working on these delicate points close to the eyes, be careful to avoid heavy pressure and irritant substances that may be harmful to the eyes, such as vacha oil, mustard oil, eucalyptus oil and Tiger Balm®. It is safe to apply plain **ghee, coconut oil, castor oil** or **brahmī oil** to these marmāni. Bhru marmāni are treated in conjunction with Ashrū marmāni (page 94). All six points parallel to the eyebrow can be massaged simultaneously by sliding the fingers laterally. This repetitive motion is wonderful for relieving stress, anxiety and insomnia. The entire eyebrow and supraorbital ridge can be massaged with **jatamāmsī oil** for insomnia.

Corresponding Acupoint

None

Close to BL 2, Zanzhu (Gathered Bamboo), Yuyao (Fish Waist) and SJ 23, Sizhukong (Silken Bamboo Hollow)

Although there are no acupoints at these precise locations, three points are extremely close. Bhrūh Antara is superior to BL 2, Bhrūh Madhya is superior to extra point Yuyao, and Bhrūh Agra is superior to SJ 23. All three acupoints are located on the eyebrow, just below the corresponding marmāni. They treat a range of eye disorders as well, but have no connection to the secretion of tears or to suppressed emotions. BL 2 is indicated for facial paralysis and nasal disorders such as congestion; SJ 23 treats dizziness.

Commentary

Bhrūh is translated as eyebrow, *antar* as medial or close to the midline, *madhya* as middle, and *agra* as lateral or outer. The names directly correlate with the locations of the marmāni. Bhrūhu marmāni above the right eyebrow are connected to the liver and gallbladder, while those above the left eyebrow are associated with the spleen and pancreas. (Bhrūhu is the plural form of Bhrūh.)

The ancient Ayurvedic art of facial diagnosis involves closely examining features such as lines, creases, prominences and discolorations that correlate to various regions of the body, indicating disturbance. For example, because the area below the eyes is associated with the kidneys, dark circles there are generally a sign of low kidney energy. Marmāni on the face can be similarly used for diagnostic purposes. The region of the eye located below the Bhrūhu marmāni and above the eye itself corresponds to the liver. Hence, Bhrūhu marmāni become sensitive whenever the liver is toxic.

If Bhrūh Antara is under stress, it creates a line that rises vertically from the medial border of the eyebrow. Similarly, if Bhrūh Madhya is under stress, it results in a worry line that runs parallel to the upper border of the eyebrow. These lines indicate a high degree of stress and anxiety in a person's life.

Bhrūhu marmāni are linked to the sinuses, lacrimal glands and lacrimal secretions (tears). Treatment here benefits the eyes by relieving eye tension and retrobulbar pressure. Gentle pressure on these marmāni may improve the circulation to the frontal lobe of the brain and the aqueous and vitreous humors (the fluids within the eyeball). These marmāni are indicated for sinus

7. Bhrūh Antara

Zanzhu BL-2

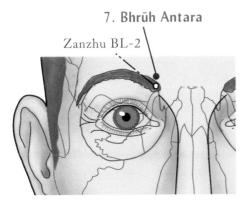

9. Bhrūh Agra

Sizhukong SJ-23

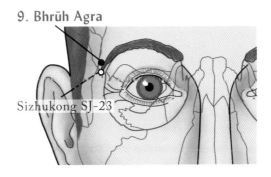

headaches as well as ophthalmic migraines and frontal headaches.

Subdoshas affiliated with the Bhrūhu points are ālochaka pitta (related to vision), sādhaka pitta (associated with unprocessed emotions) and vyāna vāyu (governing the movement of the eyelids). Pressure at these points stimulates the secretion of tears. Āyurveda describes the significance of tears as the grosser, physical manifestation of subtle emotions.

The Bhrūhu marmāni are differentiated according to the three doshas and the various emotions connected to each one. Bhrūh Antara is associated with vāta emotions such as grief, sadness, anxiety, fear and loneliness. Tears that descend from the inside corner of the eye, directly below the marma, are tears of grief. They are astringent and pungent to the taste. Bhrūh Madhya is related to pitta type emotions such as anger, frustration and rejection. Tears that drop directly below the pupil are tears of anger; they are hot, sour and bitter to the taste.

Kapha predominant emotions such as joy, love and compassion are linked to Bhrūh Agra. When these positive qualities are experienced in excess, they may be released in the form of tears that fall from the lateral corner of the eye, or directly below Bhrūh Agra. They are scanty, cool to the touch and sweet to the taste.

8. Bhrūh Madhya

Yuyao (M-HN-6)

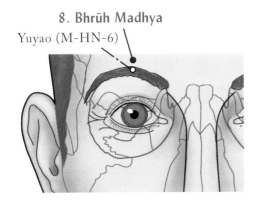

*Face
Head*

Ashrū Antara / Ashrū Madhya / Ashrū Agra

• • • • • • • • • • • • • • • • • • • •

Location
On the supraorbital ridge, just below the eyebrows. Ashrū Antara is directly below Bhrūh Antara. Ashrū Madhya is directly below Bhrūh Madhya. Ashrū Agra is directly below Bhrūh Agra.

Actions
♦ Stimulates lacrimal secretion
♦ Releases suppressed emotions
♦ Relieves headaches
♦ Benefits eyes
♦ Relieves stress, calms the mind, balances emotions

Associated Doshic Subtypes
Ālochaka Pitta, Sādhaka Pitta, Vyāna Vāyu, Tarpaka Kapha

Indications
♦ Supraorbital pain, frontal headaches
♦ Stress, insomnia
♦ Releases a wide range of vata, pitta, and kapha related emotions

Treatment
Ashrū marmāni are treated in conjunction with Bhrūhu marmāni. See Treatment section under Bhrūhu marmāni for more detail.

Corresponding Acupoint
None

Close to BL 2, Zanzhu (Gathered Bamboo), Yuyao (Fish Waist), and SJ 23, Sizhukong (Silken Bamboo Hollow). Refer to Bhrūhu marmāni corresponding acupoint section, page 92.

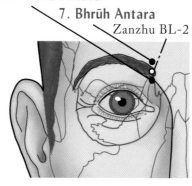

10. Ashrū Antara
7. Bhrūh Antara
Zanzhu BL-2

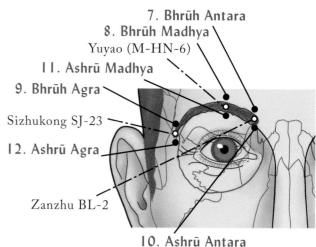

7. Bhrūh Antara
8. Bhrūh Madhya
Yuyao (M-HN-6)
11. Ashrū Madhya
9. Bhrūh Agra
Sizhukong SJ-23
12. Ashrū Agra
Zanzhu BL-2
10. Ashrū Antara

Commentary
Ashrū is translated as tears and these marmāni stimulate lacrimal secretions, which helps to release tears of unexpressed emotions. Depending on where these tears are released, they are affiliated with suppressed emotions that are vāta, pitta or kapha in nature. Refer to the Commentary under Bhrūhu marmāni for more detail. The Ashrū marmāni are sometimes included as part of the Bhrūhu marmāni in some references. Marmāni located between the eyebrow and the eye are related to the liver. If there is a slight yellowish tinge in the sclera (white of the eye) and Ashrū marmāni are sensitive, it may indicate liver toxicity. This is true of the Bhrūhu marmāni as well.

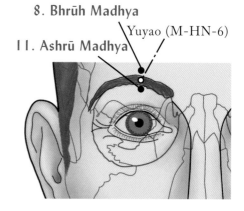

8. Bhrūh Madhya
Yuyao (M-HN-6)
11. Ashrū Madhya

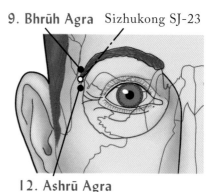

9. Bhrūh Agra   Sizhukong SJ-23
12. Ashrū Agra

Kanīnaka

• •

Location
Immediately above the inner canthus of the eye.

Actions
♦ Benefits the eyes, improves vision
♦ Enhances circulation of aqueous and vitreous humor
♦ Relieves headaches
♦ Opens nasolacrimal duct, relieves nasal congestion
♦ Relieves stress and tension

Associated Doshic Subtypes
Ālochaka Pitta, Pāchaka Pitta, Prāna Vāyu, Vyāna Vāyu, Tarpaka Kapha

Indications
♦ Frontal headaches, ophthalmic migraines
♦ Blurry vision, diminution of vision
♦ Night blindness, color blindness
♦ Glaucoma, photophobia, eye strain
♦ Excessive lacrimation
♦ Sinus congestion or stuffy nose
♦ Painful, red, itching, inflamed, swollen, or dry eyes
♦ Burning sensation in the eyes due to hyperacidity
♦ Stress and tension

Treatment
When treating Kanīnaka and other delicate points around the eyes, take care to avoid heavy pressure and irritant substances that may be harmful to the eye, such as vacha oil, mustard oil, eucalyptus oil and Tiger Balm®. Gently massage Kanīnaka along with all marmāni surrounding the eye. Start with Bhrūhu and Ashrū marmāni near the eyebrow, followed by Kanīnaka, Apānga and Vartma marmāni.

Netra basti is a treatment used in pañchakarma that involves surrounding the eye with whole wheat dough shaped in the form of a donut. The eye is then immersed in freshly prepared lukewarm, liquid ghee, while the wheat "doughnut" prevents the ghee from spreading. It is a wonderful lubricant for the eyes and effectively treats numerous eye conditions. Ghee promotes prāna, tejas and ojas related to the eyes.

Corresponding Acupoint
BL 1, Jingming (Eye Brightness)

The name Jingming, translated as eye brightness, reflects this point's ability to maintain eye luster. BL 1 is the premiere acupoint utilized for all eye disorders.

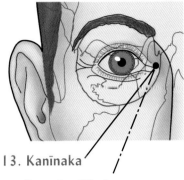

I 3. Kanīnaka

Jingming BL-1

Many of its functions and indications match those of Kanīnaka. All the yang channels in the Chinese meridian system, except the large intestine meridian, converge at BL 1. This site, as the confluence of yang energies, is a highly effective point to decrease yang in the form of heat, corresponding to Kanīnaka's ability to decrease excess pitta. Thus, heat therapy (moxibustion) is contra-indicated on this point or near any points close to the eye.

Commentary
Kanīnaka is translated as the inside of the eye. The prefix *ka* also means water and *ni* means control. The marma regulates water in terms of lacrimation, as well as the fluid within the eyeballs. Gentle pressure here improves circulation of the vitreous humor. Kanīnaka maintains normal intraocular pressure. Hence, it may be used in glaucoma, a predominantly kapha imbalance. When tears are formed, they drain via the nasolacrimal duct. Kanīnaka facilitates this drainage, relieving nasal congestion and sinus infections. It also alleviates headaches in the frontal region, especially when there is pain in the supraorbital area.

Kanīnaka specifically balances ālochaka pitta, the subdosha that governs optical function. In the embryo, the eyes are derived from the tejas aspect of pitta. It stimulates tejas, maintaining the luster and brightness of the eyes. Kanīnaka is quite effective for numerous inflammatory eye conditions that are all due to increased pitta dosha. Likewise, stress and tension often accrue from excess pitta and can be pacified through this marma. Kanīnaka on the right corresponds to the liver and on the left with the spleen.

Apānga

Location
Lateral to the outer canthus of the eye in a prominent depression.

Actions
♦ Benefits the eyes, improves vision
♦ Relieves headaches
♦ Enhances circulation of aqueous and vitreous humor
♦ Opens nasolacrimal duct, relieves nasal congestion
♦ Relieves stress and tension behind the eyes
♦ Pacifies pitta dosha
♦ Can help to control lacrimation in patients with Bell's palsy

Associated Doshic Subtypes
Ālochaka Pitta, Udāna Vāyu, Apāna Vāyu, Tarpaka Kapha

Indications
♦ Temporal headaches, supraorbital pain
♦ Blurry vision, diminution of vision
♦ Poor night vision and color blindness
♦ Eye strain
♦ May be helpful for glaucoma
♦ Puffiness of lower eyelid
♦ Excessive lacrimation
♦ Allergic itching

Treatment
Refer to Treatment section under Kanīnaka marma, page 95.

Corresponding Acupoint
GB 1, Tongziliao (Pupil Crevice)

GB 1 is located approximately 0.5 cun lateral to the outer canthus of the eye. It has similar functions and indications as Apānga. TCM describes the acupoint as eliminating Wind, which is similar to pacifying vāta, and clearing heat, which can be equated with pacifying pitta. GB 1 is also mentioned for deviation of the mouth and eye leading to Bell's palsy. It treats throat obstruction, correlating to Apānga's ability to regulate udāna vāyu.

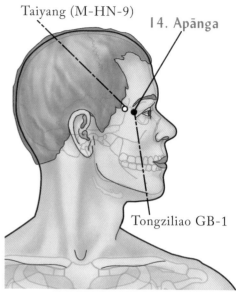

Taiyang (M-HN-9)   14. Apānga

Tongziliao GB-1

Commentary
Apānga means outer corner or angle of the eye. Its functions and indications are almost identical to Kanīnaka marma. While Kanīnaka benefits frontal headaches, Apānga addresses those in the temporal region. Unlike Kanīnaka, Apānga regulates udāna vāyu activity.

Apānga is functionally related to the kidneys, adrenals and colon. Apānga on the right is connected to the right kidney and ascending colon. The marma on the left is associated with the left kidney and descending colon. The eyes release a mucoid discharge near the marma when there are toxins in the colon. When kidney energy is low, the lower eyelids may become puffy, especially in the region of Apānga marma.

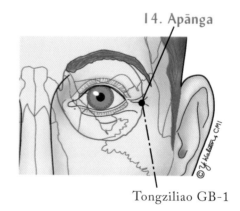

14. Apānga

Tongziliao GB-1

Antara Vartma / Madhya Vartma / Bāhya Vartma

16. Madhya Vartma
15. Antara Vartma / Chengqi ST-1
Qiuhou (M-HN-8) 17. Bāhya Vartma

Face
Head

Location

All three are located inferior to the eye. *Antara Vartma* is inferior to the inner canthus of the eye on the infraorbital ridge. *Madhya Vartma* is directly below the pupil between the eyeball and the infraorbital ridge, midway between Antara Vartma and Bāhya Vartma. *Bāhya Vartma* is inferior and slightly medial to the outer canthus of the eye, above the infraorbital ridge and midway between Madhya Vartma and Apānga.

Actions
♦ Benefits the eyes and nose
♦ Enhances circulation of aqueous and vitreous humor
♦ Lubricates and decongests nasal passages
♦ Regulates lacrimation
♦ Releases suppressed emotions
♦ Improves kidney and adrenal functions

Associated Doshic Subtypes
Ālochaka Pitta, Sādhaka Pitta, Tarpaka Kapha

Indications
♦ Allergic manifestation such as painful, red, itching, inflamed, swollen, or dry eyes
♦ Glaucoma, increased pressure within the eye
♦ Diminution of vision, night blindness
♦ Twitching or fluttering of the eyelids
♦ Excessive lacrimation, unresolved grief and sadness
♦ Puffiness of lower eyelids
♦ Nasal congestion, dryness of the nose
♦ Allergic rhinitis
♦ Kidney and adrenal stress
Madhya Vartma specifically:
♦ Anxiety
♦ Chronic indigestion

Treatment
Refer to Kanīnaka Treatment section, page 95.

Corresponding Acupoint
Antara Vartma: None, Close to ST 1 and BL 1, Jingming (Bright Eyes)

Madhya Vartma: ST 1, Chengqi (Container of Tears)

Bāhya Vartma: None, Close to Qiuhou (Behind the Ball) and GB 1, Tongziliao

Antara Vartma has no corresponding acupoint, but is located midway between ST 1 and BL 1, two crucial points for treating eye problems because they strongly stimulate qi and blood locally.

Madhya Vartma corresponds directly to ST 1, called the "container of tears" because it treats excessive lacrimation. These points are located directly below the pupil when the eyes are looking straight ahead. An influential point on the Stomach meridian, ST 1 does not address chronic indigestion, according to classical TCM literature, although Madhya Vartma does. It also differs from the marma in that it does not treat kidney and adrenal stress.

In addition to the functions of Madhya Vartma, ST 1 clears Wind and heat. Wind resembles high vāta and heat is excess pitta. Wind manifests as twitching of the eyelids or visual dizziness. Heat is expressed through redness, swelling and pain. Other indications include deafness, tinnitus, deviation of the mouth and eye, and inability to speak.

Bāhya Vartma is extremely close to an extra point named Qiuhou, which treats all eye disorders and has the same functions and indications as Bāhya Vartma, except it does not treat the kidneys or adrenal stress. However, it is used in TCM facial diagnosis to determine low Kidney Qi. It is also clost to GB 1. Refer to Apānga Commentary for more information on GB 1, page 96.

Commentary

Vartma translates as eyelid, antara means medial, madhya means middle and bāhya means outer. These names describe the marmāni locations on the lower rim of the eye socket, under the lower eyelid. The Vartma marmāni benefit the eyes and nose, addressing many similar conditions to Kanīnaka and Apānga. Because they are connected to the nasolacrimal gland and lacrimal duct, they benefit allergies, rhinitis and sinusitis. They lubricate and decongest the nasal passages. Pressure on Vartma marmāni releases repressed grief and sadness and reduces excessive accumulation of tears. These marmāni

are affiliated with ālochaka pitta, the subdosha governing the eyes and vision.

The lower eyelid region is connected to the kidneys.
Often a kidney disturbance will lead to puffiness and
sometimes a blackish discoloration of the lower eyelid.
The Vartma marmāni may improve kidney and adrenal
energy; they present as tender when there is stagnation in
the liver. Madhya Vartma specifically treats anxiety and
chronic digestive disorder.

15. Antara Vartma

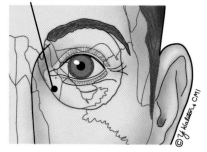

16. Madhya Vartma
Chengqi ST-1

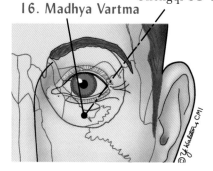

17. Bāhya Vartma

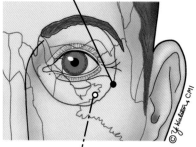

Qiuhou (M-HN-8)

Nāsā Mūla

● ●

Location

At the glabella, the midpoint between the eyebrows, one angula below Ājñā.

Actions

♦ Calms the mind, balances emotions
♦ Relieves headaches
♦ Regulates prāna
♦ Benefits eyes and nose
♦ Pacifies pitta dosha

Associated Doshic Subtypes

Prāna Vāyu, Sādhaka Pitta, Tarpaka Kapha, Apāna Vāyu

Indications

♦ Migraines, frontal headaches
♦ Glaucoma, increased eye pressure condition
♦ Runny nose
♦ Stuffy sinus, dry nasal passages causing scanty blood in the nose
♦ Snoring
♦ Difficulty breathing
♦ Emotional disturbances
♦ Difficulty falling asleep
♦ Stress
♦ Prostatic dysfunction, discomfort in prostate gland
♦ Dysfunction or discomfort of cervix

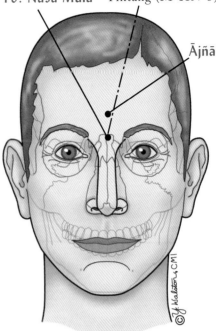

18. Nāsā Mūla   Yintang (M-HN-3)

Ājñā

Treatment

Brahmī and **jatamāmsī oils** have a cooling, tranquilizing effect on the mind. An application of one drop of **vacha oil** to the marma point may open the nasal passage. Gently massaging all nasal marmāni together is much more effective than treating one individually. A sequential gentle massage starting from Nāsā Agra, followed by Nāsā Madhya, Nāsā Mūla and ending at Ājñā, is particularly relaxing and calming to the mind. This should be followed by Nāsā Puta, Ūrdhva Ganda, Adhah Ganda and Kapola Nāsā, to open the sinuses.

Corresponding Acupoint

Yintang (Hall of Impression)

Yintang is an extra point with similar functions and indications as Nāsā Mūla. It is a cardinal acupoint to calm the mind and balance the emotions. Both points treat headaches due to heat. Āyurveda attributes this to high pitta and TCM to excess Liver fire or Liver yang. Unlike the marma, Yintang also treats hypertension and

facial pain. It expels excess Wind that has taken the form of dizziness and infantile convulsions. This function can also be ascribed to its location on the pathway of the GV meridian, which is known for its calming energetics.

Commentary

Nāsā means nose and *mūla* means root; thus Nāsā Mūla is "the root of the nose." Because it is close to Ājñā, both marmāni share similar energetics. They are considered the meeting point of the īdā and pingalā nādīs, the two principal channels of subtle energy that open into the right and left nostrils. Hence, they have a remarkable ability to regulate prāna. Nāsā Mūla and Ājñā calm the mind, significantly decreasing stress, insomnia and emotional disturbances, especially those due to sādhaka pitta disorders. Nāsā Mūla pacifies vāta imbalances such as emotional insecurity, fear and anxiety, as well as pitta flare-ups manifesting in anger, rage and agitation.

Because of its location, Nāsā Mūla also addresses several nasal conditions; pressure here has similar action to pressing Ājñā marma. By balancing tarpaka kapha, it relieves congestion and sinus drainage. By pacifying pitta dosha, it may help to alleviate migraines, rhinitis, prostatitis and cervicitis. Nāsā Mūla is associated with the cervix in females and prostate in males. Thus, it can be helpful for diagnosing and treating disorders of those organs.

Nāsā Madhya

Location
At the junction between the nasal cartilage and bony skeleton of the nose, midway between Nāsā Mūla (Yintang) and Nāsā Agra (GV 25).

Actions
♦ Benefits nose
♦ Relieves congestion
♦ Calms the mind

Associated Doshic Subtypes
Prāna Vāyu, Sādhaka Pitta, Tarpaka Kapha

Indications
♦ Allergies, sinus congestion, nosebleeds, may be helpful for rhinitis
♦ Difficulty breathing
♦ Snoring
♦ Anger, aggressiveness, overly competitive behavior

Treatment
Refer to Nāsā Mūla marma Treatment section, page 99.

Corresponding Acupoint
None

Close to Yintang (Hall of Impression)

Close to GV 25, Suliao (White Crevice)

Nāsā Madhya is located midway between Nāsā Mūla, which corresponds to the acupoint Yintang, and Nāsā Agra, corresponding to acupoint GV 25. See commentaries for Nāsā Mūla and Nāsā Agra for further discussion of the acupoints.

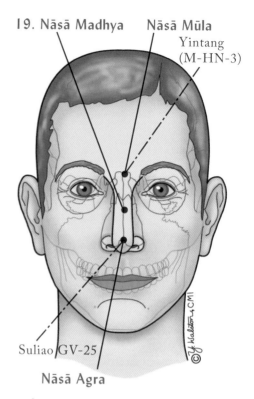

19. Nāsā Madhya   Nāsā Mūla
Yintang (M-HN-3)

Suliao GV-25

Nāsā Agra

Commentary
Nāsā means nose and madhya means middle. The marma is located midway between Nāsā Mūla (root of the nose) and Nāsā Agra (tip of the nose). All three marmāni effectively treat a number of nasal conditions, as described above (Nāsā Mūla).

On a subtler, more refined level, the Nāsā marmāni are connected to the sushumnā nādī that runs through the center of the body. The sushumnā courses from the base of the spine to the topmost point of the cranium, passing through all seven chakras. The nose can be viewed as a microcosm of the chakra system. Nāsā Agra, at the tip of the nose, corresponds to mūlādhāra chakra, located at the base of the spine. Nāsā Madhya relates to the solar plexus, while Nāsā Mūla is equivalent to the third eye or Ājñā chakra. Nāsā Madhya's connection to the solar plexus and its ability to calm the mind allows it to treat mental imbalances such as anger, aggressiveness and overly competitive behavior provoked by excess pitta.

Nāsā Agra

Location
On the tip of the nose.

Actions
♦ Benefits the nose and lungs
♦ Restores consciousness in case of fainting
♦ Regulates prāna and apāna vāyu

Associated Doshic Subtypes
Prāna Vāyu, Vyāna Vāyu, Apāna Vāyu, Avalambaka Kapha

Indications
♦ Bronchial asthma, bronchitis
♦ Nasal irritation
♦ Rhinitis, sinusitis, nosebleed (epistaxis), anosmia
♦ Hemorrhoids
♦ Cervical and prostate dysfunction
♦ Syncope (transient loss of consciousness)

Treatment
In addition to stimulation of Nāsā Agra, syncope can be treated successfully by inhalation of **fresh onion juice** or using a few drops as a nasya (medication administered through the nose). This remedy has instantaneous action. **Vacha oil** applied to the marma and then put into the nose can help to open the nasal passages. Refer to Nāsā Mūla marma Treatment section, page 99.

Corresponding Acupoint
GV 25, Suliao (White Crevice)

GV 25, which corresponds directly to Nāsā Agra, benefits the nose in a similar way. It has a wider range of action, also treating nasal obstruction, nasal sores, polyps and copious nasal discharge. In addition, it addresses hypotension and dyspnea (shortness of breath). Unlike Nāsā Agra, it is not indicated for hemorrhoids or dysfunction of the cervix and prostate.

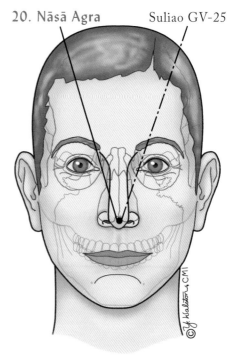

20. Nāsā Agra   Suliao GV-25

Commentary
Nāsā Agra is considered the door to the nose and the opening of prāna vaha srotas (respiratory channels). *Nāsā* is translated as nose and *Agra* as tip. It is used for many nasal disorders, similar to other Nāsā marmāni. In cases of syncope (fainting), it restores consciousness by stimulating prāna vāyu.

In females, the marma is related to the cervix and in males to the prostate and rectum. Nāsā Agra benefits apāna vāyu disturbances such as cervical and prostate dysfunction, and hemorrhoids. According to facial diagnosis, a groove on the tip of the nose is highly suggestive of an individual being prone to hemorrhoids.

Nāsā Agra can produce extraordinary sense perception, particularly the sense of smell. This ability can be developed by a technique that involves converging the eyes to look at this point in meditation. Some yogis and Ayurvedic physicians possess this *siddhi* (power) to the extent that they can detect various diseases through the sense of smell.

Nāsā Puta

Location
In the groove at the center of each nasal ala (nostril).

Actions
♦ Benefits the nose
♦ Enhances functional capacity of the lungs
♦ Stimulates ovaries, benefits ārtava dhātu

Associated Doshic Subtypes
Prāna Vāyu, Apāna Vāyu

Indications
♦ Allergic rhinitis, epistaxis (nosebleeds), sinusitis, anosmia
♦ Breathlessness, lung congestion, difficulty breathing, may be helpful for emphysema and asthma
♦ Sinus congestion, diminished sense of smell

Treatment
Refer to Nāsā Mūla Treatment section, page 99.

Corresponding Acupoint
None

Nāsā Puta is close to Nāsā Agra marma at the tip of the nose, which correlates to acupoint GV 25. See commentary under Nāsā Agra for further discussion of the acupoint.

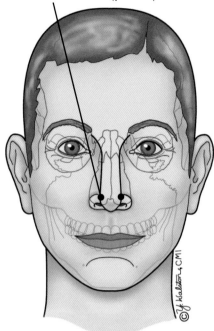

21. Nāsā Puta (paired)

Commentary
Nāsā means nose and *puta* is translated as door or petal. Nāsā Puta is the doorway to the nose or the nose petal. It is related functionally to the nasal mucus membrane, lungs, bronchi, and reproductive organs. Nāsā Puta is used to treat asthma and emphysema by enhancing lung capacity. Stimulating the marma also activates the mediastinal lymph nodes and maintains pulmonary immunity.

Indian women pierce their nose at the location of this marma, a cultural custom based on the marma's energetics. Nāsā Puta is connected to the ovaries, fallopian tubes and ārtava dhātu, the female reproductive tissue. It is believed a nose ring here stimulates the flow of energy to the ovaries. More specifically, a diamond nose ring is recommended because of the gem's strong affinity to ārtava dhātu.

Ūrdhva Ganda

Location
Immediately lateral to the edge of the nose, level with Nāsā Madhya.

Actions
♦ Enhances flow of prāna vāyu and relieves respiratory stress
♦ Benefits the nose, relieves congestion
♦ Relieves headaches
♦ Opens sinuses, facilitates bronchodilatation
♦ Releases suppressed emotions
♦ Relieves colon dysfunction

Associated Doshic Subtypes
Tarpaka Kapha, Avalambaka Kapha, Prāna Vāyu, Apāna Vāyu

Indications
♦ Sinus headache, sinus pain and congestion, postnasal drip
♦ Runny nose
♦ Asthma, shortness of breath
♦ Nosebleed (epistaxis)
♦ Unresolved grief and sadness
♦ Colon dysfunction

Treatment
Applying **vacha oil** to Ganda marmāni opens the nasal passages and facilitates bronchodilatation. Vacha nasya, a medicated oil administered through the nose, has an instantaneous action to open the nasal passages.

Corresponding Acupoint
None

Superior to Bitong. See Commentary under Adhah Ganda.

Commentary
Ganda means maxilla or maxillary bone and *urdhva* is translated as upward. Hence, it is located at the upper end of the maxillary bone. Gentle pressure at the marma enhances the flow of prāna, benefiting the nose and sinuses, as well as promoting bronchodilatation. Ūrdhva Ganda is related to the upper and middle lobes of the lung, while Adhah Ganda (see below) is related to the lower lobes. Thus, these marmāni can help to alleviate many lung conditions.

Stimulating marmāni close to the nose, the door of prāna, has a direct and immediate influence on thought

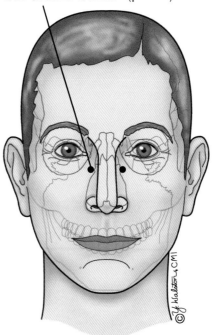

22. Ūrdhva Ganda (paired)

and emotion. Thus, the Ganda marmāni can be used to help release unresolved emotions such as grief and sadness. As all readers who have practiced yoga or meditation have discovered, there is a deep connection between the breath and thoughts, which move together. Thinking is the psychological counterpart of breathing, breathing the physical part of thinking. If the mind and thoughts are scattered, the breath will be shallow and uneven. Shallow and/or rapid breathing tend to generate thoughts of the same nature. Calming the mind through meditation, for example, or concentrated focus, immediately results in more regular and smooth breathing, and vice versa: regulating or quieting the breath settles the mind. Patañjali, traditionally hailed as the founder of Yoga, discussed the science of breath at great length and with deep yogic insight.

Ūrdhva Ganda is connected to the absorption of minerals in the colon and treats colon dysfunctions. This demonstrates the inherent link between prāna and apāna vāyu. Prāna vāyu governs respiration, the inward flow of energy, and resides in the lungs. Apāna vāyu, located in the colon, controls elimination and the outward flow of energy. A similar link is found in TCM, where the Lung and Large Intestine are paired meridians of the Metal element, with an extremely close connection.

Adhah Ganda

Location
Immediately lateral to the edge of the nose, level with the midpoint between Nāsā Madhya and Nāsā Agra. Inferior to Ūrdhva Ganda.

Actions
♦ Enhances flow of prāna vāyu and relieves respiratory stress
♦ Benefits the nasal passage, relieves congestion
♦ Promotes bronchodilatation
♦ Opens sinus cavities
♦ Helps relieve headaches
♦ Releases suppressed emotions
♦ Relieves congestion of oral mucus membrane

Associated Doshic Subtypes
Tarpaka Kapha, Avalambaka Kapha, Prāna Vāyu, Bodhaka Kapha

Indications
♦ Sinus headache, sinus pain and congestion, postnasal drip
♦ Runny nose
♦ Shortness of breath, snoring, nosebleeds
♦ Pulmonary congestion
♦ Unresolved grief and sadness
♦ Oral mucus congestion, toothache

Treatment
Refer to Ūrdhva Ganda Treatment section, page 103.

Corresponding Acupoint
Bitong (Penetrating the Nose)

Bitong is a modern addition to TCM's collection of extra points. It shares Adhah Ganda's ability to alleviate many nasal disorders. The acupoint is commonly used in connection with LI 20 (Kapola Nāsā). Often needling from LI 20 to Bitong can significantly open the nasal passages. Bitong also pacifies nosebleeds. Unlike Adhah Ganda, Bitong is not typically employed by practitioners to release suppressed emotions. Yet all acupoints located on or near the nose are related to the lungs, which are the storehouse of grief and sadness according to TCM. Thus, it can be reasoned that stimulating Bitong would release these suppressed emotions.

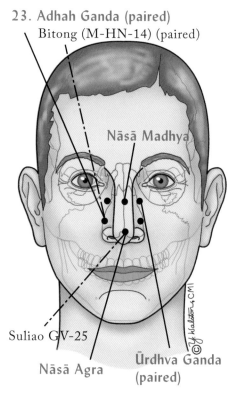

23. Adhah Ganda (paired)
Bitong (M-HN-14) (paired)
Nāsā Madhya
Suliao GV-25
Nāsā Agra
Ūrdhva Ganda (paired)

Commentary
Adhah Ganda is translated as downward maxillary bone, describing its location at the descending aspect of the maxillary bone. Like Ūrdhva Ganda, the marma is functionally related to the sinuses and colon. It also has some relationship to the pancreas. Unlike Ūrdhva Ganda, this marma affects bodhaka kapha, present in the oral cavity and saliva. It can effectively treat toothache and oral mucus congestion. Refer to the commentary under Ūrdhva Ganda for more information.

Kapola Nāsā

Location
Immediately lateral to each side of the nostril in the nasolabial groove

Actions
♦ Benefits nose, relieves congestion
♦ Opens nasal passages and sinuses
♦ Enhances flow of prāna vāyu and benefits respiration
♦ Improves functional capacity of the lung
♦ Benefits the face
♦ Calms the mind, balances emotions

Associated Doshic Subtypes
Prāna Vāyu, Tarpaka Kapha, Avalambaka Kapha

Indications
♦ Poor sense of smell (anosmia), nosebleed
♦ Naso-sino-bronchial congestion
♦ Respiratory allergy, asthma and breathlessness
♦ "Low lung energy," emphysema, shortness of breath
♦ Bell's palsy (facial paralysis)
♦ Unresolved grief and sadness

Treatment
Refer to Nāsā Mūla marma Treatment section, page 99.

Corresponding Acupoint
LI 20, Yingxiang (Welcome Fragrance)

LI 20 is one of the premiere points to treat all nasal disorders. It expels Wind manifesting as deviation of the mouth, itching and facial swelling. Like Kapola Nāsā, it also treats Bell's palsy. LI 20 clears excess heat that manifests symptomatically as red eyes or pain and swelling of the lip.

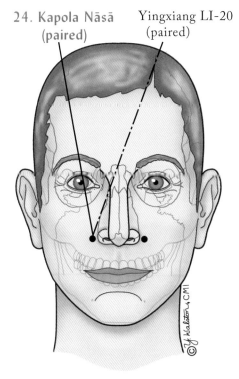

24. Kapola Nāsā (paired) Yingxiang LI-20 (paired)

Commentary
Kapola means cheek and nāsā is translated as nose. Kapola Nāsā is the marma point that is located roughly between the cheek and the nose. Similar to all Nāsā marmāni, it treats a variety of nasal conditions. Like Nāsā Puta, this marma also enhances the vital capacity of the lungs by stimulating prāna. The vital life force enters into the body and nourishes life through respiration. The dynamic relationship between the nose, lungs and prāna means the associated marmāni are inherently connected. In addition, Kapola Nāsā benefits facial paralysis.

Kapola Madhya

Location
A depression on the cheek that is felt when the teeth are clenched. At the midpoint of the anterior border of the masseter muscle.

Actions
♦ Regulates salivary secretion
♦ Enkindles agni
♦ Promotes digestion of carbohydrates
♦ Improves absorption and assimilation in the colon
♦ Stimulates the parotid gland
♦ Benefits face, relieves local pain
♦ Improves color complexion

Associated Doshic Subtypes
Bodhaka Kapha, Apāna Vāyu, Samāna Vāyu, Kledaka Kapha, Pāchaka Pitta

Indications
♦ Excess salivation, toothaches
♦ Malabsorption, loose stools, ulcerative colitis and pain in the colon
♦ Mumps (parotitis) and ear disorders
♦ Bell's palsy (facial paralysis), trigeminal neuralgia, TMJ pain

Treatment
Massaging this marma with **brahmī ghee** pacifies pitta conditions. **Camphor oil** may be used for both vāta and pitta disorders. **Nutmeg oil** has a calming effect on the digestive system and may be used for vāta disorders.

Corresponding Acupoint:
None

Close to ST 5, Daying (Great Welcome) and ST 6, Jiache (Jaw Bone)

Although there is no corresponding acupoint for Kapola Madhya, close by are a number of Stomach meridian points. The passage of this meridian through this area may help to explain the marma's influence on digestion and agni.

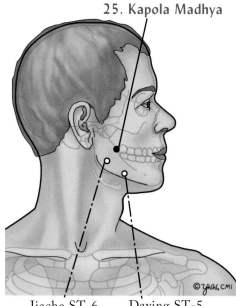

25. Kapola Madhya

Jiache ST-6   Daying ST-5

Commentary
Kapola is translated as cheek and madhya as middle. Kapola Madhya is therefore the middle of the cheek. The salivary duct opens into the oral cavity close to the marma. Kapola marma helps to regulate salivary secretions by stimulating deficient secretions or reducing excess salivation. The sphere of influence for Kapola Madhya is digestion and it especially promotes the digestion of carbohydrates. It enkindles agni (gastric fire) and improves absorption and assimilation in the colon. Kapola Madhya on the right side is connected to the ascending colon and on the left side with the descending colon. The marma may become sensitive when there are toxins in the colon, and in the presence of inflammatory conditions or other pathology involving either the small or large intestines. Locally, the marma is an effective point for treating facial paralysis. Because of its influence on the eustachian tube, it also treats ear disorders.

Oshtha

Location
On the midline of the philtrum (central groove between the nose and the upper lip), one-third of the distance between the nose and the upper lip.

Actions
♦ Restores consciousness in case of fainting
♦ Enhances cerebral circulation
♦ Improves concentration and mental alertness
♦ Enkindles agni, improves digestion
♦ Coordinates balance between prāna and udāna vāyu
♦ Improves color complexion of the face

Associated Doshic Subtypes
Prāna Vāyu, Udāna Vāyu, Tarpaka Kapha, Bodhaka Kapha, Pāchaka Pitta

Indications
♦ Syncope, coma, vertigo
♦ Cerebral ischemia (decreased blood supply to the brain)
♦ Hypoxia (decreased oxygen supply to the brain)
♦ Seizure disorder
♦ Headache
♦ ADHD, poor concentration
♦ Bell's palsy (facial paralysis), trigeminal neuralgia
♦ Toothaches, nosebleed
♦ Speech disorders

Treatment
Vacha oil is best for syncope (fainting or temporary loss of consciousness) and speech disorders. **Sandalwood oil** may be used for dizziness.

Corresponding Acupoint
GV 26, Renzhong (Middle of Person)

GV 26 is located at the junction of the upper one-third and lower two-thirds of the philtrum. According to TCM theory, it is the most vital point to restore consciousness and re-establish balance between yin and yang energies. It forcefully expels excess Wind manifesting as a distortion of the face and mouth and thus treats Bell's palsy. Similar to Oshtha, GV 26 has a strong influence to calm the mind. However, Oshtha focuses more on concentration, while GV 26 treats a wide range of psycho-emotional disorders, such as mania and depression.

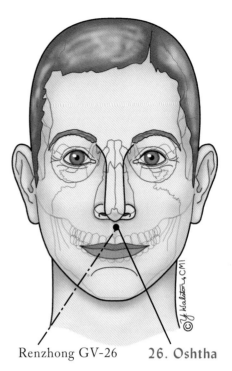

Renzhong GV-26   26. Oshtha

Unlike Oshtha, the acupoint is not used in order to influence digestion and appetite. But, it is interesting to note that GV 26 is the point where the GV channel intersects with the Stomach meridian. And the name Renzhong also means middle of a person, referring to its connection with the central part of the body. This could offer a possible explanation for Oshtha's functions and indications. In addition, GV 26 is indicated for edema and hypertension. It is especially effective for low back pain, because the GV meridian ascends along the spine. Points at one end of a meridian can often influence imbalances at the other end of the channel.

Commentary
There are a number of translations for the name *oshtha*. The most literal is "upper lip," which describes its location. Another meaning is "self-expression" and the lips are indeed one of the primary instruments we use to express ourselves. The marma activates the normal functioning of udāna vāyu, which is responsible for speech, and coordinates balance between udāna and prāna vāyu. Hence, it benefits speech disorders such as stuttering, aphasia (loss of speech) and dysarthria (slurred speech) resulting from a stroke. The third meaning of oshtha is energy rising to the brain. Oshtha is considered a gateway of prāna, making it a crucial point for maintaining vitality and consciousness. It improves concentration and alertness and has proven successful in helping children with ADHD.

Pressure at the marma regulates pranic flow to the brain and regularizes brain activity. Oshtha enhances cerebral circulation by virtue of its functional relation-

107

ship to major cerebral vessels, such as the middle cerebral artery. Disruption of the flow of prāna to the brain can result in stroke-related paralysis, loss of consciousness, and seizure disorder in which disturbed prāna vāyu leads to abnormal brain activity. Cerebral ischemia or hypoxia may result when there is a decreased blood or oxygen supply to the brain. Oshtha is an effective marma in treating these disorders.

The marma, which lies between two incisors, is helpful for relieving toothaches. Due to its close proximity to the mouth, Oshtha is connected to bodhaka kapha, which is located in the throat and tongue. It improves digestion and appetite by kindling the gastric fire and it is believed to stimulate the secretion of hydrochloric acid in the stomach.

Oshtha is a *snāyu marma,* which has an influence on the oral and cerebral blood vessels.

Hanu

Location
In a depression between the chin and the lower lips at the labiomental sulcus.

Actions
♦ Regulates bodhaka kapha and salivary secretion
♦ Relieves pain
♦ Improves color complexion of the face and tone of the facial muscles
♦ Regulates apāna vāyu
♦ Relieves stress and unresolved emotions

Associated Doshic Subtypes
Bodhaka Kapha, Apāna Vāyu, Sādhaka Pitta

Indications
♦ Excess salivation
♦ TMJ pain, pain in lower incisors
♦ Bell's palsy (facial paralysis), trigeminal neuralgia
♦ Temporal headaches, stress
♦ Hormonal imbalance
♦ Cervical pain, testicular pain, prostatitis
♦ Sexual dysfunction, hemorrhoids
♦ Emotional disturbances

Treatment
Hanu should be held with firm pressure for one to two minutes. **Brahmī, jatamāmsī** or **sandalwood oil** can soothe pitta and relax the mind.

Corresponding Acupoint
CV 24, Chengjiang (Container of Fluids)

The name "container of fluids" reveals the point's ability to regulate saliva and control drooling. Like Hanu, it treats facial disorders attributed to excess Wind, such as Bell's palsy and trigeminal neuralgia. Wind creates pain, numbness and swelling of the face. When severe, it will manifest as a stiff neck, facial nerve paralysis, tetany, hemiplegia and seizure disorder. Other local conditions that are commonly treated by CV 24 include dry mouth, sudden loss of voice, gum pain and nosebleeds. It can also be stimulated to help relieve psychoemotional conditions such as depression and mania. Similar to the marma's ability to address pelvic conditions, CV 24 is indicated for dark urine and abdominal masses in females.

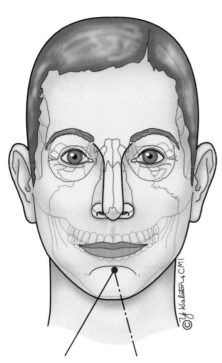

In Hinduism, Hanuman is a deity in the form of a monkey who is the son of the God of Wind. He is the embodiment of strength and courage. Hanuman symbolizes prāna and is deeply connected to Rāma, the pure consciousness that dwells within us. This consciousness manifests in the form of prāna or the breath. Mastering prānāyāma, control of the breath, is like attempting to catch the tail of Hanuman. Once the difficult task of catching the tail is accomplished, one is led towards Rāma, the highest consciousness, and Sītā, inner peace.

27. **Hanu**   Chengjiang CV-24

Commentary

Hanu is translated as mandible or chin, and also as pride. Pride is related to the marma's ability to elicit courage and self-confidence. Under the sway of these qualities, posture is affected. By standing straight and proud, the chin is held more erectly. This courage and confidence translates into a positive attitude and reduces stress and tension. Thus, Hanu is an integral point to use for stress management. Stress may be due to pitta emotions such as anger, pride and overconfidence, kapha emotions such as attachment, greed and melancholy, or vata emotions such as fear, loneliness, grief and sadness.

By regulating bodhaka kapha, it controls drooling, especially in children. Hanu is related functionally to the two lower incisors and relieves localized pain and congestion in the sublingual and submandibular salivary glands. The marma can also relieve TMJ pain, temporal headaches, and low back pain. Gentle pressure on Hanu allows the jaw to relax and significantly diminishes tension and stress.

Hanu marma is functionally related to the posterior pituitary, colon and lumbosacral area. Consequently, it helps to alleviate any dysfunction in these areas that is governed by apāna vāyu. It addresses reproductive disturbance, specifically that affecting the prostate in males and the cervix in females. According to facial diagnosis, a cleft chin on a male may indicate prostate dysfunction and a deep groove on a woman may be indicative of cervical weakness.

Chibuka

Face Head

Location
Half an angula lateral to the angle of the mouth.

Actions
♦ Regulates bodhaka kapha and salivary secretions
♦ Promotes appetite and improves digestion
♦ Improves facial color complexion, relieves facial pain
♦ Balances apāna vāyu

Associated Doshic Subtypes
Bodhaka Kapha, Prāna Vāyu, Apāna Vāyu

Indications
♦ Excessive salivation
♦ Low digestive energy, lack of appetite
♦ TMJ pain, toothache
♦ Bell's palsy, trigeminal neuralgia
♦ Sexual dysfunction

Treatment
Brahmī oil or **tikta ghrita ghee** can be applied to the marma. Tikta ghrita stimulates agni (digestive fire).

Corresponding Acupoint
ST 4, Dicang (Earth Granary)

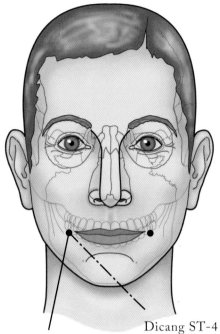

28. Chibuka (paired)   Dicang ST-4 (paired)

Commentary
Chi means prāna and *buka* means oral cavity. The name is translated as prāna of the oral cavity. Chibuka is related to the oral mucus membrane and sublingual salivary glands. It promotes salivary secretions by regulating bodhaka kapha. It improves digestion by kindling the appetite. It is interesting to note that if *jāthara agni* (central gastric fire) is extremely low, a whitish secretion may appear at the corner of the mouth that is a sign of āma (toxins) in the GI tract. Locally, Chibuka relieves toothaches, TMJ pain and facial paralysis.

The name Chibuka derives from the root *chibu*. Chibu, or the word *chumbana*, translates as kiss. Thus, it is affiliated with shukra and ārtava vaha srotas, the channels related to the male and female reproductive systems respectively. The marma corresponds to the ovaries in females and testicles in males. In facial diagnosis, one can detect sexual dysfunction manifesting as impotence by a deepening of the nasolabial groove at this marma.

ST 4 is located 0.4 cun lateral to the angle of the mouth. It is one of the principal acupuncture points to expel Wind from the face in disorders of facial paralysis, trigeminal neuralgia, numbness and deviation of the mouth. Like Chibuka, the acupoint can give relief of toothaches and local pain. Its location on the Stomach meridian may suggest why both Chibuka and ST 4 are used therapeutically to improve digestion and stimulate the appetite. Unlike the marma, ST 4 benefits the eyes; it can soothe itching eyes, ceaseless movement of the eyeballs, inability to close the eyes, and night blindness.

Marma Head and Facial Massage

• •

If you are not very experienced with Ayurvedic marma therapy, before attempting the following procedure please review chapter 8, especially "Guidelines for Touch and Pressure" on page 75 that offers specific information about massaging marmāni. Appendix C has the series of marma massage directions and illustrations starting on page 284.

The instructions here refer to the drawings on these pages. The numbers are for use with these massage drawings only; they are different from the numbering system for the marma points used throughout the book. To look up details on a particular marma point, refer to the beginning of this chapter, page 81, to the tables that reference all the marma points and their page numbers.

Apply a few drops of essential oil to the tips of the fingers. Start with gentle pressure on the marma points, and gradually increase according to the capacity of the individual. If you use too much pressure, the person will show facial expressions, such as wrinkling of the face. Pressure on all marmāni should be held for approximately one to two minutes. If you feel that stronger pressure is needed, you can apply it when the patient exhales.

A. Ask the patient to lie in supine position and be at the head end of the patient. Begin with gentle pressure on Mūrdhni marma **(1)** with both thumbs. Then move up towards Brahma-randhra **(2)**, 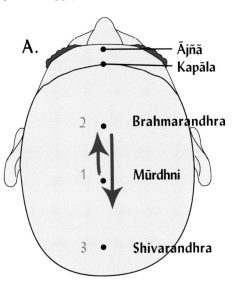 back to Mūrdhni and then to Shivarandhra **(3)**, applying pressure on each point for one minute.

B. Next, massage Kapāla marma **(4)** on the forehead with both thumbs. Massage the entire midline of the scalp from Kapāla all the way to Shivarandhra **(3)**. Give emphasis to Kapāla **(4)** briefly again and then move down the forehead to Ājñā marma **(5)** and apply pressure.

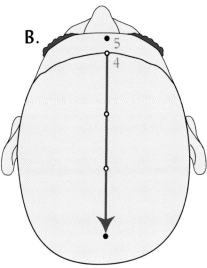

C. Repeat this motion three times, then move from Ājñā **(5)** to Bhrūh Antara **(6)** above the eyebrows, then Bhrūh Madhya **(7)**, all the way across to Bhrūh Agra **(8)**. Repeat this gentle, relaxing motion three times. Sweep the fingers from Ājñā **(5)** across the eyebrows until the thumbs land in a natural depression at Shankha marma **(9)**. Pressure should be held longer here, with a gentle counterclockwise rotation done to pacify pitta individuals.

Note: Here and in other instances, some people may not feel comfortable using the thumb; in that case, they may use the index or middle finger.

Next, apply light pressure on Kanīnaka **(10)** directed towards the inner side of the eyeball, then gradually move the fingers along the eye orbit. Then pinch the eyebrows at the medial end and release, repeating this technique towards the 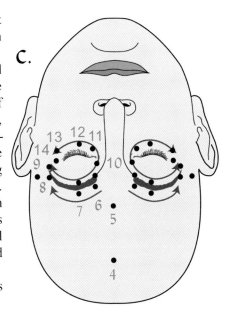 lateral end of the eyebrows to stimulate all Bhrūhu **(6, 7, 8)** and Ashrū marmāni **(inner 6, 7, 8)** simultaneously. This technique can be repeated several times. Use caution not to pull the eyelid or place pressure on the eyeball.

Gently move downwards from Kanīnaka **(10)** to the Vartma marmāni **(11, 12, 13)**, applying very light pressure to avoid discomfort. Start at the medial point and move laterally from the Vartma marmāni to Apānga **(14)** and then to Shankha **(9)**. With both middle fingers stimulating Shankha **(9)**, place the thumbs on Ājñā marma **(5)**, followed by Kapāla **(4)**. Pressure should be held for a slightly longer duration if the patient has a vāta constitution.

D. From Ājñā **(5)** move downwards to Nāsā Mūla **(15)**, Nāsā Madhya, Nāsā Agra **(16)** and Nāsā Puta, applying extremely light pressure. Then move to Kapola Nāsā **(17)**, followed by pressure on Ganda marmāni. Next, move the thumbs from Ganda marmāni downwards, until they fall in the natural groove at Kapola Madhya, followed by Chibuka **(18)**. Stimulate Oshtha with the thumb and then circle the fingers around the mouth, giving emphasis to Chibuka again.

Move to Hanu marma **(19)** at the chin and apply firm deep pressure with both thumbs. Grasp the chin between the thumbs and the index fingers and move from Hanu along the length of the mandible. Repeat this motion three times. After the last repetition, gently move upwards towards Shankha and hold. From Shankha return to Ājñā and hold the pressure for one minute. From Ājñā, let both thumbs slide upwards and hold Mūrdhni. Then move the fingers from the midline to the side of the head to complete the facial massage.

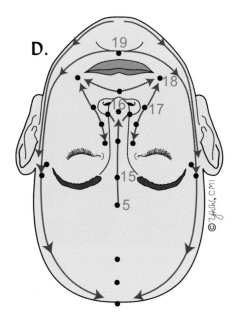

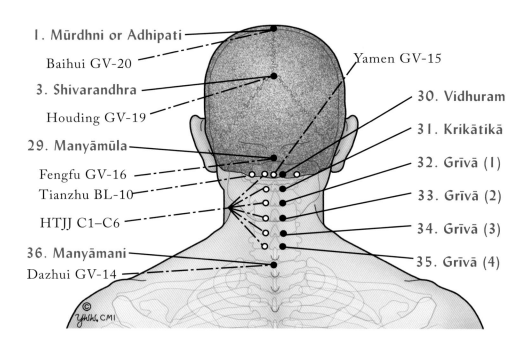

1. Mūrdhni or Adhipati
Baihui GV-20
Yamen GV-15
3. Shivarandhra
30. Vidhuram
Houding GV-19
31. Krikātikā
29. Manyāmūla
32. Grīvā (1)
Fengfu GV-16
33. Grīvā (2)
Tianzhu BL-10
HTJJ C1–C6
34. Grīvā (3)
36. Manyāmani
35. Grīvā (4)
Dazhui GV-14

Shiro (Back of Head) and Grīvā (Neck) Marmāni (5)

#	Marma Points	Page	Acupoint
29	Manyāmūla	116	GV 16
30	Vidhuram	118	HTJJ C1
31	Krikātikā	120	HTJJ C2
32	Grīvā (1)	121	HTJJ C3
33	Grīvā (2)	121	HTJJ C4
34	Grīvā (3)	121	HTJJ C5
35	Grīvā (4)	121	HTJJ C6
36	Manyāmani	122	GV 14

Shiro (Head), Grīvā (Neck) and Karna (Ear) Marmāni

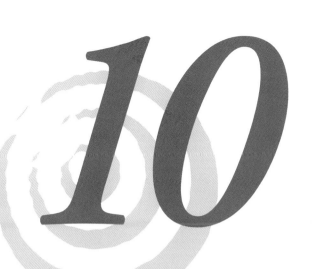

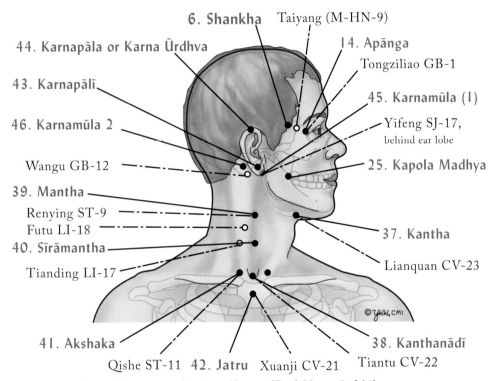

6. Shankha   Taiyang (M-HN-9)

44. Karnapāla or Karna Ūrdhva

14. Apānga

Tongziliao GB-1

43. Karnapālī

45. Karnamūla (1)

46. Karnamūla 2

Yifeng SJ-17, behind ear lobe

Wangu GB-12

25. Kapola Madhya

39. Mantha

Renying ST-9

Futu LI-18

37. Kantha

40. Sīrāmantha

Tianding LI-17

Lianquan CV-23

41. Akshaka

38. Kanthanādī

Qishe ST-11   42. Jatru   Xuanji CV-21   Tiantu CV-22

Jatru Ūrdhva (Front of Neck) Marmāni (6)

#	Marma Points	Page	Acupoint
37	Kantha	123	CV 23
38	Kanthanādī	124	CV 22
39	Mantha	125	ST 9
40	Sīrāmantha	126	≈LI 17, LI 18
41	Akshaka	127	ST 11
42	Jatru	128	CV 21

Karna (Ear) Marmāni (4)

#	Marma Points	Page	Acupoint
43	Karnapālī	130	Eye point on ear
44	Karnapāla or Karna Ūrdhva	131	Ear apex point
45	Karnamūla 1	132	SJ 17
46	Karnamūla 2	132	≈GB 12

Manyāmūla

Location
In a depression immediately below the occipital protuberance.

Action
♦ Enhances cerebral blood circulation and circulation of cerebrospinal fluid (CSF)
♦ Enhances lymphatic circulation
♦ Relieves neck tension and headaches
♦ Improves coordination and equilibrium
♦ Stimulates agni (digestive fire) of stomach and pancreas

Associated Doshic Subtypes
Prāna Vāyu, Samāna Vāyu, Apāna Vāyu, Sādhaka Pitta, Tarpaka Kapha, Pāchaka Pitta, Rañjaka Pitta

Indications
♦ Increased intracranial pressure
♦ Disorders of posterior cranial fossa
♦ Disequilibrium, vertigo, fainting
♦ Lymphatic congestion in the neck and shoulder blade area
♦ Neck pain, occipital headaches
♦ Postural hypotension (sudden drop in blood pressure when changing positions)
♦ Chronic indigestion, toxins in descending colon
♦ Hypoglycemia, pancreatic dysfunction

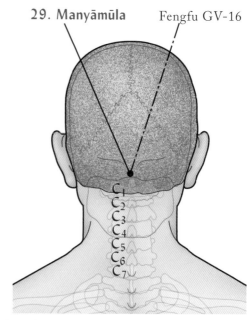

29. Manyāmūla   Fengfu GV-16

Treatment
The marma should be gently stimulated with **vacha** or **nutmeg oil**. Nutmeg has a mildly narcotic action. Using mustard oil may help to decrease intracranial pressure. **Sandalwood oil** and **khus oil** pacify pitta conditions because of their cooling properties. For severe neck tension, **mahānārāyana oil** is a strong analgesic that penetrates deeply to soothe the muscles.

Corresponding Acupoint
GV 16, Fengfu (Palace of the Wind)

GV 16 is located below the occiput and approximately one cun above the posterior hairline. It shares with Manyāmūla the ability to address stiffness of the neck and occipital headaches. However, GV 16 does not have similar functions to enkindle agni and affect the digestive system or pancreas. It principally benefits the head and neck in conditions such as blurry vision, nosebleed, sudden loss of voice and difficulty breathing. The

acupoint also addresses mania, whereas Manyāmūla is not known for any psycho-emotional functions.

GV 16 is one of the foremost acupoints to expel excess Wind (*feng*) in the body, specifically in conditions such as visual dizziness, hypertension, hemiplegia and numbness in the legs. Although none of these indications are listed for Manyāmūla, the marma treats other conditions that TCM would attribute to Wind pathologies, such as vertigo, disequilibrium and stroke paralysis. Āyurveda attributes these wind pathologies to disturbances in prāna vāyu. This is another example of how, despite differences in terminology, both systems often describe the same phenomena.

Commentary
Manyāmūla is translated as the beginning of the neck. *Mūla* means root and *manya* means neck. It is a notable marma for helping to relieve neck tension and increasing the neck's range of motion and can be used effectively for addressing headaches in the occipital region. Sushruta describes alternate locations for Manyāmūla as both the depression below the occiput and the bony protuberance of the occiput itself. This originates from his tendency to sometimes describe marmāni in terms of an area as much as several anguli wide, rather than simply a specific point.

Manyāmūla is functionally related to the posterior cranial fossa, posterior cerebral artery and occipital bone. This marma can be stimulated to enhance cerebral blood circulation and the circulation of CSF, especially to the occipital lobes. Like Shivarandhra, it treats posterior cranial fossa dysfunction. It aids in recovery of muscle strength and coordination in stroke patients. For vertigo or disequilibrium, this marma helps to ground and balance the individual.

Manyāmūla is connected to the hypothalamus, considered in Āyurveda to be the seat of fire in the brain. According to modern medicine, within the hypothalamus is a thermal center that regulates body temperature. Highly skilled yogis can increase their body temperature by focusing awareness on this marma, while holding the head in a chin lock and the hands together in a position known as *agni vārdhini mūdra*.

The connection with fire is reflected in this marma's ability to enkindle agni (the fire principle) in the stomach and pancreas. Thus, it can be helpful in treatment of chronic indigestion, hypoglycemia and pancreatic dysfunction. In addition, Manyāmūla becomes sensitive if there is chronic constipation or toxins in the descending colon because the occipital area is associated with apāna vāyu.

Vidhuram

Location
On the posterior aspect of the neck, level with the lower border of the spinous process of C1 (atlas) vertebra. One angula on each side from the midline.

Action
♦ Promotes tarpaka kapha health and function
♦ Relieves headaches and neck pain
♦ Relieves meningeal irritation
♦ Reduces stress
♦ Regulates rakta dhātu (blood)
♦ Benefits liver and spleen
♦ Benefits eyes

Associated Doshic Subtypes
Prāna Vāyu, Udāna Vāyu, Tarpaka Kapha, Ālochaka Pitta, Rañjaka Pitta

Indications
♦ Migraines, occipital headache
♦ Headache related to cervical spondylosis
♦ Neck pain and stiffness, decreased range of motion
♦ Stress and tension in the shoulder
♦ Nosebleed, raised blood pressure, recurrent bleeding
♦ Liver and spleen pain
♦ Disequilibrium, vertigo
♦ Visual disturbances, blurry vision

Treatment
Vacha oil can reduce neck rigidity due to vāta dosha. **Mahānārāyana oil** effectively balances stress and tension in the neck area. **Khus oil** pacifies pitta, thereby alleviating most nosebleeds.

Corresponding Acupoint
Huatuojiaji (HTJJ) extra points (C1)

Close to BL 10, Tianzhu (Celestial Pillar)

Close to GV 15, Yamen (Gate of Muteness)

Vidhuram corresponds to the Huatuojiaji points level with C1. They are both indicated for local pain and stiffness. See the Huatuojiaji section in appendix B for additional information regarding the Huatuojiaji points that run parallel to the spine. Vidhuram is also located midway between two influential points: BL 10 and GV 15. GV 15 is located below the spinous process of the first cervical vertebrae, while BL 10 is 1.3 cun lateral

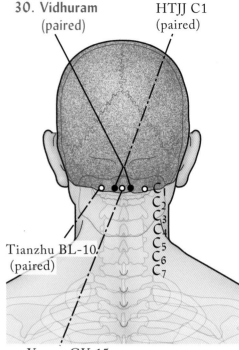

30. Vidhuram (paired)   HTJJ C1 (paired)

Tianzhu BL-10 (paired)

C1
C2
C3
C4
C5
C6
C7

Yamen GV-15

to GV 15. These acupoints, along with Vidhuram, treat headaches and stiffness of the neck, and like the marma, BL 10 is healing to various conditions of the eyes. Both acupoints calm the spirit, addressing mania and epilepsy. Each benefits the head and treats dizziness and a feeling of heaviness of the head. Neither has any connection to the liver, spleen or raised blood pressure. However, GV 15 is indicated for nosebleeds that do not stop, analogous to Vidhuram. In addition, GV 15 is connected to the tongue and can help treat loss of voice or muteness.

Commentary
The translation of *Vidhuram,* literally "that which holds the skull," beautifully describes the marma's location. The name derives from the Sanskrit root *dhru,* which means to hold. Vidhuram can also be translated as that which holds consciousness. These names elegantly depict the marma's ability to anchor the mind and make it more stable. Holding head, neck and trunk in a straight line helps to make the mind stable—which is why it is good to meditate with an erect posture.

Locally, Vidhuram relieves occipital headaches and neck rigidity. It has an influence on the eyes and helps with ophthalmic migraines. Like Shivarandhra marma, it may relieve meningeal irritation. Sushruta classified it as a vital marma because powerful impact or trauma here can lead to quadriplegia or blindness.

Vidhuram's ability to regulate the blood is due to its affiliation with rakta dhātu and the spleen, which is the root of rakta vaha srotas (channels of blood). The marma on the right side of the head is connected to the liver and that on the left to the spleen. It can address pain or dysfunction in either of these organs. Because it promotes tarpaka kapha, Vidhuram arrests most nosebleeds, but does not treat nosebleeds due to bleeding disorders. Nasal bleeding can be due to high blood pressure in the cerebral artery; gentle pressure on this marma can be effective to reduce blood pressure. Vidhuram may also be beneficial when there is repeated or persistent bleeding of the nose due to trauma or sunstroke.

Krikātikā

Location
On the posterior aspect of the neck, level with the lower border of the spinous process of C2 (axis) vertebra. One angula on each side from the midline, directly inferior to Vidhuram.

Action
♦ Benefits the head, neck and ears
♦ Relieves pain locally, relieves headaches
♦ Relieves tension, stress, and emotions
♦ Benefits the lungs and stimulates bronchodilatation

Associated Doshic Subtypes
Prāna Vāyu, Udāna Vāyu, Kledaka Kapha, Avalambaka Kapha

Indications
♦ Tension headache, occipital headaches
♦ Neck pain and stiffness, decreased range of motion
♦ Paresthesia (tingling and numbness), radiculopathy (pinched nerve)
♦ Stress related to emotional turbulence
♦ Middle ear infection, tinnitus, Ménière's syndrome
♦ Asthma, unresolved grief

Treatment
Nutmeg or **mahānārāyana oil** relieves stress, tension and local pain. A gentle upward pull of the head when the person is lying in supine position stretches all the marmāni of the neck, including Krikātikā, and induces deep relaxation. By sitting in the yoga posture *vajrāsana,* performing chin lock with the chin close to the chest, and doing *bhrāmāri prānāyāma* (humming breath), tension in the neck is relieved.[2]

Corresponding Acupoint
Huatuojiaji extra points (C2)

Krikātikā corresponds to the Huatuojiaji points level with C2. They are both indicated for addressing pain and stiffness locally. See the Huatuojiaji section in appendix B for additional information regarding these extra points that run parallel to the spine. See the Huatuojiaji section in Appendix B for additional information regarding these extra points that run parallel to the spine.

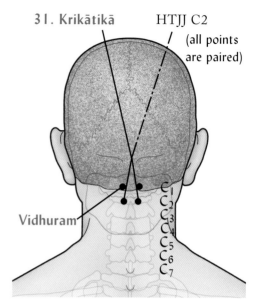

31. Krikātikā   HTJJ C2
(all points are paired)
Vidhuram
C1 C2 C3 C4 C5 C6 C7

Commentary
Krikātikā means axis: that which facilitates the rotation of the skull. It is located one angula laterally from C2, known as the axis. Krikātikā can also be translated as responsibility. When "carrying the weight of the world" on one's shoulders, tensions tend to collect in this area, and the trapezius muscle may become stiff and rigid. Tenderness may also be felt if there is dysfunction in the pancreas, since this marma is related to the head of the pancreas.

Krikātikā is functionally related to the hypothalamus, medulla oblongata and all intraspinal nerves. It is a delicate area; a severe trauma at the level of this marma can damage the spinal cord and result in quadriplegia. Krikātikā alleviates neck pain and stiffness resulting from cervical spondylosis as well as symptoms of a pinched nerve. This condition, termed *avabāhuka* in Sanskrit, results in pain from the base of the neck radiating down the arm to the fingers.

Krikātikā is also associated with the upper lobes of the lungs. Applying pressure at the marma stimulates bronchodilatation and helps to relieve asthma. The lungs are the storehouse of grief and related to avalambaka kapha, and Krikātikā may be tender if there is unresolved grief. This marma also treats Ménière's disease (due to vāta pushing pitta in the middle ear) characterized by periods of tinnitus, vertigo and diminished hearing.

---

2. Yoga postures are shown in chapter 18. Bhrāmāri prānāyāma is described in *The Complete Book of Ayurvedic Home Remedies,* chapter 6, "Breathing Techniques."

Grīvā (4)

Location
Four paired points on the back of the neck, level with the lower border of the spinous process of C3 – C6 vertebrae. One angula on each side from the midline, inferior to Krikātikā.

Action
♦ Relieves pain locally, relieves headaches
♦ Relieves stress and tension
♦ Enhances circulation of plasma and lymphatic fluid
♦ Benefits the throat
♦ Regulates thyroid and parathyroid functions

Associated Doshic Subtypes
Tarpaka Kapha, Bodhaka Kapha, Kledaka Kapha, Udāna Vāyu, Apāna Vāyu, Samāna Vāyu, Pāchaka Pitta

Indications
♦ Occipital headaches
♦ Neck pain and stiffness, decreased range of motion
♦ Radiculopathy (pinched nerve)
♦ Stress and tension
♦ Enlargement of cervical lymph node
♦ Pharyngeal and laryngeal congestion, enlarged tonsils
♦ Toxins in the colon
♦ Thyroid and parathyroid dysfunction

Treatment
Refer to Krikātikā Treatment section, page 120.

Corresponding Acupoint
Huatuojiaji extra points C3 – C6

Grīvā marmāni correspond to the Huatuojiaji points level with C3 – C6. All address pain and stiffness locally. See the Huatuojiaji section in appendix B for additional information regarding these extra points that run parallel to the spine.

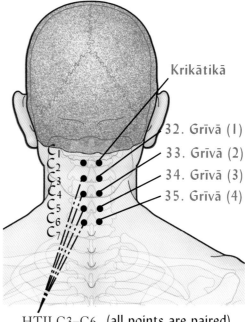

Krikātikā

Head
Neck

32. Grīvā (1)
33. Grīvā (2)
34. Grīvā (3)
35. Grīvā (4)

HTJJ C3–C6   (all points are paired)

Commentary
Grīvā can be translated as neck or pride. People with power, prestige and position tend to hold their neck straight and their head up high. Pitta-natured individuals often fit this image because they are confident, ambitious, driven and goal-oriented. When pitta is out of balance, an individual may become egotistical, fanatical and over-ambitious, and this may increase tension in the Grīvā marmāni.

Grīvā's sphere of action is locally on the cervical vertebrae as well as on the small intestine, colon and appendix. They relieve congestion of the cervical lymph nodes and the respiratory system. Grīvā marmāni have different functions, depending on the specific cervical vertebrae they correspond to. Grīvā marmāni located at the level of C3 are related to the thoracic duct, vocal cord and cerebrospinal meninges. They may be helpful in cases of pharyngitis, tonsillitis and laryngitis. They are associated with bodhaka kapha and udāna vāyu disorders. Marmāni at the level of C4 and C5 correspond to the thyroid and parathyroid. Pressure here will help to regulate the thyroid. Marmāni level with C6 are associated with the trachea, thymus, small intestines and colon. These are related to samāna vāyu and apāna vāyu dysfunction. They address chronic āma or toxins in the intestines. If there is high pitta in the intestines, Grīvā marmāni at C6 may become sensitive and cause neck pain.

Manyāmani

Location
On the midline at the base of the neck, in a depression inferior to the spinous process of C7.

Action
♦ Relieves neck pain
♦ Helps regulate pituitary, thyroid and parathyroid functions
♦ Relieves stress

Associated Doshic Subtypes
Prāna Vāyu, Vyāna Vāyu, Apāna Vāyu, Udāna Vāyu

Indications
♦ Neck pain and stiffness, decreased range of motion
♦ Pituitary dysfunction, thyroid and parathyroid disorders
♦ Paresthesia (tingling and numbness) in the upper extremities
♦ Radiculopathy (pinched nerve)
♦ Scoliosis
♦ Cervical spondylosis
♦ Stress

Treatment
Refer to Krikātikā Treatment section, page 120.

Corresponding Acupoint
GV 14, Dazhui (Great Vertebrae)

GV 14 is the meeting point of the GV meridian, which ascends the spine with the six yang channels of the body. Therefore, it is an influential point to clear pathogens and excess yang heat, and to tonify qi and yang. Unlike Manyāmani, GV 14 is a principal point for malaria and sweating disorders. The acupoint is also indicated for epilepsy, insomnia, hypertension, vomiting blood, incessant nosebleed and throat obstruction.

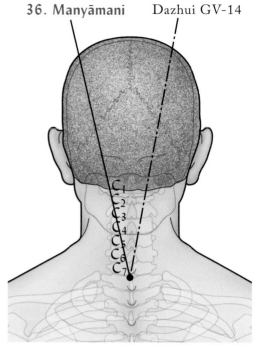

36. Manyāmani   Dazhui GV-14

Commentary
Manyāmani means "jewel of the neck," because a woman's necklace will often touch the skin at this precise spot. Sushruta described the location of this marma as both below C7 and on the spinous process of C7 itself, due to his observation that a marma could encompass more than one precise spot. Manyāmani is functionally related to the pituitary, heart, lower segment of the spinal cord and the corresponding intervertebral spinal nerves. During myocardial infarctions, severe chest pain could radiate to the intrascapular region and to this marma. Due to its relation to the thyroid, the marma may be sensitive in the presence of thyroid disorders.

Manyāmani is very reactive to stress and tension. One of the most common musculoskeletal conditions in the modern world is pain and stiffness in the cervical area. These symptoms may be a result of pinched nerve or myofascial tightness, a term used by many practitioners of musculoskeletal medicine. This tension can be relieved by stretching the neck. As described above, a gentle upward pull of the head when the person is lying in supine position stretches all the marmāni of the neck and induces deep relaxation. A pinched cervical nerve can result in tingling and numbness of the upper extremities. This marma can be used effectively for all of the above conditions.

Kantha

• •

Location
On the anterior midline of the neck, in a depression above the hyoid bone.

Action
♦ Regulates thyroid and parathyroid function
♦ Enkindles agni and eliminates āma (toxicity)
♦ Regulates udāna vāyu, benefits speech
♦ Benefits lungs, pharynx, larynx, trachea
♦ Calms respiration, stimulates bronchodilatation
♦ Regulates expression of thought, feeling and emotion through speech
♦ Releases suppressed emotions

Associated Doshic Subtypes
Prāna Vāyu, Udāna Vāyu, Bodhaka Kapha, Avalambaka Kapha, Sādhaka Pitta

Indications
♦ Goiter, hypothyroidism, hyperthyroidism
♦ Hoarseness of voice, speech disorders
♦ Dysphagia (difficulty in swallowing)
♦ Gastroesophageal reflux disease (GERD)
♦ Asthma, chronic cough, difficulty breathing, hiccups
♦ Emotional disturbances

Treatment
All marmāni of the throat region are very sensitive and require gentle pressure. **Vacha** or **cinnamon oil** applied externally benefits speech disorders and hoarseness of voice. An **herbal paste of jaggary and lime** taken internally may revive the voice. **Camphor oil** applied externally has a penetrating action as a bronchodilator. For inflammatory conditions, **khus oil** is effective. Hypothyroidism due to excess kapha is pacified by **hina, ginger** or **vacha oil** applied with clockwise rotation. Hyperthyroidism resulting from excess pitta is counteracted by **khus, sandalwood** or **jasmine oil** applied with counterclockwise rotation. In chromotherapy (color therapy), one can shine blue light on the marma to help heal the above conditions. Refer to chapter 7 for more information on chromotherapy.

Corresponding Acupoint
CV 23, Lianquan (Corner Spring)

CV 23 has similar functions and indications to Kantha. It regulates qi, in the same way that the corresponding marma regulates udāna vāyu. Since the point is

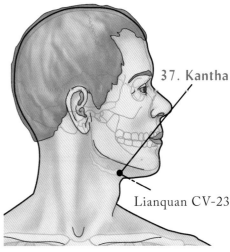

37. Kantha

Lianquan CV-23

located at the root of the tongue, it benefits the tongue, implying its application for speech disorders. Unlike the marma, CV 23 is also indicated for dry mouth, thirst, mouth ulcers, lockjaw and difficulty breathing. It is not, however, used for thyroid dysfunction or suppressed grief.

Commentary
Kantha, translated as throat, is intimately related to vishuddhi chakra, the throat chakra. Vishuddhi means purity of emotions. It is largely through the voice and speech that we express thoughts and emotions. Thus, this chakra is one of the main sites where unexpressed emotions accumulate. Kantha marma can help to release these unexpressed emotions and relieve emotional disturbances, especially when they are due to increased vāta or kapha dosha. It is helpful in the treatment of speech disorders, since it is the seat of udāna vāyu and functionally related to the vocal cords and larynx. Injury here can fracture the trachea and vocal cord, ultimately leading to suffocation and death. This marma also has a strong local action to benefit the lungs, serving as a bronchodilator. Thus, it is helpful for treating asthma, cough and shortness of breath. By regulating udāna vāyu, it can also help to relieve symptoms of GERD.

Kantha marma enhances metabolism through its action on the thyroid gland and by eliminating āma (toxins). Thyroid hormones T3 and T4 maintain cellular metabolic activity, equivalent to the Ayurvedic concept of cellular agni (*pīlu agni* and *pithara agni*). Thus, the marma addresses thyroid dysfunctions. Yogis perform chin lock and meditate deeply at this marma to improve thyroid functioning. Shiva, the Hindu deity of destruction, is called Nīla Kantha, which means blue throat. In a traditional story, his throat becomes blue when he must hold all the poison of the universe in his throat. Mystically, this marma is thought to "burn poison."

Kanthanādī

Location
On the anterior midline of the neck, in the center of the suprasternal fossa.

Action
♦ Benefits lungs, pharynx, larynx, trachea
♦ Calms respiration, stimulates bronchodilatation
♦ Benefits speech
♦ Regulates thyroid and parathyroid functions
♦ Improves metabolism
♦ Regulates cardiac functions
♦ Releases suppressed emotions

Associated Doshic Subtypes
Prāna Vāyu, Udāna Vāyu, Vyāna Vāyu, Sādhaka Pitta, Avalambaka Kapha

Indications
♦ Asthma, chronic cough, difficulty breathing, hiccups
♦ Laryngitis, tonsillitis
♦ Hoarseness of voice, speech disorders
♦ Dysphagia (difficulty in swallowing)
♦ Gastroesophageal reflux disease (GERD)
♦ Palpitations, cardiac arrhythmias
♦ Goiter, hypothyroidism, hyperthyroidism
♦ Emotional disturbance

Treatment
Refer to Kantha Treatment section, page 123.

Corresponding Acupoint
CV 22, Tiantu (Celestial Chimney)

CV 22 has many functions and indications similar to Kanthanādī, benefiting the throat and treating loss of voice. It descends Lung Qi, so it is useful for conditions such as asthma, chronic cough and hiccups. Unlike the marma, the acupoint treats dryness, swelling, obstruction or phlegm in the throat, and it does not affect the heart or thyroid. CV 22 also relieves congestion in the chest that may manifest as tightness or constriction.

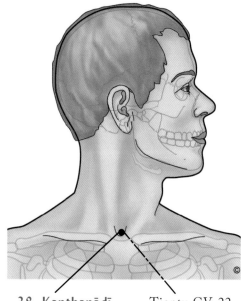

38. Kanthanādī   Tiantu CV-22

Commentary
Kanthanādī means channel of the throat. It is located on the anterior midline of the neck, on a line traced downward from Kantha marma. It is functionally related to the tracheal plexus, thyroid, heart and bronchi. Its sphere of action is almost identical to Kantha (see above) but, in some cases, it is more powerful. It can be a vital, life-saving marma when stimulated with gentle pressure during acute asthma attacks. Pressure here relieves wheezing, bronchial spasms and hiccups caused by a disturbance of udāna vāyu. In addition, Kanthanādī regulates vyāna vāyu, which can become impaired in many cardiac disorders.

Mantha

Location
On the anterior border of the sternocleidomastoid muscle (SCM), level with Kantha (CV 23). At the junction between the upper one-third and lower two-thirds of the sternocleidomastoid muscle.

Action
♦ Regulates thyroid and parathyroid functions
♦ Enhances cervical lymphatic circulation
♦ Regulates blood pressure and cardiac functions
♦ Benefits pharynx and larynx
♦ Relieves neck tension
♦ Clears the mind

Associated Doshic Subtypes
Prāna Vāyu, Udāna Vāyu, Vyāna Vāyu, Sādhaka Pitta, Tarpaka Kapha

Indications
♦ Goiter, hypothyroidism, hyperthyroidism
♦ Cervical lymph adenopathy, lymph congestion
♦ High or low blood pressure
♦ Fainting (syncope or transient loss of consciousness)
♦ Palpitations, cardiac arrhythmia
♦ Hoarseness of voice, difficulty swallowing (dysphagia)
♦ Emotional disturbance, especially confusion, depression
♦ Vertigo

Treatment
Deer musk oil has an affinity to the heart and dilates the coronary artery. To enhance clarity, pressure can be applied on the marma while the patient simultaneously performs *ujjayi prānāyāma*.[3] Refer also to Kantha Treatment section, page 123.

Corresponding Acupoint
ST 9, Renying (Man's Welcome)

Although the location of the two points is identical, how they are used differs. Similar to Mantha, the acupoint benefits the neck and throat to alleviate pain, treat vertigo and regulate blood pressure in cases of hypertension and hypotension. ST 9 does not share Mantha's ability to treat emotional disturbances or thyroid disor-

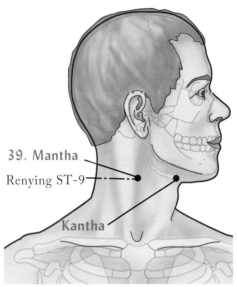

39. Mantha
Renying ST-9
Kantha

ders with the exception of goiter. And, unlike Mantha, ST 9 is indicated for headaches, asthma, shortness of breath and lumbar pain.

Commentary
Mantha is derived from *manthana*, which means churning. This refers to the marma's ability to facilitate movement of the head, allowing it to shift from right to left. Mantha also stimulates the mind, creating freshness and alertness. It churns consciousness to bring forth the butter of wisdom. Pressure here will expel doubt and confusion from the mind by enhancing clarity, a function of udāna vāyu. Mantha is functionally related to the cervical lymph nodes, cervical plexus, ciliary plexus and vagus nerve. It benefits the heart, thyroid, brain and throat, especially in conjunction with Sīrāmantha (see page 126).

---

3. To learn how to do ujjayi prānāyāma, please refer to *The Complete Book of Ayurvedic Home Remedies*, pages 74–75.

Sirāmantha

Location
On the anterior border of the sternocleidomastoid muscle, at the junction between the upper two-thirds and lower one-third of the sternocleidomastoid muscle. Inferior to Mantha.

Action
♦ Regulates thyroid and parathyroid functions
♦ Enhances cervical lymphatic circulation
♦ Regulates blood pressure and cardiac functions
♦ Relieves neck tension
♦ Benefits pharynx and larynx

Associated Doshic Subtypes
Prāna Vāyu, Udāna Vāyu, Vyāna Vāyu, Rañjaka Pitta, Sādhaka Pitta

Indications
♦ Goiter, hypothyroidism, hyperthyroidism
♦ Cervical lymph adenopathy, lymph congestion
♦ High or low blood pressure
♦ Cardiac conditions: angina, arrhythmia, palpitations
♦ Neck pain and stiffness, decreased range of motion
♦ Hoarseness of voice, dysphagia (difficulty swallowing)
♦ Vertigo

Treatment
Refer to Mantha Treatment section, page 125.

Corresponding Acupoint
None

Close to LI 17, Tianding (Heaven's Tripod)

Close to LI 18, Futu (Support the Prominence)

LI 17 and 18 are 1 cun apart and located on the posterior border of the sternocleidomastoid muscle, between the sternal and clavicular heads of the SCM. Both acupoints benefit the throat, but traditionally do not address thyroid, heart and blood pressure concerns, as does Sīrāmantha.

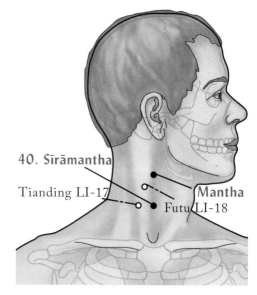

40. Sīrāmantha

Tianding LI-17

Mantha

Futu LI-18

Commentary
The translation of *sīrāmantha* is "a rope that does churning." It is located below Mantha marma on the neck and shares many similar functions. Sīrāmantha is functionally related to the carotid artery, cervical plexus, phrenic nerve and vagus nerve. Stimulating the marma helps to regulate heart rate and blood pressure. It is used for angina and arrhythmias. Compared to Mantha, Sīrāmantha's influence is slightly stronger. Refer to Commentary under Mantha for more detail.

Akshaka

· ·

Location
Superior to the medial border of the clavicle, between the sternal head and clavicular head of the sternocleidomastoid muscle.

Action
♦ Regulates cardiac functions
♦ Calms respiratory distress
♦ Enhances cervical lymphatic circulation
♦ Regulates the functions of liver and spleen
♦ Improves health of the eyes, benefits vision

Associated Doshic Subtypes
Prāṇa Vāyu, Udāna Vāyu, Vyāna Vāyu, Rañjaka Pitta, Sādhaka Pitta, Ālochaka Pitta

Indications
♦ Cardiac arrhythmia, palpitations, angina
♦ Difficulty breathing, hiccups, laryngeal congestion
♦ Cervical lymph adenopathy, lymph congestion
♦ Nausea and vomiting
♦ Dysfunction of spleen, liver or gallbladder
♦ Eye strain and pain
♦ Emotional disturbance, especially pitta: excessive judgment, criticism, pride

Treatment
Refer to Mantha Treatment section, page 125.

Corresponding Acupoint
ST 11, Qishe (Abode of Qi)

ST 11 is principally used for regulating respiration and descending rebellious Qi. Rebellious Qi is a TCM term for energy that is moving in an improper direction. (In Āyurveda, this is described as a disturbance of Udāna Vāyu, which is responsible for the upward movement of energy.) This can manifest as difficulty breathing or hiccups. ST 11 does not share Akshaka's function to benefit the heart, spleen or liver.

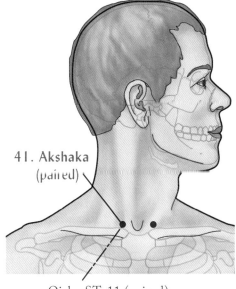

Head
Neck

41. Akshaka (paired)

Qishe ST-11 (paired)

Commentary
Akshaka means that which makes the eyes bright. It is derived from *aksha*, eyes. Pressure on this marma stimulates tejas, which enhances the light and luster of the eyes. If there is a slight yellowish tinge to the eyes, indicating disturbance of the liver caused by excess pitta, apply gentle pressure on this marma to relieve the pitta. It calms respiratory distress by stimulating proper flow of prāṇa vāyu. It pacifies hiccups by regulating udāna vāyu.

Akshaka on the right is affiliated with the left arm, left side of the heart, spleen and gallbladder. On the left, it is related to the right arm, right side of the heart and liver. (There is a criss cross effect.) Tenderness may reflect disturbance in any of these organs, such as liver toxicity or gallbladder dysfunction. If the gallbladder is congested, there may be stagnant bile or blood. Pressure on these marmāni can reduce hepato-splenic dysfunction and relieve nausea and vomiting.

Jatru

Location

On the midline of the manubrium sterni, slightly below the suprasternal notch and Kanthanādi.

Action

♦ Maintains immunity and stimulates ojas
♦ Stimulates dhātu agni and eliminates dhātu āma (toxicity)
♦ Regulates respiration
♦ Benefits lungs and throat
♦ Regulates thyroid and parathyroid functions
♦ Enhances lymphatic circulation in the chest
♦ Enhances communication
♦ Benefits spleen
♦ Releases suppressed emotions

Associated Doshic Subtypes

Prāna Vāyu, Udāna Vāyu, Avalambaka Kapha, Sādhaka Pitta, Tarpaka Kapha

Indications

♦ Low immunity
♦ Fatigue
♦ Asthma, difficulty breathing, hiccups
♦ Recurrent respiratory infections, laryngitis, pharyngitis
♦ Laryngeal congestion
♦ Gastroesophageal reflux disease (GERD)
♦ Hyperthyroidism, hypothyroidism, goiter
♦ Speech disorders
♦ Emotional disturbance

Treatment

A **paste of jaggary and ginger** applied here can treat cold, congestion or cough. To deepen devotion, apply **sandalwood oil** or **gopichandana** (a fragrant clay from India). **Turmeric** has an antibacterial action, though it will temporarily color the skin yellow. Refer also to Kantha Treatment section, page 123.

Corresponding Acupoint

CV 21, Xuanji (Jade Pivot)

CV 21 shares with Jatrū the ability to help relieve respiratory dysfunction caused by descending qi (or prāna). However, it is not known to possess the same capacity to influence the thyroid, nor provide any effect on immunity. It also does not have any of the spiritual indications mentioned for Jatrū. Unlike the marma,

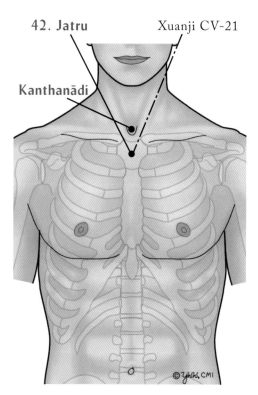

42. Jatru   Xuanji CV-21

Kanthanādi

CV 21 is a strong point to dispel abdominal fullness as the CV meridian runs down the central midline of the body through the abdominal region.

Commentary

Jatrū means to preserve or maintain. Health is preserved and maintained through strong and vital immune function, known in Āyurveda as *vyādhi kshamātva*. A central role in maintaining immunity is attributed to ojas, the superfine essence of all bodily tissue and the sap of kapha, which nourishes all tissues and is responsible for immunity on a cellular level. Jatrū is situated in front of the thymus, which can be poetically called *ojo granthi*, the seat of ojas. Stimulating Jatrū marma enhances immune response to bacteria and viruses. Tap lightly several times on this marma to awaken immune function.

Autoimmune disease occurs when the immune system is triggered to produce antibodies that act against the body's own tissues. Āyurveda describes this as an impairment of pīlu agni, or cellular intelligence, which produces antibodies that start destroying the neighboring cells. Intelligence is blocked by stagnant toxins at the cellular level due to impairment of dhātu agni (tissue metabolism). Jatrū marma activates normal functioning of dhātu agni, which burns āma (toxins) and promotes cellular intelligence. It can be quite beneficial in cases of low immunity, autoimmune disorders and chronic fatigue syndrome, when ojas is reduced.

Jatrū is functionally related to the trachea, bronchi, suprasternal notch, cardiac plexus, tracheal plexus and thyroid. It shares similar indications with other nearby marmāni to benefit the throat, promote respiration and address thyroid dysfunction. It is a delicate marma; an injury here can lead to serious conditions. One has to treat it gently.

Spiritually, Jatrū helps to maintain longevity and unfold bhakti (devotion) in the heart. A tulsi mala (necklace) worn around the neck should touch the skin at this precise spot to enhance its effectiveness. Jatrū also enables communication and expression. It is through speech that the inner world meets with the outer world.

Jatrūrdhva granthi is the term for the thyroid gland. Its functions are similar to Jatrū marma, primarily strengthening immunity through ojas and regulating respiration through the flow of prāna. It also promotes cellular metabolic activity. The thyroid gland is the bridge between the *bhūta agni,* the fire or digestive components present in the liver, and *dhātu agni,* the fire component of the tissues. It stimulates cellular metabolic activity through pīlu agni and pithara agni, the fire components present within the cell membrane and nucleus respectively.

Karnapālī

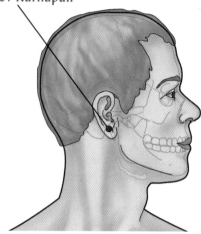

43. Karnapālī

Location
At central part of lower ear lobule.

Action
♦ Benefits eyes and stimulates vision
♦ Relieves headaches
♦ Helps to relieve ear congestion
♦ Calms hyperactivity of the mind, ADHD
♦ Relieves stress

Associated Doshic Subtypes
Prāna Vāyu, Ālochaka Pitta, Sādhaka Pitta

Indications
♦ Eye disorders: blurry vision, poor eyesight
♦ Migraines, periorbital headache, temporal headache
♦ Ear disorders including earaches, tinnitus
♦ Hyperactive mind, ADHD
♦ Vertigo
♦ Stress and anxiety

Treatment
Brahmī oil and **vacha oil** are applied to Karnapālī because they have an affinity for majjā dhātu (nervous system). Brahmī oil calms the nervous system while vacha oil is more stimulating. Ghee should not be applied to the inner ear because it will coagulate and lead to clogging in cold weather. The marma may be pierced with a red coral earring for children suffering from ADHD. (From an astrological point of view, ADHD is due to the affliction of Mars in the second or twelfth house.)

Corresponding Acupoint
Acupoint on the ear corresponding to the eye

The point is needled when treating various eye disorders, especially acute conjunctivitis. The Chinese representation of the ear is identical to the Ayurvedic model, representing an upside down fetus, as illustrated in appendix C, page 269.

Commentary
Karnapālī is located at the center of the ear lobule, where the ears are generally pierced. This point is known as *daiva kruta chidra,* which means, "fortunate, nature-made point to pierce." Nature has "designed" this as a place where there are no capillaries; piercing here causes little bleeding. In India, this is typically done at a young age, because stimulating—or piercing—Karnapālī enhances eyesight and immunity. The ear is a microcosm of the human body and in both Āyurveda and TCM it is compared to an upside down fetus.[4] In this representation, the eyes of the fetus correspond directly with this marma.

Karnapālī also benefits the ears and can be used for tinnitus and vertigo due to inner ear dysfunction. Gently pulling the ear lobe downwards helps to descend energy to relieve headaches and migraines. This action also aids in stress management and quieting children who are hyperactive. Another reason the marma has this tranquilizing effect is because of its functional connection with higher cerebral activity, which promotes tranquility and bliss.

---

4. Please see the diagram of the ear as a microcosm of the body in appendix C, page 269.

Karnapāla or Karna Ūrdhva

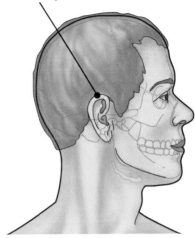

44. Karnapāla or Karna Ūrdhva

Location
At the apex of the ear.

Action
♦ Benefits the ears
♦ Relieves pain in low back, face and neck
♦ Stimulates the awakening of kundalinī energy
♦ Calms hyperactivity of the mind
♦ Stimulates mental alertness

Associated Doshic Subtypes
Prāna Vāyu, Apāna Vāyu

Indications
♦ Ear disorders including earaches, tinnitus
♦ Cervical lymph adenopathy
♦ Vertigo
♦ TMJ pain, mumps (parotitis)
♦ Low back pain, sciatica
♦ Hyperactive mind, ADHD

Treatment
Brahmī and **vacha oil** calm the mind and act on majjā dhātu (nervous tissue).

Corresponding Acupoint
Ear apex point

The ear apex point is often bled in TCM for excess yang energy that can manifest as heat, hypertension, hyperactivity or fever. It is also indicated for acute conjunctivitis. The acupoint does not have any of the marma's spiritual indications.

Commentary
Karnapāla is also called Karna Ūrdhva, translated as the pinnacle or top of the ear. The point is located at the apex of the ear. Pressure here automatically creates alertness and sharpness of mind. Yogis sometimes wear a pearl earring here to enhance wisdom. In ancient Vedic schools, a pearl earring was worn as a reward for academic excellence. The guru can apply pressure on this marma to awaken kundalinī energy and supreme intelligence. Karnapāla is functionally related to the lumbosacral spine and mūlādhāra chakra, where the kundalinī resides until it awakens and rises up the spine.

From an Ayurvedic perspective, hyperactive mind is a condition in which kundalinī energy is shaky and unstable. Gentle massage at Karnapāla and Karnapālī helps to soothe and quiet the mind of hyperactive individuals, both children and adults. In many respects, these two marmāni have similar spheres of influence.

Tenderness here may indicate an ear infection. The marma benefits cervical lymph adenopathy and the early stages of mumps. Karnapāla stabilizes prāna that is out of balance in cases of vertigo due to inner ear dysfunction. The marma is also connected to the coccyx and the colon, sites that are governed by apāna vāyu. In the representation of an upside down fetus, this part of the ear directly corresponds to the lumbosacral area. Thus, Karnapāla is effective in the treatment of low back pain and sciatica.

Karnamūla (2)

Location
Two points behind the ear.
Karnamūla 1 is in a depression between the tip of the mastoid process and the posterior margin of the ramus of the mandible.
Karnamūla 2 is in a depression at the posterior aspect of the mastoid process.

Action
♦ Benefits facial nerves, especially in cases of Bell's palsy
♦ Relieves pain and headaches
♦ Enhances kidney function

Associated Doshic Subtypes
Prāna Vāyu, Apāna Vāyu, Sādhaka Pitta, Tarpaka Kapha

Indications
♦ Ear disorders including earaches, tinnitus, poor hearing
♦ Bell's palsy (facial paralysis), TMJ pain, trigeminal neuralgia
♦ Mastoid infection, toothache
♦ Headaches (periorbital and suboccipital)
♦ Vertigo
♦ Kidney dysfunction or infection

Treatment
Refer to Karnapālī Treatment section, page 130.

Corresponding Acupoint
Karnamūla 1: SJ 17, Yifeng (Wind Screen)

Karnamūla 2: Close to GB 12, Wangu (Mastoid Process)

Yifeng SJ 17 benefits the ear for the same indications as Karnamūla 1. The acupoint addresses facial paralysis, toothache, trigeminal neuralgia and mumps. In TCM, many of these conditions are attributed to excess heat and Wind. Wangu GB 12 benefits the head and neck and treats headaches, stiff neck, toothache, deviation of the mouth and eye. It also calms the mind and treats insomnia and mania. Unlike the marmāni, these acupoints have no relation to the kidneys.

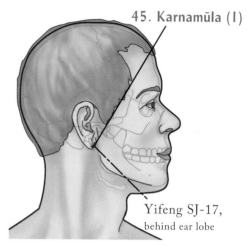

45. Karnamūla (I)

Yifeng SJ-17,
behind ear lobe

Commentary
Karnamūla is translated as the root of the ear. Both of these marmāni are beneficial in treatment of numerous ear disorders. They effectively treat facial paralysis and TMJ pain because of their proximity to the facial nerve. By balancing prāna vāyu, Karnamūla can alleviate vertigo. Karnamūla 1 is indicated for periorbital headaches and Karnamūla 2 for suboccipital headaches. They are useful in resolving kidney dysfunction including infection. Strong pressure here can lead to unconsciousness—a person can pass out.

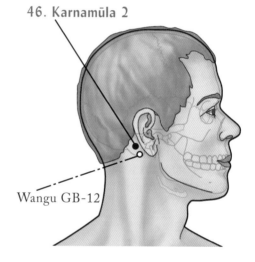

46. Karnamūla 2

Wangu GB-12

Marma Massage for Back of the Head and Neck

If you are not very familiar with Ayurvedic marma therapy, before attempting the following procedure please review chapter 8, especially "Guidelines for Touch and Pressure" on page 75 that offers specific information about massaging marmāni. Appendix C has the series of marma massage directions and illustrations starting on page 284.

The instructions here refer to the drawings on these pages. The numbers are for use with these massage drawings only; they are different from the numbering system for the marma points used throughout the book. To look up details on a particular marma point, refer to the beginning of this chapter, page 115, to the tables that reference all the marma points and their page numbers.

Apply a few drops of essential oil to the tips of the fingers. Start with gentle pressure on the marma points, and gradually increase according to the capacity of the individual. If you use too much pressure, the person will show discomfort through facial expressions, such as wrinkling of the face. Pressure on all marmāni should be held for approximately one to two minutes. If you feel that stronger pressure is needed, you can apply it when the patient exhales.

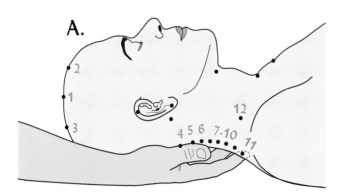

A. Let the patient lie in the supine position with the practitioner at the head. Begin by applying gentle pressure on Mūrdhni marma **(1)** at the crown with both thumbs. Then move up to Brahmarandhra **(2)**, back to Mūrdhni, and then Shivarandhra **(3)**, applying pressure on each marma for one minute. From here, apply pressure down the midline until Manyāmūla **(4)** at the base of the occiput. Move the fingers to Vidhuram **(5)** on each side of C1, then to Krikātikā **(6)** at C2, followed by Grīvā marmāni **(7–10)** from C3 to C6. Steady pressure should be held at each pair for roughly one minute, or longer if there is tenderness. Return to Manyāmūla and repeat this sequence a second time, until reaching Manyāmani **(11)** at C7, applying clockwise or counterclockwise pressure

according to need. Generally, clockwise pressure increases pitta and relieves kapha and vāta, while counterclockwise pressure increases vāta and kapha and relieves or pacifies pitta. If the pain is pitta type, massage with a counterclockwise motion, and if it is vāta and kapha type, the motion should be clockwise. After massaging the back of the neck, stimulate Ūrdhva Skandha.

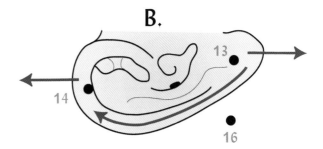

B and C. To massage the ears, begin at Karnapālī **(13)**. Squeeze the ear lobes between the thumbs and index fingers and gently pull them downwards. Then slowly massage along the ear lobes towards Karnapāla **(14)** at the apex and pull upwards. This sequence can be repeated several times. From the apex, move to Karnamūla marmāni, which are posterior to the ear. From Karnamūla 1 **(15)** move the fingers along the posterior border of the sternocleidomastoid muscle, activating Mantha **(16)**, then Sīrāmantha **(17)** and then Akshaka **(18)**. Repeat this sequence three times.

When the patient is in the supine position, the marmāni on the front of the neck can be gently stimulated. This is an extremely sensitive area and should be handled delicately. Lightly touch Kantha **(20)**, followed by Kanthanādī **(21)** and then Jatrū marma **(22)**.

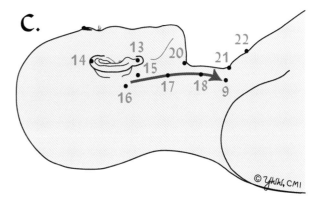

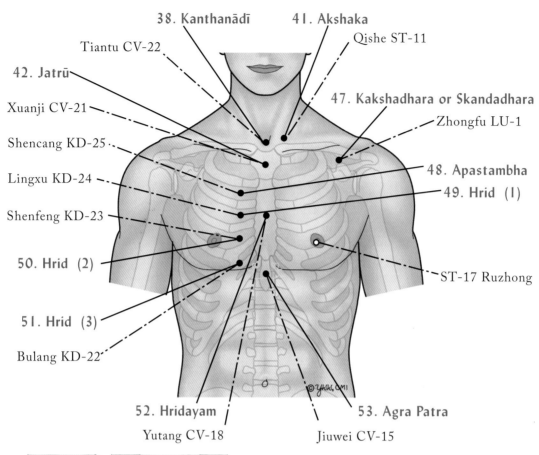

38. Kanthanādī
41. Akshaka
Tiantu CV-22
Qishe ST-11
42. Jatrū
47. Kakshadhara or Skandadhara
Xuanji CV-21
Zhongfu LU-1
Shencang KD-25
Lingxu KD-24
48. Apastambha
Shenfeng KD-23
49. Hrid (1)
50. Hrid (2)
ST-17 Ruzhong
51. Hrid (3)
Bulang KD-22
52. Hridayam
53. Agra Patra
Yutang CV-18
Jiuwei CV-15

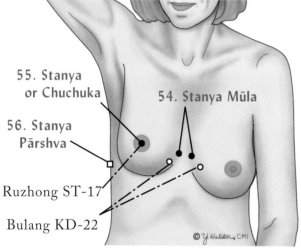

55. Stanya or Chuchuka
54. Stanya Mūla
56. Stanya Pārshva
Ruzhong ST-17
Bulang KD-22

Urah (Chest) Marmāni (11)

#	Marma Points	Page	Acupoint
47	Kakshadhara or Skandadhara	136	LU 1
48	Apastambha	137	KD 25
49	Hrid 1	138	KD 24
50	Hrid 2	138	KD 23
51	Hrid 3	138	KD 22
52	Hridayam	140	CV 18
53	Agra Patra	141	CV 15
54	Stanya Mūla	142	≈KD22
55	Stanya/Chuchuka	143	ST 17
56	Stanya Pārshva	144	SP 21
75	Pārshva Sandhi	145	LR 13

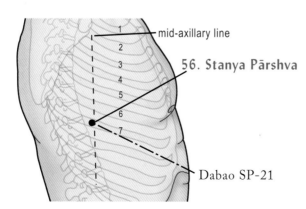

mid-axillary line
56. Stanya Pārshva
Dabao SP-21

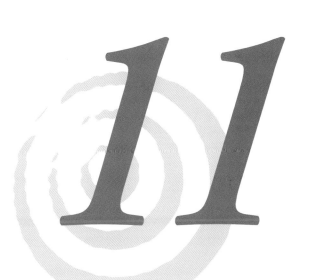

Antaradhi (Chest and Trunk) Marmāni

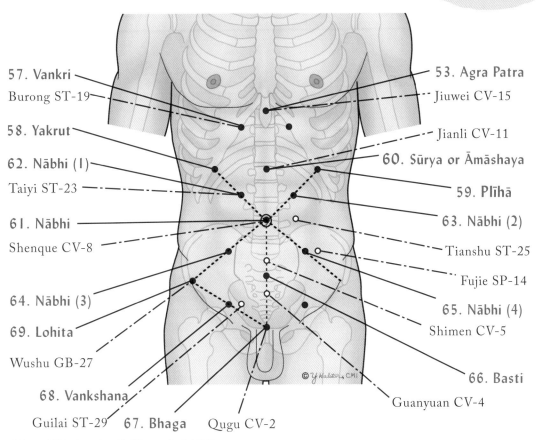

57. Vankri
Burong ST-19

58. Yakrut

62. Nābhi (1)

Taiyi ST-23

61. Nābhi

Shenque CV-8

64. Nābhi (3)

69. Lohita

Wushu GB-27

68. Vankshana

Guilai ST-29   67. Bhaga   Qugu CV-2

53. Agra Patra
Jiuwei CV-15

Jianli CV-11

60. Sūrya or Āmāshaya

59. Plīhā

63. Nābhi (2)

Tianshu ST-25

Fujie SP-14

65. Nābhi (4)
Shimen CV-5

66. Basti

Guanyuan CV-4

© Y Walston, CMI

Udara (Abdominal) Marmāni (12)

#	Marma Points	Page	Acupoint	#	Marma Points	Page	Acupoint
57	Vankri	146	ST 19	66	Basti	152	≈CV 4, CV 5
58	Yakrut	147	----------	67	Bhaga	153	CV 2
59	Plīhā	148	----------	68	Vankshana	154	≈ST 29
60	Sūrya/ Āmāshaya	149	CV 11	69	Lohita	155	GB 27
61	Nābhi	150	CV 8				
62	Nābhi 1	150	ST 23				
63	Nābhi 2	150	ST 23				
64	Nābhi 3	150	≈SP 14				
65	Nābhi 4	150	≈SP 14				

Kakshadhara or Skandadhara

Location
In the deltopectoral groove, at the level of the first intercostal space, 7 anguli lateral from the sternum.

Action
♦ Enhances lung capacity and flow of prāna
♦ Relieves tightness in chest and bronchospasm
♦ Relieves pulmonary congestion
♦ Relieves shoulder and arm pain
♦ Pacifies aches and soreness in the breasts

Associated Doshic Subtypes
Prāna Vāyu, Vyāna Vāyu, Udāna Vāyu, Sādhaka Pitta, Rañjaka Pitta, Avalambaka Kapha

Indications
♦ Asthma, chronic cough, shortness of breath
♦ Bronchitis, pleuritic pain, chest pain
♦ Congestion in diaphragm, lungs, lymph nodes
♦ Tremors of hands and peripheral neuropathy of upper extremities
♦ Adhesive capsulitis (frozen shoulder), bursitis, brachial plexopathy (impaired movement or sensation in the arm or shoulder)
♦ Shoulder pain, forearm pain
♦ Cold hands, poor circulation
♦ Fibrocystic changes in the breast

Treatment
Massaging the breasts with **castor oil** helps to decrease fibrocystic changes. Combine the castor oil with **flax seed oil** and **corn oil** in equal proportions for more potent results. Deep massage with **mahānārāyana oil** or **Tiger Balm®** relieves local pain and stiffness and soothes the muscles.

Corresponding Acupoint
LU 1, Zhongfu (Middle Palace)

LU 1 is the first point on the Lung meridian and one of the foremost acupoints for treating all lung disturbances. Identical to Kakshadhara in location, it is 6 cun lateral from the midline at the first intercostal space. Like Kakshadhara, LU 1 is used to treat shoulder and chest pain. It also addresses stomach conditions such as difficult ingestion, vomiting and abdominal distention, which the marma does not.

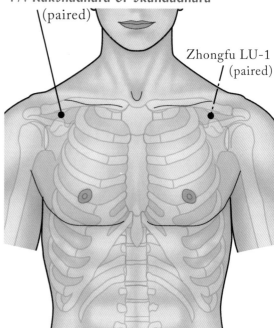

47. Kakshadhara or Skandadhara (paired)

Zhongfu LU-1 (paired)

Commentary
Skandadhara can be translated as that which holds the shoulder or the shoulder joint. (The verb *dhārana* means to hold.) The marma is more commonly referred to as Kakshadhara, implying a bridge between the upper extremities and the chest. This marma, along with other Skandha marmāni, helps to relieve disturbances of the shoulder, arm and hand.

Kakshadhara is functionally related to the brachial plexus, axillary artery and vein, and axillary and mediastinal lymph nodes. It benefits the lungs and bronchi by promoting expansion of the chest and increased circulation within the mastic tissue and pectoralis muscles. It also regulates venous circulation, governed by vyāna vāyu. Stagnation in the mastic tissue can lead to fibrocystic changes. Kakshadhara decreases congestion in the lymph nodes, diaphragm, lungs and mastic tissue precipitated by elevated kapha dosha. Tenderness at Kakshadhara may be indicative of pulmonary congestion or lung pathology.

Apastambha

· ·

Location
On both sides of the chest, one angula lateral from the midline of the chest in the second intercostal space.

Action
♦ Regulates respiration and relieves bronchospasms
♦ Facilitates optimal function of lungs and airways
♦ Relieves congestion in lungs and airways
♦ Benefits the heart and regulates cardiac activity
♦ Releases suppressed emotions

Associated Doshic Subtypes
Prāna Vāyu, Udāna Vāyu, Vyāna Vāyu, Avalambaka Kapha, Sādhaka Pitta

Indications
♦ Chronic cough, hiccup, shortness of breath
♦ Bronchial asthma, bronchitis, pleural and pericardial effusion
♦ Pleuritic pain, chest pain
♦ Palpitations, cardiac arrhythmia
♦ Hypertension
♦ Emotional disturbances

Treatment
Gentle pressure on the marma with **tulsi oil** unfolds love and compassion. **Tulsi** and **cinnamon oils** act on the heart and lungs. Internally, **licorice tea with ten drops of mahānārāyana oil** is an effective bronchodilator. One sip of the tea taken every ten minutes brings results that are similar to stimulating Apastambha marma.

Corresponding Acupoint
None

Close to KD 25, Shencang (Spirit Storehouse)

Shencang KD 25 is located 2 cun lateral from the midline and lateral to Apastambha. Both points benefit the lungs and chest for cough, asthma and shortness of breath. In TCM, these conditions are termed "rebellious qi," where qi flows in a retrograde direction. Unlike Apastambha, the acupoint also treats rebellious Stomach Qi that manifests as vomiting. Shencang KD 25 does not have any association with heart disturbances or emotions.

Commentary
The name Apastambha is derived from the root *sthambha*, which means a pillar that supports or stabilizes.

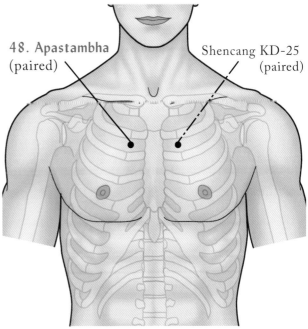

48. Apastambha (paired)   Shencang KD-25 (paired)

Chest Trunk

The marma is a pillar of support for both the heart and lungs by its action of stabilizing the flow of prāna. Apastambha on the right side of the body is functionally related to the aortic valve, sinoatrial node and right bronchus. On the left side, it corresponds to the pulmonary valve and left bronchus.

Pressure on the marma helps to alleviate all respiratory conditions, including the sensation of "air hunger" during acute asthmatic exacerbation. The lungs and chest are the primary sites for avalambaka kapha. Excess avalambaka kapha leads to mucus in the airways, difficulty breathing, palpitations, asthma and chronic cough. Massage of Apastambha helps to disperse excess kapha from the chest and relieves any blockage in the airways.

Apastambha marma is also helpful for numerous heart conditions, such as irregular heart rhythm and impaired circulation, caused by disturbed prāna vāyu, vyāna vāyu or sādhaka pitta. All three subdoshas are present in the heart and maintain normal cardiac activity.

Applying pressure, or focusing attention on the marma during meditation, calms any negative surge of emotion, especially sadness. Statues of the Buddha pointing to the chest draw attention specifically to this marma and its effectiveness in calming the mind. Ayurvedic physicians believe the right chamber of the heart is connected to the origin of emotion as a pure neuro-electrical impulse, which occurs before it becomes a psychological phenomenon. These impulses transform into feeling and then emotion. Āyurveda encourages us to witness emotions as they blossom, which helps to transform them into compassion. In Āyurveda, emotion is said to be the creation of an unsettled, unsteady mind while compassion is born of a calm, peaceful mind.

Hrid Marmāni (3)

Location
Three paired points just inferior to Apastambha; on each side of the sternum.

Hrid 1 is 2 anguli lateral from the midline in the third intercostal space.

Hrid 2 is 2 anguli lateral from the midline in the fourth intercostal space.

Hrid 3 is 2 anguli lateral from the midline in the fifth intercostal space.

Action
♦ Regulates cardiac function and heart rate
♦ Improves coronary circulation
♦ Maintains optimal function of lungs and airways
♦ Relieves congestion in breast tissue
♦ Enhances lymphatic circulation in chest area
♦ Calms mind, balances emotions, relieves stress

Associated Doshic Subtypes
Prāna Vāyu, Vyāna Vāyu, Udāna Vāyu, Sādhaka Pitta, Avalambaka Kapha

Indications
♦ Heart dysfunction, angina, palpitations
♦ Cardiac arrhythmia, bradycardia, tachycardia
♦ Non-cardiac chest pain
♦ Asthma, chronic cough, difficulty breathing
♦ Congested lymphatic or breast tissue
♦ Emotional disturbance

Treatment
The area near the heart is delicate and vital, so heat and moxibustion are contraindicated. ***Shringa shunthi lepa,*** a paste made of dried deer horn ash and ginger, is effective to enhance coronary circulation and treat anginal pain. **Dashamūla oil** alleviates pain that is vāta in nature. **Vacha, camphor or mahānārāyana oil** benefits the heart and lungs. All three marmāni are usually treated together.

Corresponding Acupoint
Hrid 1: KD 24, Lingxu (Spirit Ruin)

Hrid 2: KD 23, Shenfeng (Spirit Seal)

Hrid 3: KD 22, Bulang (Walking Corridor)

These three acupoints on the kidney meridian match the Hrid marmāni and have a similar influence on the respiratory system. Unlike the Hrid marmāni, they are

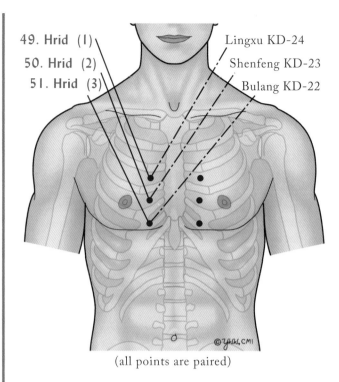

49. Hrid (1)
50. Hrid (2)
51. Hrid (3)

Lingxu KD-24
Shenfeng KD-23
Bulang KD-22

(all points are paired)

also indicated for vomiting. Shenfeng KD 23 and Lingxu KD 24 are recommended for the breasts, specifically in the treatment of breast abscesses. Lingxu KD 24 is the only one mentioned for relieving palpitations.

Commentary
Hrid means heart. These marmāni are connected to the cardiac plexus (heart chakra) and exert a strong influence upon the heart. In addition to its vital role in physical health and functioning, the heart is a deeply spiritual and mystic organ. It is the seat of compassion, love and devotion. It regulates prāna, the life force, and is the seat of vyāna vāyu, which governs circulation.

The heart is considered the seat of emotion. Sādhaka pitta is the subdosha that resides in the heart and is responsible for processing feelings and emotions. Stimulating Hrid marmāni enlivens sādhaka pitta and allows repressed emotions to surface.

Since the heart is connected to awareness and supreme intelligence, these marmāni can promote these qualities. Sushruta illustrated the spiritual depth of these marmāni by describing them as the seat of sattva, rajas and tamas—the three gunas (qualities) that pervade the universe (see gunas, page 8). All marmāni associated with the heart are sattvic in nature.

Hrid marmāni may be gently massaged for any heart problem due to doshic imbalance. Arrhythmia is due to vāta imbalance. Pitta aggravation is responsible for all inflammatory conditions of the heart. Bradycardia, a pulse rate less than 60 beats per minute, generally results from a kapha disorder, though highly trained athletes may have a resting pulse as low as 40. Treatment at these marmāni can benefit coronary circulation and help to relieve chest pain. Hrid marmāni also enhance lung capacity and treat respiratory dysfunction, manifesting as asthma, chronic cough and shortness of breath.

Hrid 1 is functionally related to the bronchi, pericardium, myocardium and aortic valves. The marma on the right side of the body corresponds to the right atrium and aortic valve, and on the left side with the left atrium and pericardium. Hrid 1 promotes the circulation of *āhāra rasa* (end product of digested food or chyle) through the thoracic duct. Āhāra rasa is the part of rasa dhātu that governs nutrition and nourishment.

Hrid 2 on the right corresponds to the right ventricle and tricuspid valve, and on the left to the left ventricle and mitral valve. Hrid 2 and 3 are connected to the cardiac apex, diaphragm and interventricular septum. Hrid 3 is also functionally related to the lower border of the heart.

Hridayam

*Chest
Trunk*

Location
On the anterior midline, at the level of the third intercostal space.

Action
♦ Regulates cardiac function and heart rate
♦ Improves coronary circulation
♦ Maintains optimal function of lungs and airways
♦ Benefits stomach, decreases acidity
♦ Calms mind, balances emotions, relieves stress

Associated Doshic Subtypes
Prāna Vāyu, Vyāna Vāyu, Udāna Vāyu, Sādhaka Pitta, Pāchaka Pitta, Avalambaka Kapha

Indications
♦ Heart dysfunctions: angina, palpitations, cardiac arrhythmia
♦ Pain in the pericardium, chest pain
♦ Asthma, chronic cough, difficulty breathing
♦ Peptic ulcer, gastritis
♦ Gastroesophageal reflux disease (GERD)
♦ Emotional disturbances

Treatment
Refer to Hrid Treatment section, page 138.

Corresponding Acupoint
CV 18, Yutang (Jade Hall)

CV 18 does not have the same action on cardiac function as Hridayam marma. It does share the similar function of benefiting the lungs and airways to treat difficulty in breathing, coughing, wheezing and obstruction in the throat. It is also used locally for pain of the chest and sternum. Like Hridayam marma, CV 18 benefits the digestive system and can be used for treatment of difficult ingestion and vomiting. CV 18 does not have the same range of action for emotional disturbances. CV 17, however, is a more frequently used acupoint located 1 cun below CV 18 that shares Hridayam's ability to calm the mind and harmonize emotional disturbances.

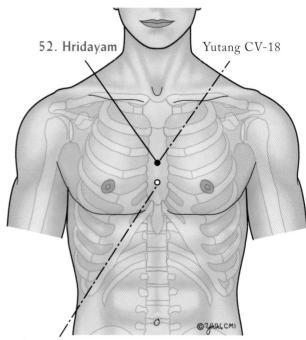

52. Hridayam   Yutang CV-18

Shanzhong CV-17

Commentary

Hridayam, a synonym for the name Hrid, is translated as heart. Refer to the Hrid marmāni Commentary for discussion about the heart, page 138. This marma is functionally related to the right side of the heart, including the right atrium, right ventricle and pericardium. It is also associated with the esophagus, trachea, bronchi and interventricular septum. Its action on the heart and lungs is identical to Hrid marmāni. They all relieve stagnant prāna in the chest that is the result of impaired vyāna vāyu and unresolved emotions.

Two special *mālā* (necklaces) have a salutary effect on the heart when they touch Hridayam marma and possibly Agra Patra marma as well (see page 141). The physical contact of a tulsi or *rudraksha* necklace with this marma can help to balance the energy of the heart chakra. A tulsi mālā is a necklace made of tulsi beads (holy basil). Rudraksha is the seed from a rudraksha tree, which can be strung on a thread to form a mālā. The prefix *ru* means crying and *dra* is derived from the verb *dravana* that means to liquefy. An ancient story tells that Lord Shiva, emerging from long meditation, was so moved by the sorrows and suffering of humanity that tears came to his eyes; the first tear that fell became the seed of the rudraksha tree. Wearing rudraksha around the heart facilitates the letting go of unexpressed emotions. Every unresolved emotion must liquefy like Shiva's tears so that it may be transformed into compassion.

Agra Patra

. . . .

Location
At the center of the xiphoid process, inferior to Hrldayam.

Action
♦ Regulates cardiac function and heart rate
♦ Enhances lung functions
♦ Relieves pain locally
♦ Releases suppressed emotions

Associated Doshic Subtypes
Prāna Vāyu, Udāna Vāyu, Vyāna Vāyu, Pāchaka Pitta, Sādhaka Pitta

Indications
♦ Heart dysfunctions: palpitations, cardiac arrhythmia
♦ Asthma, hiccups, pleuritic pain
♦ Nausea, anorexia, vomiting
♦ Gastritis, peptic ulcer, duodenal ulcer
♦ Gastroesophageal reflux disease (GERD)
♦ Emotional disturbances

Treatment
Refer also to Hrid Treatment section, page 138. Agra Patra, the terminal part of the leaf, looks like the tiny tail of the turtle, which breathes very quietly. If a person is having breathing distress, applying a little **vacha oil** to Agra Patra and gently stimulating this marma will quiet the breathing, and the person will breathe like a turtle.

Corresponding Acupoint
CV 15, Jiuwei (Turtledove Tail)

CV 15 regulates the heart and calms the spirit, thus having a similar range of action as Agra Patra to help heal heart dysfunction, chest pain and emotional disturbances. CV 15 also enhances lung function and removes blockages in the chest area thus treating coughing, wheezing and throat obstruction. Although it is not used specifically for gastritis and ulcer, as is Agra Patra, it does help alleviate stomach reflux.

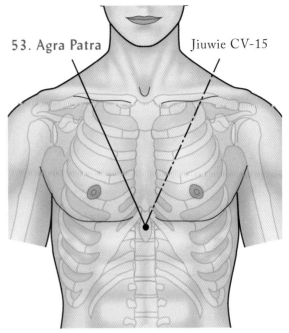

53. Agra Patra   Jiuwie CV-15

Chest Trunk

Commentary
Agra patra is translated as the front or terminal part of a leaf, poetically illustrating its location at the distal part of the sternum. It influences prāna, udāna and vyāna vāyus because of its functional relationship to the diaphragm, heart, mitral and tricuspid valves. It is also related to the esophageal orifice and fundus of the stomach. Agra Patra can treat nausea, vomiting, ulcers, gastritis and GERD because of its action on the stomach and ability to pacify pāchaka pitta. It also balances primarily pitta types of emotions. Similar to Hridayam and Hrid marmāni, Agra Patra is related to the pericardium and shares their capacity to treat respiratory and cardiac disturbances.

Stanya Mūla

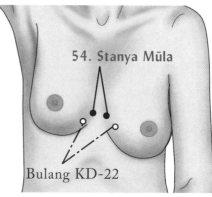

54. Stanya Mūla

Bulang KD-22

Location
Slightly superior to the xiphisternal junction and 1 angula lateral from the midline, on each side.

Action
♦ Benefits the breasts
♦ Regulates lactation
♦ Relieves congestion in breast tissue
♦ Enhances lymphatic circulation

Associated Doshic Subtypes
Vyāna Vāyu, Udāna Vāyu, Avalambaka Kapha

Indications
♦ Painful, tender breasts
♦ Breast tissue congestion, mastitis
♦ Breast abscess, cysts
♦ Fibrocystic changes in the breast
♦ Insufficient lactation
♦ Pleuritic pain
♦ Indigestion, nausea, vomiting
♦ Congestion or stagnation in liver or spleen

Treatment

Daily self-massage of the breasts with **castor oil** helps to relieve fibrocystic changes in breast tissue. During PMS or ovulation, when the breasts are tender or swollen, apply a little **castor** or **vacha oil**, using gentle circular movements, first five times clockwise and then five times counterclockwise. Castor oil can also be combined in equal proportions with **flax seed oil** and **corn oil**. To increase the growth of breast tissue, use shatāvarī ghrita. It can be applied locally and taken internally, one teaspoon once a day with a cup of milk. Massage Stanya Mūla first, then Stanya Pārshva, page 144, followed by Kakshadhara, page 136.

Corresponding Acupoint:
None

Close to KD 22, Bulang (Walking Corridor)

The acupoint's primary functions are to open the chest and descend Rebellious Qi that manifests as cough, wheezing, asthma, shortness of breath, vomiting and nausea. Stanya Mūla is also indicated for nausea, vomiting and indigestion. KD 22 does not share the same functions to benefit the breasts as Stanya Mūla.

Commentary

Stanya Mūla is translated as the root of the breast. This marma helps maintain the tone of the breast tissue. It can also be useful in treating various breast disorders, including infection, difficulties with lactation and congestion. Pain or discomfort in the breasts is often associated with the onset of menstrual periods. Sensitivity may also be due to fibrocystic changes in the breast caused by stagnation and solidification of kapha. To prevent such stagnation from building up, it is helpful for women to perform a routine self-massage of the breast. (See below under Treatment.)

In addition to excess kapha, impairment of vyāna vāyu may also lead to stagnation and congestion in the chest and breast area. Massage to Stanya Mūla enhances lymphatic circulation by stimulating vyāna vāyu, and thus can help reduce the congestion.

Breast tissue is a by-product of rasa dhātu. If rasa dhātu agni is low then there is undue production of raw breast tissue, which may lead to unduly enlarged breasts. If rasa dhātu agni is high, then the mastic tissues do not develop, and the chest becomes flat. Stimulation of Stanya Mūla marma normalizes the dhātu agni and maintains normal healthy development.

The marma on the right is affiliated with the liver and on the left with the spleen. Gentle massage here relieves congestion and stagnation in both these organs as well as the breast tissue. Stanya Mūla is functionally related to the heart and stomach and gentle pressure here benefits indigestion, nausea and vomiting.

Stanya or Chuchuka

• •

Location
The center of the nipple.

Action
♦ Regulates lactation
♦ Stimulates uterine contractions during childbirth

Associated Doshic Subtypes
Vyāna Vāyu, Apāna Vāyu, Prāna Vāyu, Avalambaka Kapha

Indications
♦ Insufficient lactation
♦ Difficult uterine contractions

Treatment
Generally, Stanya is used only for self-treatment by the patient for lactation difficulties. It also stimulates uterine contractions and can be used to ease pain during menstruation, or labor. Stanya may be massaged by the midwife or the patient herself. Use **castor oil** applied gently.

Note: It is not necessary for the practitioner to touch a patient's Stanya marma. If you feel that using Stanya is beneficial for treatment, you can verbally instruct the client and demonstrate on yourself.

Corresponding Acupoint
ST 17, Ruzhong (Middle of the Breast)

The Stomach meridian runs 4 cun lateral from the midline traversing through the nipples. ST 17 is merely a landmark on the meridian and is not used for treatment purposes. It is contraindicated for needling and moxibustion.

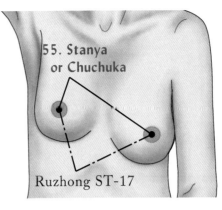

55. Stanya or Chuchuka

Ruzhong ST-17

Chest Trunk

Commentary
Stanya is translated as breast. An alternate name for the marma is Chuchuka, derived from the Sanskrit root *chusna,* meaning "to suck." Chuchuka is that which babies suckle for nourishment. This is a highly sensitive marma, especially during ovulation and menses. It is the opening of *stanya vaha srotas,* the female reproductive channels, through which breast milk flows. Hence, it can be used for resolving difficulties with lactation. (These channels are activated only in postpartum women.) Stanya corresponds to shukra and ārtava dhātu, the male and female reproductive tissues respectively. It is related to the clitoris, ovaries (*antah phala*) and fallopian tubes in the female, and to the spermatic cord, testicles and glans penis in the male. Stanya is connected to sexual energy and love. In Tantra, an esoteric spiritual tradition, sexual energy is awakened through the prāna nādī that includes the lips, nipples and genital area. Stanya marmāni are also well known to stimulate uterine contractions during childbirth.

Stanya Pārshva

Chest
Trunk

Location
On the midaxillary line, in the seventh intercostal space.

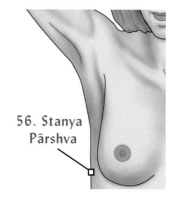

56. Stanya Pārshva

Action
♦ Benefits the breasts
♦ Regulates lactation
♦ Relieves congestion in breast tissue
♦ Enhances lymphatic circulation

Associated Doshic Subtypes
Vyāna Vāyu, Avalambaka Kapha, Udāna Vāyu, Rañjaka Pitta

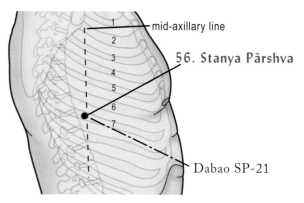

mid-axillary line

56. Stanya Pārshva

Dabao SP-21

Indications
♦ Painful, tender breasts
♦ Congestion in breast tissue
♦ Breast abscess, cysts
♦ Fibrocystic changes in the breast
♦ Insufficient lactation
♦ Congestion or stagnation in the liver or spleen

Treatment
Refer to Stanya Mūla Treatment section, page 142.

Corresponding Acupoint
SP 21, Dabao (Great Wrapping)

Dabao SP 21 opens the chest and promotes the flow of qi in the lateral costal region. It treats pain in the chest, lateral costal region and the entire body. It is not used to treat or benefit the breasts.

Commentary
The meaning of Stanya Pārshva is the side of the breast. It shares the same indications as Stanya Mūla. The marma on the right side of the body is connected to the liver and right chamber of the heart, and the marma on the left side with the spleen and left chamber of the heart. Refer to Stanya Mūla Commentary for more discussion of Stanya marmāni, page 142.

Pārshva Sandhi

Location
At the tip of the eleventh (floating) rib.

Action
♦ Enhances flow of prāna
♦ Benefits lungs and respiration
♦ Benefits liver, spleen and kidney function
♦ Relieves pain locally

Associated Doshic Subtypes
Prāna Vāyu, Udāna Vāyu, Sādhaka Pitta, Rañjaka Pitta, Avalambaka Kapha

Indications
♦ Asthma, hiccups, chronic cough
♦ Pleuritic pain, chest pain
♦ Intercostal pain
♦ Pain in liver or spleen area
♦ Congestion of liver and spleen
♦ Renal colic (kidney pain), kidney stones
♦ Abdominal pain

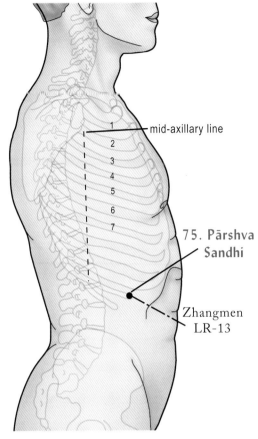

Chest
Trunk

mid-axillary line

75. Pārshva Sandhi

Zhangmen LR-13

Treatment
Kewrā is used for the liver and **kadamba oil** for the spleen. Deep massage with **mahānārāyana oil** penetrates into the muscles and relieves local pain.

Corresponding Acupoint
LR 13, Zhangmen (Completion Gate)

LR 13 shares similar functions with Pārshva Sandhi to benefit the chest and treat coughing and wheezing. It's more powerful sphere of action, however, is to harmonize the liver and spleen due to its classification as the Mu point of the Spleen. Both points treat disturbance of these organs, abdominal pain and distention. LR 13 does not have any influence on the kidneys. It is an important point on the Liver meridian to help with regulating stagnation of Liver qi that is responsible for fiery emotions such as anger.

Commentary
Pārshva is translated as rib or side and *sandhi* as joint. These words together represent the side of the ribs or the joint between the ribs and the side of the body. Pārshva Sandhi's function is to relieve pain in the ribs, chest, intercostal and abdominal regions. It is functionally related to the pleura, the delicate tissue that protects and cushions the lungs. The marma on the right side of the body corresponds to the liver and on the left to the spleen. It is affiliated with rakta vaha srotas, because these organs are the root of that channel system. Treatment here can alleviate pain, congestion and inflammation of these organs. Pārshva Sandhi is also functionally related to the kidneys and reduces kidney pain and stones. Similar to Bruhatī marma, pressure on Pārshva Sandhi increases the flow of prāna to the lungs and treats lung dysfunction.

Vankri

Location
Lies on the costal margin, level with the tip of the xiphoid process.

Action
♦ Benefits liver, gallbladder, spleen and pancreas
♦ Relieves pain locally
♦ Regulates digestion and acid secretion
♦ Maintains tone of diaphragm muscle
♦ Regulates lactation

Associated Doshic Subtypes
Samāna Vāyu, Udāna Vāyu, Vyāna Vāyu, Rañjaka Pitta, Pāchaka Pitta, Kledaka Kapha

Indications
♦ Liver and gallbladder dysfunction
♦ Peptic ulcer
♦ Gastroesophageal reflux disease (GERD)
♦ Anorexia
♦ Insufficient lactation
♦ Epigastric pain, pleuritic pain, intercostal pain
♦ Pain in right and left upper quadrants of abdomen

Treatment
Sandalwood oil pacifies pitta conditions where there is inflammation or sharp pain. In cases of anorexia, massaging Vankri with **vacha oil** may be helpful. **Jasmine** or **camphor oil** may be used for gastric conditions such as ulcers, gastritis and abdominal pain.

Corresponding Acupoint
ST 19, Burong (Not Contained)

Like Vankri, ST 19 also benefits digestion and treats epigastric pain and nausea. It is also helpful for relief of vomiting and abdominal distention. Unlike Vankri, ST 19 pacifies coughing and difficulty breathing.

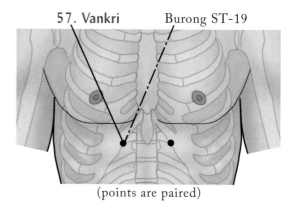

57. Vankri   Burong ST-19

(points are paired)

Commentary
Vankri is translated as curved bone or bony curvature. It is located along the costal margin where the bone appears to be curved. Its action benefits several major organs. The marma on the right is functionally related to the liver, gallbladder, head of the pancreas, duodenum and lesser curvature of the stomach. On the left, it corresponds to the spleen, tail of the pancreas, and greater curvature of the stomach. Vankri is effective for disorders of all these organs.

Its action on the stomach pacifies pāchaka pitta in the treatment of peptic ulcer and GERD. Vankri stimulates digestion and may be helpful in treating anorexia. Its close proximity to the breasts allows it to regulate lactation in conjunction with other Stanya marmāni. Vankri maintains the tone of the diaphragm muscle that is governed by udāna vāyu. It relieves pain in many regions, including the lungs, abdomen, epigastric, and intercostal areas.

Yakrut

Location
The point where a vertical line drawn from the mid-clavicular point intersects the costal margin on the right side of the body.

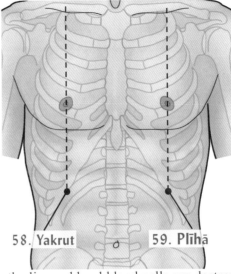

58. Yakrut   59. Plīhā

Action
♦ Regulates the function of liver and gall bladder
♦ Stimulates bhūta agni (liver metabolism) and detoxifies āma
♦ Regulates digestion and metabolism of all seven dhātus (tissues)
♦ Regulates functions of small intestine and colon
♦ Relieves pain locally
♦ Pacifies fiery emotions

Associated Doshic Subtypes
Rañjaka Pitta, Pāchaka Pitta, Samāna Vāyu, Apāna Vāyu, Kledaka Kapha

Indications
♦ Liver and gallbladder dysfunction
♦ Pain in upper right quadrant of abdomen
♦ Stagnation of bile, toxins in liver
♦ Nausea and vomiting related to liver and gallbladder dysfunction
♦ Abdominal pain and distention, epigastric pain
♦ Colon dysfunctions: diarrhea, constipation
♦ Emotional disturbance, especially pitta: anger, rage, irritability, impatience, frustration, envy.

Treatment
Massage of Yakrut marma with **bhringarāja oil** pacifies pitta disorders and benefits the liver. **Neem oil** or **tikta ghrita** (bitter ghee) can be administered orally or topically to improve liver function.

Corresponding Acupoint
None

Commentary
Yakrut, translated as liver, is the principal point for treating liver dysfunction. The prefix *ya* means circulation and *krut* means action. The liver is a vital organ with a wide range of functions. It is related to the stomach, spleen and bone marrow. The liver and spleen are both considered the root of *rakta vaha srotas*, the tissue that governs the blood. In the embryo, the liver regulates blood volume by the creation of new red blood cells, a process known as erythrogenesis.

In the liver, old red blood cells are destroyed and hemoglobin is broken down; heme is separated from globulin. The globulin becomes ojas in the liver, which has a protective, immune-enhancing function, and the heme takes part in the creation of rañjaka pitta or bile.

In addition, the liver has the important task of metabolizing fat and alcohol, and it synthesizes cholesterol into testosterone. Thus, the field of action of the liver leads up to shukra dhātu, the male reproductive tissue.

The liver is the seat of bhūta agni, the fire component of the ether, air, fire, water and earth elements. The food we eat also contains those five elements. When we eat and begin to digest our food, each bhūta agni acts on the corresponding elements in the ingested food and converts them into biological components at the cellular level. Thus, the five bhūta agnis process the organic five elements of the ingested food and convert them into the five biological components of a living cell.

Bhūta agni is the metabolic fire that fuels all the liver's activities. It is the bridge between the dhātu agni present in all seven tissues and the *jāthara agni* in the stomach. It supports the liver in digestion, metabolism and detoxification. Yakrut marma stimulates bhūta agni and thereby all the liver's diverse functions. When bhūta agni is strong, it facilitates detoxification and optimal liver function, preventing toxins from accumulating in the tissues.

Yakrut marma is functionally related to the head of the pancreas, right kidney, ascending colon, adrenal gland and the hepatic flexure. Diagnostically, palpation-induced sensitivity at the site of this marma may suggest pathology in these organs. The marma is located near the junction between the ascending colon and transverse colon. Hence, it is affected by apāna vāyu and treats gastrointestinal dysfunction. It also relieves pain locally in the epigastric area and upper right quadrant of the abdomen. Yakrut marma pacifies fiery pitta-natured emotions, which are associated with the liver.

Plīhā

Location
At a point where a vertical line drawn from the mid-clavicular point intersects the costal margin on the left side of the body.

Action
♦ Regulates spleen functions
♦ Regulates and detoxifies blood
♦ Enhances immunity
♦ Enhances lymphatic circulation
♦ Regulates functions of small intestine and colon
♦ Relieves pain locally
♦ Balances emotions

Associated Doshic Subtypes
Rañjaka Pitta, Pāchaka Pitta, Samāna Vāyu, Apāna Vāyu, Kledaka Kapha

Indications
♦ Splenic dysfunction
♦ Low immunity
♦ Lymphatic congestion
♦ Anemia, chronic fatigue syndrome
♦ Abdominal distention, epigastric pain
♦ Pain in upper left quadrant region
♦ Colon dysfunction: diarrhea, constipation
♦ Emotional disturbance

Treatment
Applying **vacha oil** here drains lymphatic congestion. **Sandalwood oil** and **brahmī oil** pacify pitta conditions. **Dashamūla oil** promotes immunity and vāta-type stress management.

Corresponding Acupoint
None

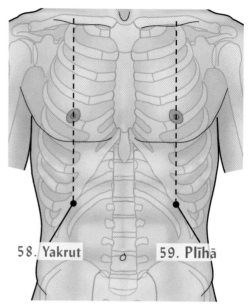

58. Yakrut   59. Plīhā

Commentary
The Sanskrit term for the spleen is *plīhā*, meaning to filtrate. The spleen and liver are the root of *rakta dhātu*, the tissue that governs the blood. This marma has a strong detoxifying action on the blood.

The spleen filters the blood through the action of rañjaka pitta, removing bacteria, parasites and other foreign bodies. Rañjaka pitta controls the production, preservation and destruction of blood cells. The spleen sends old red blood cells to the liver to process for elimination, so that they are removed from circulation. The spleen also has a role in producing white blood cells such as lymphocytes, which produce antibodies to act against bacteria and viruses. In this way, the spleen plays a major role in maintaining vitality and healthy functioning throughout the immune system. Because Plīhā marma regulates and enhances the functioning of the spleen, it can be very effective in treating conditions of low immunity.

In the embryo, the spleen produces red blood cells, but in adults, it produces only lymphocytes and monocytes (white blood cells). If the bone marrow is damaged, the spleen can come to the rescue and produce red blood cells. Also, within pockets of the spleen, it stores fresh oxygenated blood and, in times of emergency such as when a person is in shock, it will contract and release that blood into circulation. So, it acts as a kind of blood bank for emergencies.

Plīhā marma is located on the left side, while its mirror image on the right is Yakrut marma. Plīhā is functionally related to the left kidney, descending colon, tail of the pancreas and splenic flexure. Similar to Yakrut, Plīhā treats local pain and addresses colon dysfunction. While Yakrut pacifies pitta emotions, Plīhā balances kapha, in the form of attachment, greed, possessiveness and sustained depression.

Sūrya or Āmāshaya

Location
On the midline of the abdomen. The midpoint between Nābhi (umbilicus) and the tip of the xiphoid process.

Action
♦ Regulates stomach and pancreas functions
♦ Enkindles agni
♦ Relieves pain locally
♦ Regulates hydrochloric acid secretions in the stomach
♦ Pacifies pitta
♦ Harmonizes emotions

Associated Doshic Subtypes
Samāna Vāyu, Apāna Vāyu, Pāchaka Pitta, Kledaka Kapha, Rañjaka Pitta

Indications
♦ Peptic ulcer
♦ Gastroesophageal reflux disease (GERD)
♦ Epigastric pain, generalized abdominal pain
♦ Constipation, diarrhea
♦ Poor appetite, anorexia, nausea, vomiting
♦ Pancreatic dysfunction
♦ Emotional imbalance

Treatment
Use cooling, pitta-pacifying oils such as **sandalwood** or **khus** on the marma. **Jatamāmsī** may also be used; it is warming when taken internally, but externally it is cooling. **Asafoetida and garlic paste** pacify vāta and **ginger paste** reduces kapha.

Corresponding Acupoint
CV 11, Jianli (Strengthen the Interior)

Close to CV 12, Zhongwan (Middle Cavity)

CV 11, located 3 cun above the umbilicus, shares Sūrya marma's influence on stomach and digestive disturbances. CV 12, located 4 cun above the umbilicus, is considered the principal abdominal point to regulate Stomach function in TCM. Hence, it is used much more frequently than the neighboring point CV 11. The functions of CV 12 match those of Sūrya marma, except that it is not known to influence pancreatic dysfunction. Like Sūrya, CV 12 is also indicated for emotional disturbances such as anxiety and worry, which impair the functions of the Stomach.

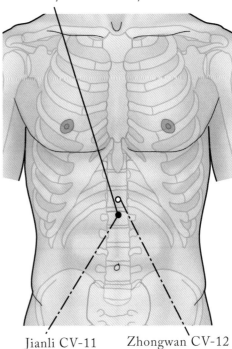

60. Sūrya or Āmāshaya

Jianli CV-11   Zhongwan CV-12

Commentary
Although this marma is commonly known as Sūrya, its full name is Sūrya Mandala. In Sanskrit, *sūrya* is the sun, the source of all heat and fire, and *mandala* means vortex. Sūrya marma represents the microcosmic sun within us, the solar plexus. It influences pitta dosha, the essence of fire and heat in the body, and it relieves pitta emotions that are fiery in nature. It also cools excess heat and inflammation, both manifestations of pitta, and alleviates hyperactive stomach, nausea and diarrhea related to anxiety and nervousness.

Sūrya enkindles all aspects of agni, particularly jāthara agni in the stomach. (Another term for the marma is *Āmāshaya,* which means stomach.) Thus, it has a strong influence on digestion and stimulates the appetite. It improves metabolism of the tissues by kindling or supporting dhātu agni. Sūrya is effective for all GI tract disturbances and for pancreatic dysfunction, as well as relieving local pain.

Samāna vāyu, pāchaka pitta and kledaka kapha are the three subdoshas present in the stomach. Samāna vāyu is responsible for the peristaltic movement of the stomach, secretion of digestive juices, and moving the food down to the cecum for further absorption. Both samāna vāyu and pāchaka pitta differentiate food into essential and non-essential products. Kledaka kapha acts in part as the mucous lining that protects the GI tract. It helps to regulate acidity and digestive enzymes that fuel the jāthara agni. Massage at Sūrya marma balances all three subdoshas and pacifies pāchaka pitta by regulating acidity and treating GERD.

Nābhi Marmāni (5)

Chest Trunk

Location

Nābhi is located at the center of the umbilicus (belly button). Four additional Nābhi marmāni surround the navel in the four abdominal quadrants:

Nābhi 1 lies in the right upper quadrant at the midpoint of a line drawn from Nābhi to Yakrut.

Nābhi 2 lies in the left upper quadrant at the midpoint of a line drawn from Nābhi to Plīhā.

Nābhi 3 lies in the right lower quadrant at the midpoint of a line drawn from Nābhi to the right anterior superior iliac spine (ASIS).

Nābhi 4 lies in the left lower quadrant at the midpoint of a line drawn from Nābhi to the left anterior superior iliac spine (ASIS).

Action

♦ Enkindles agni, regulates samāna vāyu
♦ Stimulates digestion and absorption in stomach, small intestine and colon
♦ Regulates functions of liver, gallbladder, spleen, intestines
♦ Regulates function of kidneys, pancreas, and adrenals
♦ Relieves congestion in these associated organs
♦ Relieves stagnation locally caused by vyāna vāyu
♦ Relieves abdominal pain and distention

Associated Doshic Subtypes

Prāna Vāyu, Samāna Vāyu, Apāna Vāyu, Vyāna Vāyu, Pāchaka Pitta, Ranjaka Pitta, Kledaka Kapha

Indications, all 5 Nābhi marmāni

♦ Abdominal pain, fullness, distention
♦ Low agni, impaired digestion, anorexia
♦ Immune disorders, such as chronic fatigue syndrome

Nābhi 1: hepatic dysfunction, gallbladder dysfunction, stagnant bile in gallbladder, peptic ulcer, disorders of small intestine and right kidney, pancreatic dysfunction, adrenal insufficiency

Nābhi 2: splenic dysfunction, anemia, disorders of small intestine and left kidney, pancreatic dysfunction, adrenal insufficiency

Nābhi 3: dysmenorrhea (painful menses), āma (toxins) in the colon, constipation, irritable bowel syndrome (IBS), urinary tract disorders, urinary infections, urinary retention, kidney dysfunction

Nābhi 4: same as Nābhi 3

Treatment

Nābhi marmāni may be stimulated by rubbing with oil several times. Massage all abdominal marmāni gently in a clockwise fashion. Start with marmāni on the right side of the abdomen over the ascending colon, and finish with marmāni on the left side of the abdomen over the descending colon. Use **sesame oil** for pacifying vāta dosha, **sunflower oil** for pitta and **corn** or **safflower oil** for kapha.

Corresponding Acupoint

CV 8, Shenque (Spirit Gateway)

Nābhi 1 and Nābhi 2: ST 23, Taiyi (Supreme Unity)

Nābhi 3 and Nābhi 4: None. Close to SP 14, Fujie (Abdomen Knot)

Nābhi marma, the center of the umbilicus, corresponds to CV 8. In TCM as in Āyurveda, the umbilicus is viewed as the entry and exit point of the soul or spirit. There are numerous other points in TCM that are said to treat "spirit possession." Shenque CV 8 is forbidden to needle, but moxibustion with substances such as ginger, garlic and salt may be used here. This acupoint is primarily used to increase yang energy when it is severely depleted and to warm the intestines and abdomen. CV 8 is indicated for diarrhea, rectal prolapse, periumbilical pain, abdominal distention and loss of consciousness.

Nābhi 1 and 2 match ST 23, which also treats epigastric and abdominal pain. It is not indicated for immune disorders, impaired digestion or specific actions on other organs. ST 23 is also indicated for poor appetite and diarrhea.

Nābhi 3 and 4 are slightly medial to Fujie SP 14, which is 4 cun lateral to the midline and 1.3 cun inferior to the umbilicus. The acupoint is used primarily for periumbilical pain, diarrhea and abdominal pain. It does not share other functions of the Nābhi marmāni.

Head, Heart and Hara: Some people live in their heads. They are logical, mathematical, competitive and aggressive, seeking power and position. People who live in the heart have love, compassion, forgiveness and devotion. The solar plexus is the seat of being. When you breathe into the abdomen, about two inches below the belly button at the hara, dantian or solar plexus, attention is at the seat of your being. When, during meditation, you watch your thinking, and at the same time watch the watcher, you arrive at the heart, and you experience love and compassion. Then, watch the breath go deep down, below the belly button, to the solar plexus. In this centered space, there is no fear of death.

Commentary

Nābhi means umbilicus or central part of the body. It can also be translated as center, or the place with no fear. Nābhi's role is vital because it is the seat of prāna vāyu, the life force. It is the root of 72,000 nādīs or pranic

Taiyi ST-23
61. Nābhi
62. Nābhi (1)
63. Nābhi (2)
Tianshu ST-25
64. Nābhi (3)
65. Nābhi (4)
Fujie SP-14

Shenque CV-8   (ST-23, ST-25, SP-14 paired)

energy currents in the body. Focusing the breath on the umbilicus allows prāna to go deep within the abdominal cavity and nourish these subtle channels of energy. Abdominal breathing is practiced in many traditions. The abdomen is referred to as the *hara* in Japanese medicine and the *dantian* in Chinese medicine.

During pregnancy the umbilical cord and blood vessel, which are connected to the fetus, allow the child in the mother's womb to receive oxygen and nutrients through Nābhi marma. Prāna and ojas are transported from the mother to the fetus. At this marma, the baby in the mother's womb is hanging upside down from the placenta, connected by the umbilical cord and blood vessels. The baby breathes through mother's lungs; its circulation is through mother's circulation, its nutrition through mother's nutrition.

When the baby comes out, the umbilical cord is pulsating with the heartbeat of the mother. Not until the beat becomes feeble or stops does the doctor cut the cord, which then gradually dries up. What remains, the umbilicus or belly button, is called Nābhi.

Nābhi creates raw ojas (*apara ojas*) from āhāra rasa, the end product of digested food, and circulates it throughout the body, enhancing the strength and immunity of all tissues. Hence, Nābhi is associated with boosting immunity and treating immune disorders.

All Nābhi marmāni influence digestion by kindling the agnis of the digestive organs. Nābhi is considered the seat of samāna vāyu, which in part regulates the timing of digestion and acts on meda vaha srotas (channel system for fat). Stimulating Nābhi marmāni enhances blood flow and lymphatic drainage in the abdomen.

Each Nābhi marma is functionally related to specific anatomical structures. (see table 25) When they are sensitive to palpation, it is suggestive of disturbance in the associated organs. Congestion in these organs may indicate an increase of blood flow or decreased drainage of

blood. This congestion is an impairment of vyāna vāyu in the rakta dhātu. Stimulating the Nābhi marmāni increases circulation, relieves congestion and improves digestion.

Stimulating Nābhi 1 regulates bile secretion. Nābhi 3 is also known as *Unduka* marma. Unduka means cecum. It is in close proximity to McBurney's point, well known in Western medicine as a diagnostic point for appendicitis. Nābhi 4 is traditionally called *Malāshaya* marma. Malāshaya translates as descending and sigmoid colon, including the rectum. Both Nābhi 3 and 4 regulate apāna vāyu in the colon and relieve constipation. Tenderness at these sites is a sign of stagnant apāna vāyu in the colon. These marmāni are also functionally related to pāchaka pitta, rañjaka pitta and kledaka kapha.

Table 25: Field of Action of Nābhi Marmāni

Marma	Functionally Related To
Nābhi	Small intestine, mesenteric lymph nodes, peritoneum fold (omentum), abdominal aorta
Nābhi 1	Gallbladder, liver, hepatic flexure, head of the pancreas, duodenum, right kidney, right adrenal
Nābhi 2	Tail of the pancreas, spleen, stomach, left kidney, left adrenal, transverse colon, splenic flexure
Nābhi 3	Cecum, ileocecal valve, appendix, ascending colon, right ureter
Nābhi 4	Descending colon, sigmoid colon, rectum, left ureter

According to ancient Vedic literature, such as the *Garbha Upanishad*, the spirit enters and exits the body through Nābhi (belly button). The space behind the navel is said to be the seat of the lower self (jīvātman or being), while the higher self (paramātman, total or Supreme Being) resides in the cranial cavity.

The spiritual journey corresponds to the ascension of kundalinī—the dormant energy curled like a serpent in the mūlādhāra chakra, the "root" chakra at the base of the spine—through the chakra system to the crown chakra at the top of the head. But, kundalinī is also intimately connected to Nābhi and the solar plexus. This is because, before birth, in the womb, the mother's kundalinī is connected to the baby's kundalinī through Nābhi. At birth, when the first breath is taken, kundalinī from the Nābhi coils up and moves to the root chakra.

Thus, yogis may stimulate Nābhi to awaken kundalinī. One way is by performing *Mayūrāsana* (peacock pose), which exerts direct pressure on the navel. This action strengthens the abdominal wall and activates kundalinī. Another method is *uddiyana bandha* or abdominal lock, which involves drawing the abdomen in and exerting pressure on the marma.

Basti

Location
At the midpoint of a line drawn from the umbilicus (Nābhi) to the midpoint of the superior border of the pubic symphysis (Bhaga).

Action
♦ Regulates bladder, treats genitourinary dysfunction
♦ Regulates apāna vāyu
♦ Relieves pain
♦ Increases circulation and enhances function in pelvic organs

Associated Doshic Subtypes
Apāna Vāyu, Vyāna Vāyu, Rañjaka Pitta, Kledaka Kapha

Indications
♦ Bladder pain, cystitis, urethritis
♦ Urinary tract infection (UTI)
♦ Frequent urination, enuresis (bed-wetting)
♦ Incontinence, retention of urine
♦ Burning pain on urination
♦ Lower abdominal pain, dysmenorrhea
♦ Pelvic inflammatory disease (PID), pelvic pain
♦ Fibroid tumors

Treatment
See Nābhi Treatment section, page 150.

Corresponding Acupoint
None

Close to CV 4, Guanyuan (Gate of Origin)

Close to CV 5, Shimen (Stone Gate)

Basti marma is located midway between two points on the Conception Vessel numbered CV 4 and CV 5. CV 4 is 3 cun inferior to the umbilicus, while CV 5 is 2 cun inferior. Basti marma is 2.5 cun inferior to the umbilicus in relation to these points. Both acupoints are related to the dantian, the abdominal seat of energy and reservoir of qi according to TCM.

Both acupoints are similar to Basti marma. CV 5 is the Mu point of the San Jiao, the network of organs that regulate water. Due to CV 5's effect on the bladder to transform and excrete fluids, it is an influential point to regulate water. It can treat abdominal masses, abdominal pain, and difficulty/pain with urination. Unlike Basti, both acupoints treat infertility, impotence, amenorrhea,

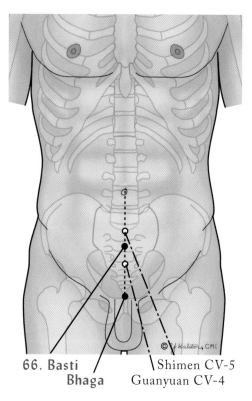

66. Basti   Shimen CV-5
Bhaga   Guanyuan CV-4

leukorrhea, edema and diarrhea. In addition, CV 4 is a principal point for strengthening the kidneys.

Commentary
Basti is translated as bladder or enema. In ancient times, the bladder of an animal was used to hold the fluid used for an enema. Basti marma is the premiere point to regulate apāna vāyu, which governs elimination. It strengthens bladder tone and function and treats various urinary disturbances including frequency, urgency, inflammation and pain. Basti enhances circulation in the pelvic organs and treats PID by balancing vyāna vāyu. The marma is functionally related to the fundus of the uterus and is used in the treatment of fibroid tumors in women. It also relieves dysmenorrhea and pain in the abdomen.

Bhaga

Location
At the midpoint of the superior border of the pubic symphysis.

Action
♦ Regulates male and female reproductive organs
♦ Enhances circulation and function in pelvic organs
♦ Relieves pelvic pain
♦ Regulates bladder and treats urinary dysfunction
♦ Stimulates sexual energy

Associated Doshic Subtypes
Apāna Vāyu, Vyāna Vāyu, Rañjaka Pitta, Kledaka Kapha

Indications
♦ Prostate dysfunction, impotence
♦ Painful coitus, low libido, decreased testosterone and estrogen
♦ Dysmenorrhea, irregular menses, ovarian disorders
♦ Pelvic inflammatory disease (PID), pelvic pain
♦ Retention of urine, enuresis (bed wetting), urethritis
♦ Frequency or urgency of urination, difficulty with urination
♦ Lower abdominal pain, fullness, distention

Treatment
Medicated ointments made of strengthening herbs such as **ashvagandha, bala** and **shatāvarī** benefit shukra and ārtava dhātu. Taking herbs such as ashvagandha and bala internally increases blood flow to the male genital organ and will produce a more dramatic effect than stimulating Bhaga marma. Refer to the Nābhi Treatment section for additional information, page 150.

Corresponding Acupoint
CV 2, Qugu (Curved Bone)

CV 2 shares Bhaga's influence on sexual, genital, urinary, lower abdominal and gynecological disorders. However, it is not mentioned for low libido. The acupoint is also known to benefit the kidneys.

Commentary
Bhaga is connected to the male and female reproductive organs and tissues (*shukra* and *ārtava dhātus,* respectively). Hence, it treats reproductive and sexual dysfunction. Some women may experience pain at the marma during ovulation. Bhaga addresses low libido resulting from a decreased supply of nutrients and blood to the genital organs. It regulates bladder function and may be sensitive to palpation in the presence of genitourinary

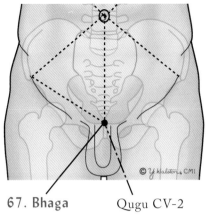

67. Bhaga   Qugu CV-2

disorders because it is affiliated with ambu vaha srotas, the channels that transport water. Bhaga pacifies apāna vāyu, thereby influencing the regulation of water and all disturbances of the pelvic cavity. Both Basti and Bhaga regulate circulation within the pelvic cavity and organs therein.

Bhaga literally means sexual pleasure and the marma is activated when there is sexual desire. *Bhagasthi* is the name of the pubic bone, which is associated with physical pleasure and sexual experience. Bhaga is derived from the root *bhoga* that means to experience or to go through.

Āyurveda holds that sexual activity should be regulated according to an individual's prakruti (constitution). Excess sexual activity can deplete ojas, the superfine essence of all dhātus that is responsible for vitality and immunity. Ideally, a vāta individual may have sex once every two weeks, pitta individuals once a week, and kapha individuals twice or three times a week. These guidelines also vary according to the seasons and to a person's age. For example, in the autumn, when vāta dosha is predominant, vāta individuals and older people should have sex only once a month. More frequent sexual activity is permissible for kapha individuals in the winter season because it may help to reduce kapha.

The Sanskrit term for sex is *mithuna,* which means balancing the polarity of male and female energy. This implies spiritual union as much as physical contact. In Āyurveda, sexual energy is closely associated with spiritual energy, because both are governed by kundalinī shakti. When kundalinī is activated at the root chakra where the sexual organs are located, it is expressed as sexual energy. When it rises to the crown chakra, superconscious energy is activated and there is complete transcendence or disappearance of sexual desire. Although many people on a spiritual path practice sexual abstinence in order to facilitate the rise of kundalinī shakti, a true *brahmacharya* is a celibate who not only renounces sexual activity, but who has mastered his/her mind and risen above all desire. Thus, spiritual awakening is the transformation of energy into supreme intelligence and pure love.

Vankshana

Location
The midpoint of a line between the superior border of the pubic symphysis (Bhaga) and the medial border of the anterior superior iliac spine (ASIS) or Lohita.

Action
♦ Regulates male and female reproductive organs
♦ Enhances circulation in pelvic organs
♦ Relieves local congestion and inflammation
♦ Regulates bladder sphincter and treats urinary dysfunction

Associated Doshic Subtypes
Apāna Vāyu, Vyāna Vāyu, Kledaka Kapha, Rañjaka Pitta

Indications
♦ Prostate dysfunction, impotence, premature ejaculation, spermatorrhea
♦ Painful coitus, low libido
♦ Leukorrhea, dysmenorrhea, uterine pain, irregular menses
♦ Ovarian disorders, fallopian tube disorders
♦ Pelvic inflammatory disease (PID), pelvic pain
♦ Lower abdominal pain, fullness, distention
♦ Retention of urine, enuresis (bed wetting), urethritis
♦ Frequency or urgency of urination, difficulty with urination
♦ Early stages of inguinal hernia

Treatment
Refer to Nābhi Treatment section , page 150.

Corresponding Acupoint
None

Close to ST 29, Guilai (Return)

Vankshana is lateral to ST 29, which also benefits the genital area and regulates menstruation. They both treat leukorrhea, irregular menstruation and other menstrual disorders. ST 29 also treats uterine masses, uterine prolapse and genital pain.

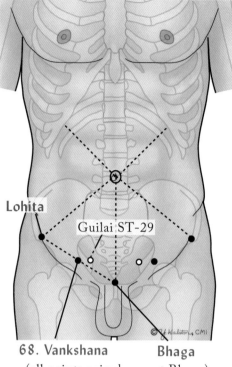

68. Vankshana
(all points paired, except Bhaga)

Commentary
The name *vankshana* means groin or joint of the thigh. It is located near Bhaga marma and shares many of the same indications for sexual and reproductive dysfunction. However, Bhaga is more influential for these indications and more commonly used. Vankshana is functionally related to the ovaries, fallopian tubes, testes, prostate, spermatic cord and inguinal ligament. Pressure on the marma relieves congestion in all these structures. Congestion results from impaired circulation of vyāna vāyu, affecting apāna vāyu in the pelvic cavity. Refer to the Bhaga Commentary for additional information, page 153.

Lohita

Location
On the medial side of the anterior superior iliac spine (ASIS).

Action
♦ Regulates the blood
♦ Enhances circulation within lower extremities
♦ Benefits pelvic area
♦ Relieves pelvic pain

Associated Doshic Subtypes
Apāna Vāyu, Vyāna Vāyu, Rañjaka Pitta

Indications
♦ Elevated blood pressure, hypertension
♦ Irregular menses, dysmenorrhea, amenorrhea
♦ Poor circulation in lower extremities, numbness, edema, cold feet
♦ Neuropathy of lower extremities
♦ Peripheral vascular disease (PVD)
♦ Pelvic inflammatory disease (PID), pelvic pain, hip pain
♦ Lymphatic obstruction
♦ Abdominal pain and distention
♦ Thrombophlebitis

Treatment
Refer to Nābhi Treatment section, page 150.

Corresponding Acupoint
GB 27, Wushu (Five Pivots)

Although GB 27 and Lohita share their location exactly, their functions widely diverge. Like Lohita, GB 27 helps to relieve abdominal pain and irregular menses. It also can be stimulated for certain conditions that Lohita does not address: uterine prolapse, constipation, tenesmus and back pain. On the other hand, GB 27 does not influence a number of conditions for which Lohita is indicated, including hypertension, lymphatic obstruction, poor circulation, neuropathy of the lower extremities and pelvic pain.

(all points paired)

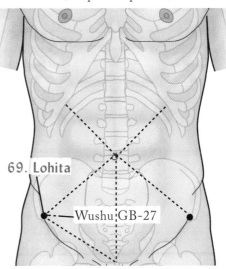

Commentary
Lohita means blood. This marma regulates the blood flow to the lower extremities and, in conjunction with Hrid and Hridayam marmāni, can be used in the treatment of various blood and circulatory disorders related to the cardiovascular system. Lohita also treats reproductive disturbances that involve blood flow, including irregular menses, dysmenorrhea and amenorrhea. In these conditions rañjaka pitta and rakta dhātu are affected. Lohita is functionally related to the femoral artery and vein, the colon, heart, and testicles. It promotes healthy circulation to the lower extremities and pelvic organs. The marma is directly affiliated with vyāna vāyu that governs circulation. Poor arterial circulation in the legs can lead to PVD, numbness and cold feet. Venous stasis (the stopping or slowing of blood flow in the veins) can cause edema of the legs.

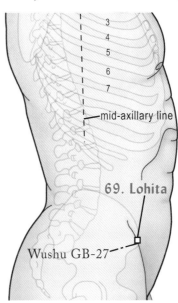

Marma Massage for the Trunk

If you are not very familiar with Ayurvedic marma therapy, before attempting the following procedure please review chapter 8, especially "Guidelines for Touch and Pressure" on page 75 that offers specific information about massaging marmāni. Appendix C has the series of marma massage directions and illustrations starting on page 284.

The instructions here refer to the drawings on these pages. The numbers are for use with these massage drawings only; they are different from the numbering system for the marma points used throughout the book. To look up details on a particular marma point, refer to the beginning of this chapter, page 135, to the tables that reference all the marma points and their page numbers.

Apply a few drops of essential oil to the tips of the fingers. Start with gentle pressure on the marma points, and gradually increase according to the capacity of the individual. If you use too much pressure, the person will show discomfort through facial expressions, such as wrinkling of the face. Pressure on all marmāni should be held for approximately one to two minutes. If you feel that stronger pressure is needed, you can apply it when the patient exhales.

A and B. Ask the patient to lie in supine position (face up) and stand at the head. Begin by stimulating Ūrdhva Skandha marma **(1)**. Then apply gentle pressure on Kakshadhara marma **(2)** with the thumbs. Both of these marmāni are often tender and require deeper stimulation if the patient can tolerate it.

Start with:
Ūrdhva Skandha

A.

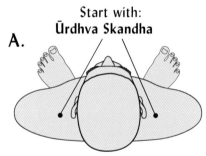

Move to the patient's side and apply pressure to Apastambha **(3)**, followed by each of the Hrid marmāni **(4–6)** for one minute. Slide from Hrid to Hridayam marma **(7)**, followed by Agra Patra **(8)**, Stanya Mūla **(9)** and then Vankri **(10)**. Move along the outer margin of the breast to Stanya Pārshva **(11)** at the lateral aspect of the breast. Repeat this sequence on the other side of the patient.

C. Next, from Agra Patra **(8)** slide along the costal margin over Vankri **(10)** towards Yakrut **(12)** and Plīhā **(13)** and apply pressure to both simultaneously. Then slide towards the midline and Sūrya marma **(14)**. From Sūrya, move outwards to Nābhi 1 and 2 **(15, 16)**, followed by

Nābhi 3 and 4 **(17, 18)**. In general, points over the descending colon should be massaged first, followed by those over the ascending colon.

Finally, stimulate Basti **(19)**, Lohita **(20)** and Vankshana **(21)** to complete the abdominal massage.

B.

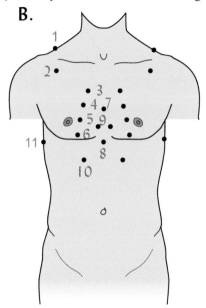

Repeat this sequence on the
left side of the patient.
(Can do both sides at the same time)

C. Follow with:

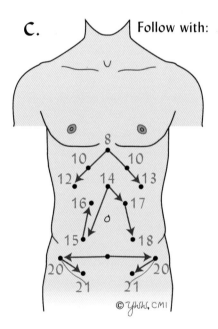

Prushtha (Back) Marmāni (10)

#	Marma Points	Page	Acupoint
70	Amsa Phalaka	160	SI 11
71	Prushtha 1	161	HTJJ T3
72	Prushtha 2	161	HTJJ T4
73	Prushtha 3	161	HTJJ T5
74	Bruhatī	162	----------
76	Vrukka	163	HTJJ T12
77	Kukundara	164	HTJJ L5
78	Kati	165	BL 31
79	Trik	166	BL 35

Prushtha (Back) Marmāni

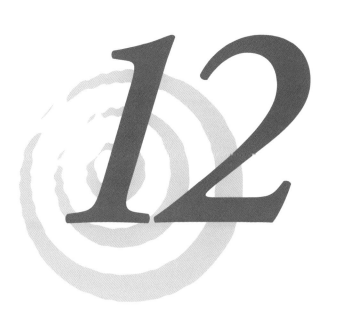

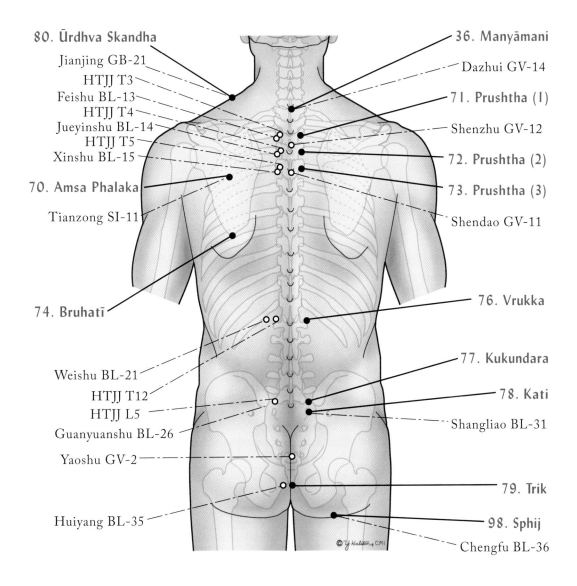

80. Ūrdhva Skandha
Jianjing GB-21
HTJJ T3
Feishu BL-13
HTJJ T4
Jueyinshu BL-14
HTJJ T5
Xinshu BL-15
70. Amsa Phalaka
Tianzong SI-11
74. Bruhatī
Weishu BL-21
HTJJ T12
HTJJ L5
Guanyuanshu BL-26
Yaoshu GV-2
Huiyang BL-35

36. Manyāmani
Dazhui GV-14
71. Prushtha (1)
Shenzhu GV-12
72. Prushtha (2)
73. Prushtha (3)
Shendao GV-11
76. Vrukka
77. Kukundara
78. Kati
Shangliao BL-31
79. Trik
98. Sphij
Chengfu BL-36

© Tj Walston, CMI

Amsa Phalaka

Location
In the infraspinous fossa at the junction of the upper one-third and lower two-thirds of a line that connects the midpoint of the scapular spine and the inferior angle of the scapula.

Action
♦ Facilitates optimal functioning of lungs and airways
♦ Enhances flow of prāna
♦ Relieves lung congestion and bronchospasm
♦ Relieves pain locally
♦ Benefits the heart
♦ Releases unresolved emotions

Associated Doshic Subtypes
Prāna Vāyu, Udāna Vāyu, Sādhaka Pitta, Avalambaka Kapha, Vyāna Vāyu

Indications
♦ Difficulty breathing, asthma, chronic cough
♦ Bronchitis, pleuritic pain
♦ Pain of upper back, neck, shoulders, interscapular area
♦ Ventricular dysfunction, palpitations
♦ Emotional disturbance, such as grief and depression

Treatment
Tulsi and **cinnamon oil** both act on the heart and lungs. Deep massage with **mahānārāyana oil** penetrates into the muscles and relieves local pain.

Corresponding Acupoint
SI 11, Tianzhong (Heavenly Gathering)

In addition to sharing the functions of Amsa Phalaka, SI 11 also benefits the breasts since it is located directly opposite them. Thus, it addresses breast abscess, insufficient lactation and pain and swelling of the breast. It is also noted for treatment of shoulder and elbow pain. SI 11 is one of the most frequently used points for scapular pain due to muscle strain, overuse and poor posture. In TCM, SI 11 treats painful obstruction due to qi and blood stagnation. This correlates to the Ayurvedic view that pain results from an obstruction in the flow of Prāna Vāyu and Vyāna Vāyu.

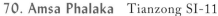

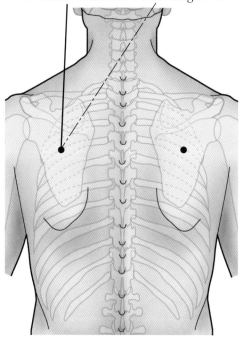

70. Amsa Phalaka   Tianzong SI-11

(points are paired)

Commentary
The term *amsa* is translated as lung and *phalak* as switchboard. The marma acts as a switchboard for the lungs, regulating the flow of pranic energy through the respiratory system. It is connected to the bronchi and pleura. Deep massage in this area releases constriction from the bronchial tree and promotes the flow of prāna. Avalambaka kapha is the subdosha related to the lungs, specifically to pleural fluid. Tenderness at the marma is diagnostic of lung pathology, or it may suggest an early sign of low pulmonary immunity. In many ways, notably its influence on respiration, Amsa Phalaka mirrors Apastambha marma on the anterior aspect of the body.

The name amsa also means fragment, part or shoulder blade. The prefix *am* literally means "to go towards." Massaging the marma and then the rest of the scapula stimulates energy flow towards the shoulder. The marma also alleviates interscapular pain and pain of the upper back, neck and shoulders. Similar to Apastambha, Amsa Phalaka benefits the heart and treats palpitations, especially the marma on the left. A chronic dull aching pain here with low grade fever and evening rise of temperature may denote tuberculosis.

Prushtha or Antar Amsa (3)

Location
3 paired points in the interscapular area.
Prushtha 1 is located one angula lateral to the lower border of spinous process of T3, on both sides.
Prushtha 2 is located one angula lateral to the lower border of spinous process of T4, on both sides.
Prushtha 3 is located one angula lateral to the lower border of spinous process of T5, on both sides.

Action
♦ Regulates functioning of heart and lungs
♦ Relieves bronchospasm and lung congestion
♦ Relieves local pain
♦ Calms the mind, releases stagnant emotions

Associated Doshic Subtypes
Prāna Vāyu, Vyāna Vāyu, Udāna Vāyu, Sādhaka Pitta, Avalambaka Kapha

Indications
♦ Asthma, chronic cough, shortness of breath
♦ Pleuritic pain, upper back pain, shoulder pain
♦ Anginal pain, cardiac pain
♦ Atrial fibrillation and flutter, palpitations
♦ Insomnia
♦ Emotional disturbance

Treatment
Prushtha marmāni are usually treated together. Refer to Amsa Phalaka Treatment section, page 160.

Corresponding Acupoint
Huatuojiaji extra points (T3, T4, T5)

Prushtha 1 – Close to BL 13, Feishu (Lung Shu)

Prushtha 2 – Close to BL 14, Jueyin Shu (Pericardium Shu)

Prushtha 3 – Close to BL 15, Xinshu (Heart Shu)

The Prushtha marmāni correspond to the Huatuojiaji extra points that are located parallel to the spine. The points from T1 to T4 treat the lungs and upper limbs, while those from T4 to T7 are indicated for the heart. This corresponds to the marmāni's affiliation with the heart and lungs. These acupoints alleviate pain and stiffness locally. Refer to appendix B for additional information regarding the Huatuojiaji points.

Prushtha marmāni are also adjacent to acupoints on the Bladder meridian that are 2 anguli or 1.5 cun lateral

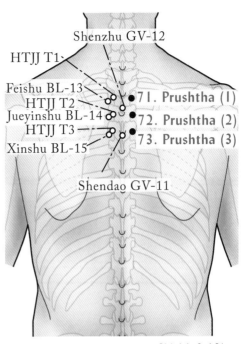

Back

(points are paired except GV 11 & 12)

from the spine. These Bladder points are 1 angula lateral to the Prushtha marmāni and are categorized as Shu points, influential points that affect the corresponding organ at the deepest level. Shu points tonify and strengthen an organ by regulating its action and can be used to treat any disturbance of the organ.

Prushtha 1 is close to BL 13, the preeminent point for all lung disorders. BL 14 corresponds to Prushtha 2 and is the back Shu point for the Pericardium, whose function is similar to that of the Heart. Prushtha 3 is near BL 15, the back Shu point for the Heart. Both BL 14 and BL 15 are indicated for benefiting the chest and heart. Like Prushtha marmāni, the three Shu points are traditionally used for emotional disturbance such as anxiety, grief, fear, disorientation, restlessness, agitation and insomnia. BL 15 is also mentioned in TCM textbooks for epilepsy, dementia, mania and depression.

Commentary
Prushtha is another name for the back. Amsa means lungs and Antar means in between, describing the location of these three paired marmāni between the lungs and the interscapular area. All of them are functionally related to the lungs and heart, regulating respiration and cardiac activity.

These marmāni are most commonly referred to as Prushtha 1, 2 or 3. Each is associated with its own specific influences. Prushtha 1 is associated primarily with the heart and lungs. Prushtha 2 is related to the trachea and bronchi. Prushtha 1 and 2 relieve asthma, chronic cough and shortness of breath by stimulating the flow of prāna to the lungs. They balance udāna vāyu, which is involved in the acts of coughing, yawning and sneezing. In addition, Prushtha 2 enkindles jāthara agni, the "fire" of the digestive system responsible for digestion and assimilation. Prushtha 3 is associated with anginal pain or pain from posterior myocardial infarction (MI) that radiates to the interscapular area. All Prushtha marmāni calm the mind and effectively treat insomnia. They release unexpressed, stagnant emotions that may be vāta or kapha in nature. Severe pain at Prushtha marma, accompanied by nausea, vomiting, and sweating, may indicate severe heart attack.

Bruhatī

Location
Immediately below the inferior angle of the scapula on both sides of the body.

Action
♦ Regulates respiration
♦ Acts on lower lobes of lungs and diaphragm
♦ Enhances flow of prāna
♦ Benefits function of the liver, gallbladder, spleen
♦ Relieves pain locally

Associated Doshic Subtypes
Prāna Vāyu, Vyāna Vāyu, Samāna Vāyu, Udāna Vāyu, Rañjaka Pitta

Indications
♦ Difficulty breathing
♦ Hepatic pain, splenic pain, intercostal pain
♦ Liver and spleen disorders, congestion in spleen
♦ Lymphatic congestion, generalized lymph adenopathy

Treatment
Kewrā is used for the liver and kadamba oil for the spleen.[5] Deep massage with mahānārāyana oil penetrates into the muscles and relieves local pain.

Corresponding Acupoint
None

74. Bruhatī (paired)

Commentary
Bruhatī means expansion to promote easy breathing. It is derived from the prefix *bru*, which means to increase or expand. Deep breathing increases diaphragmatic movement, leading to expansion of the lungs. This action stimulates the marma. Bruhatī enhances the flow of prāna vāyu that governs respiration. It is effective for shortness of breath due to anxiety or shallow breathing. Pressure on the marma soothes the respiratory system and calms the breath. Another translation for Bruhatī is support. The marma "supports" the entire scapula and alleviates local pain that can manifest in the scapular, interscapular or intercostal regions. In addition, the marma on the right reduces hepatic pain, while the marma on the left reduces splenic pain.

Bruhatī benefits the liver and spleen by alleviating inflammation or congestion of either organ. This can result from impaired vyāna vāyu, which governs circulation. Bruhatī on the left side of the body is functionally related to the mitral valve, heart and spleen, and on the right side to the liver and gallbladder. A sharp pain under the right Bruhatī marma may indicate gallstones; for sharp pain under left Bruhatī, think about splenitis.

---

5. See chapter 15 for more information on these essential oils.

Vrukka

Location
One angula lateral to the lower border of the spinous process of T12, on each side.

Action
♦ Regulates functioning of the kidneys, adrenals and bladder
♦ Regulates glomerular function (renal filtration)
♦ Pacifies renal pain and low backache

Associated Doshic Subtypes
Apāna Vāyu, Vyāna Vāyu

Indications
♦ Kidney dysfunction, renal colic, kidney stone, renal infections
♦ Adrenal pain, adrenal insufficiency
♦ Urethritis, urinary tract infection (UTI), cystitis
♦ Edema of lower extremities
♦ Low back pain, sciatica
♦ Emotional disturbance

Treatment
Pressure may be applied at the marma with **nutmeg oil**, a mild analgesic. Deep massage with **mahānārāyana oil** penetrates into the muscles and relieves local pain.

Corresponding Acupoint
Huatuojiaji extra points (T12)

Close to BL 21, Weishu (Stomach Shu)

Vrukka marma corresponds to the Huatuojiaji points that lie at the level of T12. Unlike Vrukka, the points from T10 to T12 are used to treat disorders of the spleen and stomach. For treating kidney disorders, the Huatuojiaji points that lie at the level of L1 and L2 are commonly used. Refer to appendix B for additional information regarding the Huatuojiaji points.

BL 21 lies approximately 1.5 cun lateral to T12, or 1 angula lateral to Vrukka marma. The acupoint's influence does not match Vrukka, though it is the Shu point of the Stomach meridian and treats a wide range of disorders of the stomach and digestive system.

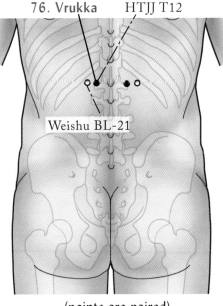

76. Vrukka   HTJJ T12

Weishu BL-21

(points are paired)

Commentary
The Sanskrit term Vrukka means organ of water filtration. The prefix *vru* means to filter and *ka* means water. The kidneys are vital organs, part of the body's water regulating system, that filter the water component from the blood. Vru also means hidden, restrained or surrounded.

Vrukka is the principal marma for treating the kidneys. If sensitive upon palpation, it may suggest kidney and adrenal gland dysfunction. It is also functionally related to the bladder and ambu vaha srotas (channels of water). As the name implies, Vrukka marma treats conditions resulting from improper filtration of water, such as edema and UTI. It is associated with apāna vāyu that governs elimination and vyāna vāyu that governs circulation. Locally, it relieves low back pain. The emotion of fear is associated with the kidneys, and can be pacified by therapeutic attention to Vrukka.

Kukundara

Back

Location
One angula lateral from the lower border of the spinous process of L5, on each side.

Action
♦ Benefits kidney and bladder functions
♦ Regulates colon activity
♦ Relieves pain locally
♦ Balances apāna vāyu

Associated Doshic Subtypes
Apāna Vāyu, Vyāna Vāyu

Indications
♦ Kidney pain, bladder pain
♦ Urethritis, ureteric pain, enuresis (bed wetting), frequent urination
♦ Chronic constipation, diarrhea
♦ Low back pain, lumbar radiculopathy (sciatica)

Treatment
Refer to Vrukka Treatment section, page 163.

Corresponding Acupoint
Huatuojiaji extra point (L5)

Close to BL 26, Guanyuanshu (Gate of Origin Shu)

The Huatuojiaji point located at the level of L5 treats disorders of the bladder, large and small intestines, uterus and lower limbs. Similarly, Kukundara acts on the bladder, colon and lower limbs. Refer to appendix B for additional information regarding the Huatuojiaji points. BL 26 is located 1.5 cun from the spine and 1 angula lateral to Kukundara marma. Similar to the marma, the acupoint is indicated for lumbar pain, constipation, diarrhea and urinary disorders. In addition, BL 26 treats abdominal distention in women.

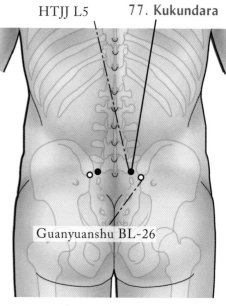

HTJJ L5   77. Kukundara

Guanyuanshu BL-26

(points are paired)

Commentary
Kukundara is translated as "that which supports the vertebral column and the back." It is a pillar of strength and support for the body. It is anatomically related to the part of the vertebral column where the lumbar spine meets the sacral spine. Lumbar pain may be due to myofascial tightness, degenerative joint disease (DJD) or even a herniated disc. In lumbar radiculopathy, pain is due to inflammation of nerve roots from the lumbar and/or sacral spine. This is commonly called a pinched nerve or sciatica.

Kukundara is functionally related to the organs of elimination including the kidneys, bladder, ureter and colon. These organs play a vital role in eliminating toxins from the body and maintaining homeostasis. Apāna vāyu governs all elimination and is balanced by applying pressure on the marma. Kukundara is also related to ambu vaha srotas and addresses urinary dysfunction.

The prefix *ku* means earth, and *ka* means water. Kapha is primarily a combination of earth and water and represents all substance and matter. It is solid, stable, grounded and supportive. This marma balances kapha.

Kati

Location
In the first posterior sacral foramen.

Action
♦ Benefits bladder
♦ Benefits ovaries and fallopian tubes
♦ Relieves inflammation
♦ Relieves local congestion
♦ Relieves pain locally

Associated Doshic Subtypes
Apāna Vāyu, Rañjaka Pitta, Kledaka Kapha

Indications
♦ Bladder pain, cystitis, kidney stones
♦ Ovarian dysfunction
♦ Low back pain, lumbar radiculopathy (sciatica)
♦ Sacroiliac joint pain
♦ Low libido, impotence

Treatment
Refer to Vrukka Treatment section, page 163.

Corresponding Acupoint
BL 31, Shangliao (Upper Crevice)

Similar to Kati, BL 31 treats urinary disturbance, impotence and low back pain. It is indicated for a number of menstrual conditions, while Kati addresses only ovarian dysfunction. BL 31 is frequently used in conjunction with BL 32, BL 33 and BL 34 located in the 2nd, 3rd and 4th posterior sacral foramen. Of these, BL 32 is the most powerful.

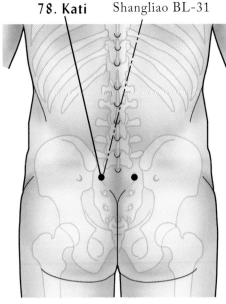

Back

78. Kati   Shangliao BL-31

(points are paired)

Commentary
The translation of *kati* is hip or waist, to both of which the marma is anatomically related. When a garment or cloth is wrapped around the hips or waist, it touches the marma. Kati is functionally related to the bladder, ovaries, testes and colon. Pain and dysfunction of these organs is due to apāna vāyu disturbance. Kati marma is related to the male and female reproductive tissues (shukra and ārtava) and addresses imbalance in these structures. Locally, it relieves low back pain, especially in conjunction with Kukundara. Kati is functionally related to the sacroiliac joint and provides stability to the lumbo-pelvic area, facilitating proper posture and locomotion. Misalignment of the sacroiliac (SI) joint precipitates several low back disorders, such as low back pain and lumbar radiculopathy (sciatica).

Trik

Location
At the tip of the coccyx.

Action
♦ Relieves pain
♦ Benefits urinary and reproductive systems
♦ Benefits pelvic floor
♦ Stimulates kundalinī energy

Associated Doshic Subtypes
Apāna Vāyu, Rañjaka Pitta, Kledaka Kapha

Indications
♦ Low back pain, pain at the coccyx
♦ Sacroiliac joint pain, pain in sacral area
♦ Lumbar radiculopathy (sciatica) (see page 164)
♦ Rectal pain, fissures, hemorrhoids
♦ Urinary retention, frequency of urination
♦ Cervical dysfunction, prostate dysfunction, impotence
♦ Low libido, pelvic floor disorders

Treatment
Castor oil, brahmī oil or **tikta ghrita (bitter ghee)** can be applied to the marma. Strong irritant oils, such as tea tree or nutmeg, should be avoided because the marma is located close to the anal orifice.

Corresponding Acupoint
None

Close to BL 35, Huiyang (Meeting of Yang)

Close to GV 2, Yaoshu (Lumbar Shu)

BL 35 is located 0.5 cun lateral to the coccyx on either side and is closer to Trik. GV 2 is on the midline of the sacrococcygeal hiatus. These acupoints, as well as the marma, are all indicated for the treatment of local pain in the sacral and lumbar area, as well as for hemorrhoids and rectal disturbance. Their sphere of influence also extends to reproductive imbalances. Trik and BL 35 both treat impotence. Trik is indicated for cervical and prostate dysfunction, low libido and pelvic floor disorders, while BL 35 addresses genital itching and leukorrhea. GV 2 can be used for irregular menses and leukorrhea. In addition, BL 35 treats diarrhea, dysentery and blood in the stools, which the other two energy points do not address.

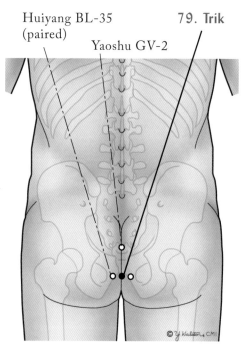

Huiyang BL-35 (paired)   Yaoshu GV-2   79. Trik

Commentary
Trik and *trikon* both mean triangle. In *trikonāsana* (triangle pose, a yoga posture), the marma is stretched and activated, thus helping to alleviate back pain. The marma's name refers to the sacral angle and the triangular tip of the coccyx. It is functionally related to the prostate and cervix. Hence, it treats many reproductive disturbances as well as shukra and ārtava dhātus, the male and female reproductive tissue. Trik addresses urinary dysfunction because of its connection to ambu vaha srotas (channels of water). It balances apāna vāyu, which governs elimination. Locally, it relieves pain in the sacral area.

Trik is a mystical marma because of its association as the seat of dormant kundalinī energy. It is intimately related to the mūlādhāra chakra located at the base of the spine. From the marma, kundalinī travels upwards to the crown chakra and Mūrdhni marma. In *padmāsana* (lotus pose, a yoga posture), both Trik and Mūrdhni marmāni are gently stimulated, activating kundalinī.

Marma Massage for the Back

If you are not very familiar with Ayurvedic marma therapy, before attempting the following procedure please review chapter 8, especially "Guidelines for Touch and Pressure" on page 75 that offers specific instructions about massaging marmāni. Appendix C has the series of marma massage directions and illustrations starting on page 284.

The instructions here refer to the drawings on these pages. The numbers are for use with these massage drawings only; they are different from the numbering system for the marma points used throughout the book. To look up details on a particular marma point, refer to the beginning of this chapter, page 159, to the tables that reference all the marma points and their page numbers.

Apply a few drops of essential oil to the tips of the fingers. Start with gentle pressure on the marma points, and gradually increase according to the capacity of the individual. If you use too much pressure, the person will show discomfort through facial expressions, such as wrinkling of the face, or by saying "Ouch!" Pressure on all marmāni should be held for approximately one to two minutes. If you feel that stronger pressure is needed, you can apply it when the patient exhales.

A. Ask the patient to lie in a prone position (face down) and stand at the head end. This massage naturally follows massaging the back of the neck. Because the muscles of the back are strong and relatively stiff, it requires deeper pressure with the thumbs.

Begin by stimulating Ūrdhva Skandha **(1)** and then slide to Amsa Phalaka **(2)**. Repeat this three times. Move medially towards Manyāmani **(3)** at C7, and then slide the thumbs down along both sides of the spine all the way to the lumbar area. Repeat this motion three times.

B. Next, apply steady pressure for one minute each from Manyāmani **(3)** to Prushtha marmāni **(4, 5, 6)** located at T3, T4 and T5. Slide the fingers along the medial border of the scapula until they reach Bruhatī marma **(7)**. Continue from Bruhatī to Pārshva Sandhi **(8)**, and from there move towards the spine and stimulate Vrukka **(9)**, then Kukundara **(10)** and Kati **(11)**. Repeat this motion two or three times. End the massage by giving added emphasis to Trik marma **(12)**.

Back

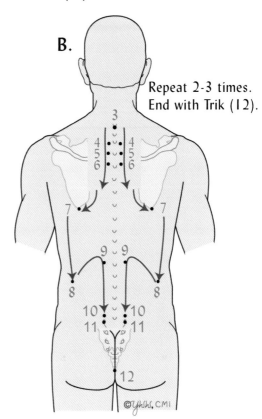

B.

Repeat 2-3 times.
End with Trik (12).

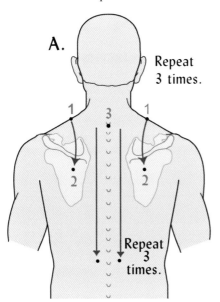

A.

Repeat 3 times.

Repeat 3 times.

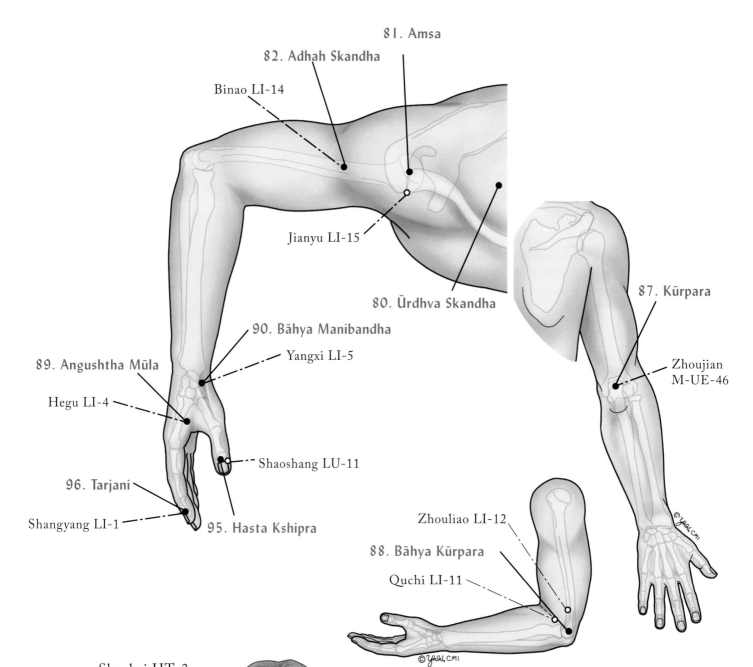

81. Amsa

82. Adhah Skandha

Binao LI-14

Jianyu LI-15

80. Ūrdhva Skandha

87. Kūrpara

Zhoujian M-UE-46

90. Bāhya Manibandha

Yangxi LI-5

89. Angushtha Mūla

Hegu LI-4

Shaoshang LU-11

96. Tarjani

Shangyang LI-1

95. Hasta Kshipra

Zhouliao LI-12

88. Bāhya Kūrpara

Quchi LI-11

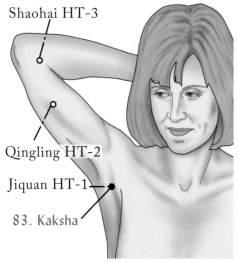

Shaohai HT-3

Qingling HT-2

Jiquan HT-1

83. Kaksha

Bahu (Arm) Marmāni (10)

#	Marma Points	Page	Acupoint
80	Ūrdhva Skandha	170	GB 21
81	Amsa	171	≈LI 15
82	Adhah Skandha	172	LI 14
83	Kaksha	173	HT 1
84	Bāhu Ūrvī	174	≈HT 2
85	Ānī	175	PC 3
86	Bāhū Indrabasta	176	≈HT 3, PC 3
87	Kūrpara	178	Zhoujian
88	Bāhya Kūrpara	179	≈LI 11

Ūrdhva Shakhah (Upper Extremities) Marmāni

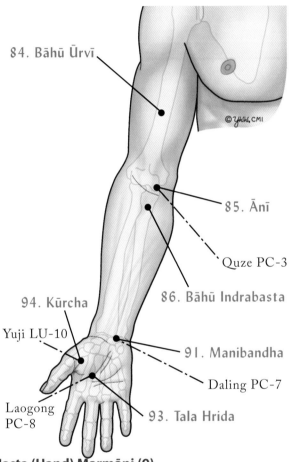

84. Bāhū Ūrvī

85. Āni

Quze PC-3

86. Bāhū Indrabasta

94. Kūrcha

Yuji LU-10

91. Manibandha

Daling PC-7

Laogong PC-8

93. Tala Hrida

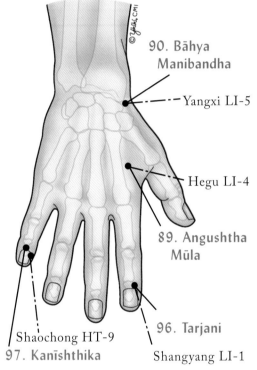

90. Bāhya Manibandha

Yangxi LI-5

Hegu LI-4

89. Angushtha Mūla

96. Tarjani

Shaochong HT-9

97. Kanīshthika

Shangyang LI-1

Hasta (Hand) Marmāni (9)

#	Marma Points	Page	Acupoint
89	Angushtha Mūla	180	LI 4
90	Bāhya Manibandha	181	LI 5
91	Manibandha	182	PC 7
92	Kūrcha Shira	183	SI 5
93	Tala Hrida	184	PC 8
94	Kūrcha	185	LU 10
95	Hasta Kshipra	186	LU 11
96	Tarjani	187	LI 1
97	Kanīshthika	188	≈HT 9

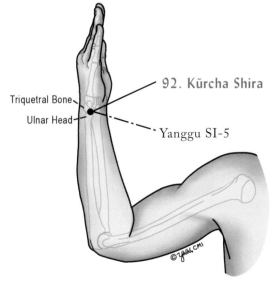

92. Kūrcha Shira

Triquetral Bone

Ulnar Head

Yanggu SI-5

Ūrdhva Skandha

Arms
Hands

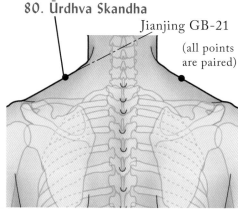

80. Ūrdhva Skandha

Jianjing GB-21

(all points are paired)

Location
At the superior aspect of the trapezius muscle, midway between the tip of the spinous process of C7 and the tip of the acromion.

Action
♦ Relieves local pain
♦ Relieves stiffness in shoulder
♦ Facilitates flow of prana into lungs and upper chest
♦ Relieves occipital headaches
♦ Relieves stress, calms the mind
♦ Releases stagnant, unexpressed emotions

Associated Doshic Subtypes
Prāna Vāyu, Udāna Vāyu, Vyāna Vāyu, Avalambaka Kapha, Shleshaka Kapha

Indications
♦ Pain, stiffness or tightness in neck and upper back
♦ Radiculopathy (pinched nerve)
♦ Interscapular pain due to muscle tightness
♦ Degenerative joint disease (DJD)
♦ Adhesive capsulitis (frozen shoulder), bursitis, shoulder pain
♦ Rotator cuff tendonitis, bicipital tendonitis
♦ Occipital headaches
♦ Shortness of breath, asthma, hiccups, bronchitis
♦ Stress, mental fatigue, insomnia

Treatment
Skandha marmāni may be massaged with **vacha** or **camphor oil**, along with other marmāni on the upper limbs. Deep massage with **mahānārāyana oil** or **Tiger Balm**® relieves pain and stiffness locally and soothes tense muscles.

Corresponding Acupoint
GB 21, Jianjing (Shoulder Well)

GB 21 is a principal acupoint on the Gallbladder meridian. It is located midway between GV 14 (which corresponds to Manyāmani at the base of C7) and the tip of the acromion. It shares the same functions as Ūrdhva Skandha for aligning the shoulders and descending "rebellious Qi," the equivalent of hyperactive udāna vāyu. Unlike Skandha marma, GB 21 is not indicated for insomnia, headaches in the occipital region, or any of the lung conditions mentioned. GB 21 also benefits the breasts for local pain, abscesses and difficulty with lacta-tion. Classical texts mention its use for uterine bleeding and phlegm accumulation into nodules.

Commentary
Two principal marma points influence the shoulder. One is Ūrdhva Skandha on the upper aspect of the trapezius muscle, and the other is Adhah Skandha on the lateral aspect of the shoulder. They can be used in conjunction with each other to relieve disturbance of the shoulder joint. The marma on the right corresponds to the liver and on the left to the spleen.

Skandha may be poetically translated as shouldering responsibility. Ūrdhva Skandha is located at a part of the body associated with support. The Grīvā marmāni located on the back of the neck are also linked with responsibility. Many individuals in modern society carry the "weight of the world" on their shoulders. As a result, they develop pain and stiffness in the neck, shoulders and upper back; commonly, the neck's range of motion also becomes limited. Pain may radiate to the occipital region of the head. Indeed, stress is one of the most common causes of occipital or tension headaches. Tension accruing in these areas also leads to mental fatigue and insomnia.

Stimulating Ūrdhva Skandha relieves these conditions and facilitates the flow of prana to the lungs and upper chest. Hence, treatment here benefits many lung conditions and may relieve hiccups, a disturbance of udāna vāyu, the upward moving energy. Pressure on Ūrdhva Skandha stimulates the downward flow of energy.

Skandha is the name of one of the sons of Lord Shiva and his wife Pārvatī, two important deities in Hinduism. (The other son is Ganesha.) In South India, the deity Skandha is also known by the names Murga, Kārttikeya and Subramanyam. He is often portrayed as a warrior armed with bow and arrow who carries tremendous responsibility. His bow rests on his shoulder and touches Skandha marma.

Amsa

Location
At the top of the shoulder at the center of the acromion.

Action
♦ Gives freedom of movement to the shoulder
♦ Relieves pain and stiffness locally
♦ Enhances flow of prāna
♦ Benefits ears
♦ Stimulates pancreatic function
♦ Relieves stress

Associated Doshic Subtypes
Prāna Vāyu, Vyāna Vāyu, Udāna Vāyu, Avalambaka Kapha, Kledaka Kapha, Shleshaka Kapha

Indications
♦ Shoulder pain, bursitis
♦ Rotator cuff tendonitis, bicipital tendonitis
♦ Adhesive capsulitis (frozen shoulder)
♦ Asthma, bronchitis
♦ Palpitations
♦ Tinnitus (ringing in the ears), earache
♦ Pancreatic dysfunction
♦ Emotional tension, stress, fatigue

Treatment
Refer to Ūrdhva Skandha Treatment section, page 170.

Corresponding Acupoint
None

Close to LI 15, Jianyu (Shoulder Bone)

LI 15 shares Amsa's ability to benefit the shoulder and arm. It dispels Wind according to TCM theory, an action similar to Amsa's ability to balance the vāyus, subtypes of vāta dosha. Unlike Amsa, LI 15 is also indicated for the treatment of goiter, seminal emission and hypertension.

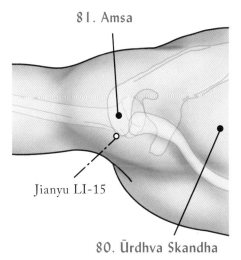

81. Amsa

Jianyu LI-15

80. Ūrdhva Skandha

Commentary
Amsa is translated as the top part of the shoulder or lung. Similar to Ūrdhva Skandha, Amsa can relieve shoulder pain and improve conditions where there is a limited range of movement. Both marmāni stimulate shleshaka kapha, which lubricates the joints and is affected whenever there are joint disorders. Both also enhance the flow of prāna to the lungs and treat asthma and bronchitis. Of the two, Ūrdhva Skandha is more effective.

Stimulating udāna vāyu via these marmāni promotes vitality and energy, thereby reducing stress, fatigue and emotional tension. Amsa calms down palpitations, a disturbance of vyāna vāyu. It also aids in balancing blood sugar and can be massaged if there is pancreatic dysfunction. The marma on the right is associated with the liver and on the left with the spleen, similar to Ūrdhva Skandha.

Adhah Skandha

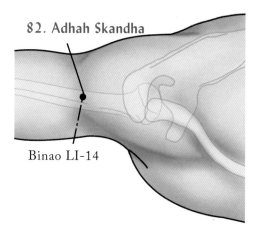

82. Adhah Skandha

Binao LI-14

Location
On the lateral side of the upper arm, in a depression between the insertion of the deltoid and brachialis muscle.

Action
♦ Benefits upper extremities and shoulders
♦ Influences lungs and stomach
♦ Relieves stress, stagnant emotions

Associated Doshic Subtypes
Prāna Vāyu, Vyāna Vāyu, Udāna Vāyu, Avalambaka Kapha, Kledaka Kapha, Shleshaka Kapha, Pāchaka Pitta

Indications
♦ Adhesive capsulitis (frozen shoulder), shoulder pain, bursitis
♦ Neuropathy of upper extremities, tremors
♦ Poor circulation, cold hands, forearm pain
♦ Lymphedema (swelling) of upper extremities
♦ Congestion in lungs, asthma, bronchitis
♦ High acidity, gastritis
♦ Emotional disturbance

Treatment
Refer to Ūrdhva Skandha Treatment section, page 170.

Corresponding Acupoint
LI 14, Binao (Upper Arm)

LI 14 benefits the shoulder, arm and neck as does Adhah Skandha. Unlike the marma, it is indicated for goiter, chest pain, and redness, swelling or pain of the eyes. It does not have the same influence on balancing emotions, or on the stomach and lungs, as the marma.

Commentary
Adhah Skandha is translated as the downward aspect of the shoulder and also means support. Along with Ūrdhva Skandha, Adhah Skandha addresses many disturbances of the shoulder. Stimulating the marma enhances circulation of prāna and thereby reduces pain. Adhah Skandha may be stimulated for referred pain from C5 to C6 and for tingling and numbness in the arms.

The marma is functionally related to the neck, and to the upper lobes of the lungs. Tenderness on palpation of this marma may suggest lung disturbance. All congestion in the lungs is associated with avalambaka kapha and this marma helps to release any excess accumulation of kapha dosha.

Adhah Skandha is also functionally related to the stomach. It is indicated in hyperacidity, gastritis and upset stomach, which are all disturbances of pāchaka pitta. However, Shankha and Sūrya marmāni are more effective for the treatment of these disturbances; Adhah Skandha pacifies primarily vāta and kapha types of emotional imbalance.

Kaksha

• • • • • • • • • • • • • • • • • • • •

Location
In the armpit, at the apex of the axillary fossa.

Action
♦ Benefits the breasts
♦ Improves lymphatic drainage of breast tissue
♦ Enhances blood and lymph circulation in upper extremities
♦ Regulates sweating
♦ Relaxes shoulder and upper extremities

Associated Doshic Subtypes
Vyāna Vāyu, Pāchaka Pitta, Shleshaka Kapha, Avalambaka Kapha

Indications
♦ Congestion in breast tissue, mastitis
♦ Pain, tenderness or swelling of the breast
♦ Fibrocystic changes in the breast, breast abscess
♦ Axillary lymph adenopathy (enlarged lymph nodes)
♦ Excessive sweating, strong acidic smell to sweat, anhidrosis (lack of sweating)
♦ Shoulder pain, rotator cuff tendonitis, brachial plexopathy (injury of plexus)
♦ Adhesive capsulitis (frozen shoulder)

Treatment
To reduce vāta-type pain, massage **nutmeg** or **vacha oil** deeply into the axilla. Pressure can also be applied at the marma with a thin rod (*shalākā*), an instrument for focusing pressure on marmāni or acupoints.

Corresponding Acupoint
HT 1, Jiquan (Summit Spring)

Similar to Kaksha, HT 1 affects the shoulder and arm. It is indicated for pain in the axilla and shoulder areas. Unlike Kaksha, the acupoint is recommended for elbow pain as well as for palpitations, shortness of breath, anxiety and sadness. The emotional indications are due to its location on the Heart meridian. HT 1 also addresses chest pain; an internal branch of the heart meridian traverses this area.

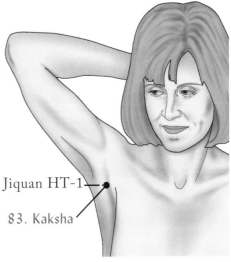

Jiquan HT-1

83. Kaksha

Arms Hands

Commentary
The name *kaksha* is translated as armpit. It is functionally related to the pectoralis major and minor muscles, similar to Kakshadhara marma (see page 136). Both of these marmāni relieve congestion, promote lymphatic drainage and alleviate pain in the shoulder, arm, breast and pectoralis muscles. Because Kaksha improves circulation to the upper extremities, a function of vyāna vāyu, it can be effective in the treatment of numerous shoulder problems. On the right side, it is connected to the right breast and lymph nodes of the right underarm; the marma on the left is affiliated with the left breast and lymph nodes of the left underarm region. Tenderness on palpation at the site of the marma may suggest pathology in the regions functionally related to it.

Bāhu Ūrvī

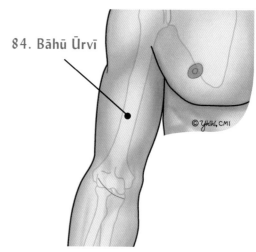

84. Bāhū Ūrvī

Location
At the center of the belly of the biceps muscle on the anterior aspect of the upper arm.

*Arms
Hands*

Action
♦ Promotes normal movement of upper extremities
♦ Relieves tremor or abnormal movement of upper extremities
♦ Increases energy and vitality
♦ Regulates udāna vāyu
♦ Promotes stomach and pancreas secretion
♦ Stimulates solar plexus

Associated Doshic Subtypes
Udāna Vāyu, Samāna vāyu, Vyāna Vāyu, Pāchaka Pitta, Kledaka Kapha

Indications
♦ Neuropathy of upper extremities, tremors
♦ Lymphedema of upper extremities
♦ Poor circulation, cold hands
♦ Chronic fatigue syndrome, myalgia (generalized muscle ache)
♦ Gastric dysfunction, nausea, vomiting
♦ Pancreatic dysfunction, hyperglycemia
♦ Colon dysfunction – flatulence, constipation, diverticulosis

Treatment
Nutmeg, vacha and **mahānārāyana oils** are effective in relieving pain and stiffness. They can be applied on Bāhu Ūrvī and then massaged along the entire length of the upper arm. Use gentle pressure at first and then steadily increase according to the patient's tolerance.

Corresponding Acupoint
None

Close to HT 2, Qingling (Green Spirit)

HT 2 is located 3 cun proximal to the medial end of the transverse cubital crease. It is approximately one cun medial and one cun posterior to Bāhu Ūrvī. It does not share many of the same actions as the marma. It is primarily used to treat pain and swelling of the arm and shoulder or difficulty in raising the arm.

Commentary
Bahu is translated as arm and *urvi* as raising energy and vitality. Stimulating the marma enlivens the upward-rising udāna vāyu, which promotes energetic effort, zeal, and motivation, and governs strength, including strength of will. Hence, this marma can be effective in treatment of chronic fatigue and generalized body ache. Bāhu Ūrvī is located on the biceps muscle, associated with strength and physical power. The marma is related to the median nerve and brachial plexus. Locally, it is useful to treat the upper extremities for limited range of movement.

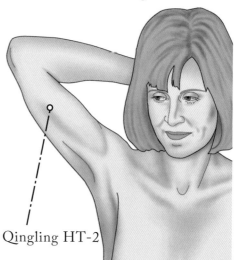

Qingling HT-2

Bāhu Ūrvī influences the solar plexus because it is functionally related to the stomach through jāthara agni and to the pancreas through kloma agni. These agnis are the metabolic components responsible for regulating these organs' activities. Pancreatic dysfunction is the result of low kloma agni, while gastric dysfunction is due to low jāthara agni. Massage of Bāhu Ūrvī also pacifies pāchaka pitta, helping to alleviate gastric conditions such as nausea and vomiting. Its strong action on vāta dosha makes it effective for colon dysfunctions like flatulence, constipation and diverticulosis.

Āni

· ·

Location
At the cubital crease of the elbow, on the ulnar side of the tendon of the biceps brachii muscle.

Action
♦ Maintains bladder tone
♦ Regulates fluids and ambu vaha srotas
♦ Treats urinary dysfunction
♦ Promotes normal range of movement of upper extremities
♦ Relieves localized pain

Associated Doshic Subtypes
Apāna Vāyu, Vyāna Vāyu, Kledaka Kapha, Shleshaka Kapha

Indications
♦ Bladder dysfunction – urinary incontinence, cystitis, bladder stones
♦ Pancreatic dysfunction
♦ Neuropathy of upper extremities, tremors
♦ Lymphedema of the upper extremities
♦ Pain in elbow and forearm, epicondylitis (golfer's elbow, tennis elbow)
♦ Carpal tunnel syndrome

Treatment
Refer to Bāhu Ūrvī Treatment section, page 174.

Corresponding Acupoint
PC 3, Quze (Marsh at the Creek)

Like Āni, PC 3 acts locally on the arm and elbow. It is associated with the stomach, while Āni exerts more influence on the pancreas. PC 3 is indicated for vomiting and diarrhea. Both points are related to water, but this is expressed differently in their actions. Āni balances and regulates water by addressing urinary disturbances that are due to an imbalance of the water element. PC 3, being the water point on the Pericardium meridian, possesses a strong ability to clear heat and is not necessarily used for water imbalances such as urinary disturbance.

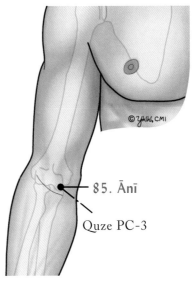

85. Āni

Quze PC-3

Commentary
The English translation of *āni* is tonification. Āni tonifies the bladder and treats bladder dysfunction. Tenderness on palpation may be felt at the marma in cases of bladder or kidney pathology, and as a precursor to cystitis. Kidney or bladder stones develop when excess kapha dosha accumulates and hardens into a stone. Āni can decrease the build up of kapha to some degree, but the most effective treatment for stones is internal administration of specific Ayurvedic herbs.

Āni regulates ambu vaha srotas, the water carrying channels, and it strengthens the function of structures related to ambu vaha srotas, such as the kidneys, bladder and pancreas. Like Bāhu Ūrvī, the marma influences pancreatic function by stimulating kloma agni.

Locally, pressure applied to Āni benefits the region of the elbow and forearm. It can pacify tingling, numbness, pain and tremors by its action on vyāna vāyu. Elbow pain may be due to epicondylitis. Lateral epicondylitis is commonly referred to as tennis elbow, and medial epicondylitis as golfer's elbow. Āni can also address carpal tunnel syndrome, especially in conjunction with Manibandha (see page 182).

Bāhū Indrabasta

Location
Two anguli below the midpoint of the cubital crease, inferior to Ānī.

Action
♦ Relieves pain locally
♦ Regulates colon functions
♦ Stimulates agni and expels toxins
♦ Stabilizes the mind
♦ Releases stagnant emotions

Associated Doshic Subtypes
Apāna Vāyu, Vyāna Vāyu, Sādhaka Pitta

Indications
♦ Neuropathy of upper extremities, tremors
♦ Lymphedema (swelling) of upper extremities
♦ Carpal tunnel syndrome
♦ Colon dysfunction: constipation, diarrhea, flatulence
♦ Irritable bowel syndrome (IBS)
♦ Inflammatory bowel disease, Crohn's disease, ulcerative colitis
♦ Menstrual cramps
♦ Emotional disturbance, especially vāta type

Treatment
Vacha oil and **sandalwood oil** pacify vāta and pitta, respectively. **Mahānārāyana oil** decreases pain and stiffness locally. Pressure should be applied on Bāhū Indrabasta and then massaged along the entire length of the upper arm.

Corresponding Acupoint
None

Close to HT 3, Shaohai (Lesser Sea)

Close to PC 3, Quze (Marsh at the Crook)

This marma does not have a corresponding acupoint but it is in close proximity to a few powerful acupoints located in the medial crease of the elbow. HT 3 is at the medial end of the transverse cubital crease while P 3 is on the ulnar side of the biceps brachii tendon located in the cubital crease. Both acupoints do also share the function of treating arm pain, tremors and swelling. Interestingly, they are also powerful points to harmonize the emotions similar to Bāhū Indrabasta.

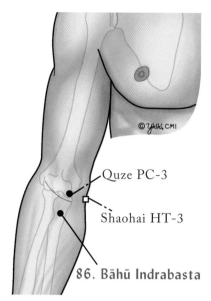

Quze PC-3
Shaohai HT-3
86. Bāhū Indrabasta

Commentary
The word *indrabasta* means the stable crown of Indra. Indra is the Lord of all the deities in the Hindu pantheon. By testing an individual's spiritual efforts (known as *tapasyā* in Sanskrit), he gauges the stability of his devotees in terms of persistent effort and dedication. Persistence in spiritual effort—or any activity in life—requires stability of mind and mastery of mental and emotional fluctuations.

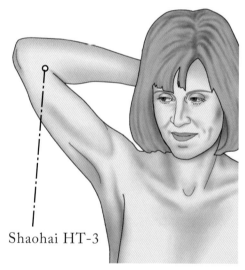

Shaohai HT-3

According to Āyurveda, there is a strong connection between the mind and the colon. Without proper elimination of the bowels, the mind becomes clogged with negative thoughts and emotions (mental āma). As a result, mental function is impaired and there is lack of clarity. That is why it is recommended to have a regular bowel movement in the early morning before commencing meditation, so that the mind is clear and still. In addition, the colon is the seat of vāta dosha. An unhealthy or clogged colon fosters fluctuations of the dosha, which unsettles the mind and leads to instability in life. Steadiness of mind, persistence, focus and the ability to sustain effort in a chosen direction are all weakened by an excess of vāta dosha.

Massage of Indrabasta marmāni helps to regulate the colon, balances vāta and thus stabilizes the mind and pacifies vāta-type emotions such as restlessness, fear, anxiety, nervousness and other qualities that disturb a person's equilibrium.

There are three Indrabasta marmāni on the extremities. Two are located on the posterior and medial aspects of the leg, while Bāhū Indrabasta is located on the arm. All three share a similar action on colon disorders such as constipation, IBS and inflammatory bowel disease. Sensitivity upon palpation of these marmāni suggests colon dysfunction and the accumulation of āma (toxins). Bāhū Indrabasta located on the left arm is functionally related to the descending colon and splenic flexure, while on the right arm it is affiliated with the ascending colon, cecum and hepatic flexure.

By stimulating vyāna vāyu, Bāhū Indrabasta also helps to relieve menstrual cramps. The marma can also be used locally to relieve arm or elbow pain.

Arms
Hands

Kūrpara

• •

Location
On the elbow, at the tip of the olecranon process of the ulna.

Action
♦ Regulates coordination of movement of upper extremities and elbow
♦ Relieves pain locally

Associated Doshic Subtypes
Vyāna Vāyu, Shleshaka Kapha

Indications
♦ Pain or restricted movement of the elbow and forearm
♦ Epicondylitis (golfer's elbow or tennis elbow)

Treatment
Refer to Bāhu Ūrvī Treatment section, page 174.

Corresponding Acupoint
Zhoujian (Elbow Tip)

Zhoujian, an extra point, is considered to have a broader range of action than Kūrpara marma. It is primarily recommended for scrofula and intestinal abscesses, because it transforms phlegm and reduces swelling. It is contraindicated for needling and is instead only treated with moxibustion.

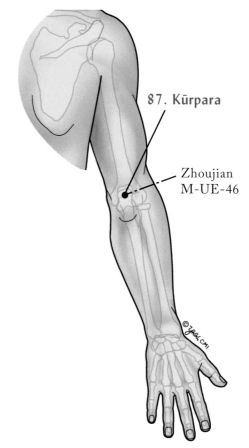

87. Kūrpara

Zhoujian
M-UE-46

Commentary
Kūrpara is named after its location, at a corner. The marma is used to locally benefit the elbow and arm. Treatment here improves the elbow's range of motion by enhancing the lubricating properties of shleshaka kapha, that fills the joint with synovial fluid. It also treats both tennis elbow and golfer's elbow. Kūrpara is classified as an asthi marma because it is located on the bone.

Bāhya Kūrpara

Location
At the elbow, on the bony protuberance of the lateral epicondyle of the humerus.

Action
♦ Harmonizes the movement of elbow and arm
♦ Relieves pain locally
♦ Improves circulation

Associated Doshic Subtypes
Prāna Vāyu, Vyāna Vāyu, Shleshaka Kapha

Indications
♦ Pain or restricted movement of the elbow and forearm
♦ Decreased circulation in the forearm
♦ Radiculopathy (pinched nerve)
♦ Upper extremity paresthesia (tingling and numbness)
♦ Lateral epicondylitis (tennis elbow)

Treatment
Refer to Bāhu Ūrvī Treatment section, page 174.

Corresponding Acupoint
None

Close to LI 11, Quchi (Pool at the Crook)

Close to LI 12, Zhouliao (Elbow Crevice)

Bāhya Kūrpara is in close proximity to two acupoints on the Large Intestine meridian. LI 11 is located at the lateral end of the transverse cubital crease and LI 12 is found in a depression 1 cun superior, lateral to LI 11. Both the marma and the acupoints benefit the elbow and arm locally to relieve pain and enhance circulation. LI 11 has a greater sphere of influence than Bāhya Kūrpara and is a commonly used acupoint to clear heat, expel Wind, drain Damp and alleviate itching. LI 11 is often used in treatment of fever, thirst, mania, hypertension and skin disorders. It can relieve abdominal pain and distention, vomiting, diarrhea and dysentery. LI 12 is not as commonly used.

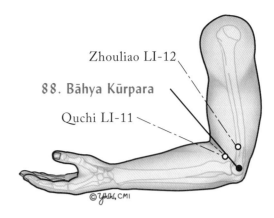

Zhouliao LI-12

88. Bāhya Kūrpara

Quchi LI-11

© Yhshi, CMI

Arms Hands

Commentary
Bāhya means external and Kūrpara means corner. It is located near Kūrpara marma and shares a similar range of action. Both benefit the elbow and arm and relieve local pain, tingling and numbness. However, while Kūrpara treats lateral and medial epicondylitis, Bāhya Kūrpara is helpful only for lateral epicondylitis, commonly called tennis elbow. Refer to the Commentary under Kūrpara (see page 178).

Angushtha Mūla

• • • • • • • • • • • • • • • •

Location
On the dorsum of the hand, in a depression between the first and second metacarpals. Level with the midpoint of the second metacarpal, on the belly of the first dorsal interosseous muscle.

Action
♦ Stimulates flow of prāna, vyāna and apāna vāyus
♦ Enhances circulation and relieves congestion
♦ Relieves pain and headaches
♦ Benefits liver and spleen functions
♦ Benefits hands
♦ Calms the mind and releases suppressed emotions

Associated Doshic Subtypes
Prāna Vāyu, Apāna Vāyu, Vyāna Vāyu, Udāna Vāyu, Rañjaka Pitta, Tarpaka Kapha

Indications
♦ Sinus congestion, lymphatic congestion
♦ Sinus headache, migraines, vertigo
♦ Liver pain, splenic pain or congestion in the spleen
♦ Pain, arthritis, tingling or neuropathy of the hand
♦ Emotional disturbance

Contraindications
♦ Pregnancy

Treatment
Nutmeg oil is effective for alleviating migraine headaches. **Vacha** and **nirgundi oils** pacify vāta and soothe pain. **Mahānārāyana oil** or **Tiger Balm®** relieves pain, numbness and stiffness in the finger joints.

Corresponding Acupoint
LI 4, Hegu (Joining Valley)

LI 4 is known as the "command point" for the face and mouth, and is widely used to address any disorder of the face, eyes, nose, mouth and ears. LI 4 is effectively used in the treatment of all types of headaches, while Angushtha Mūla specifically treats only sinus headache and migraine. Both benefit the hand and fingers. There is no mention of LI 4 having any relationship to the liver and spleen. In TCM, LI 4 is described as expelling Wind and increasing yang energy. Unlike the marma, it regulates sweating, treats hypertension and ameliorates lumbar pain. It is the premier acupoint used during pregnancy to stimulate labor and uterine contractions.

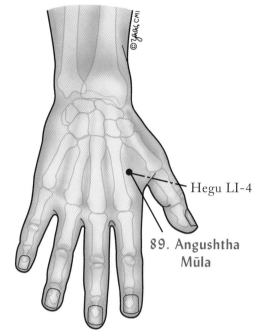

Hegu LI-4

89. Angushtha Mūla

Commentary
Angushtha Mūla is translated as the root of the thumb. It is a highly effective marma to stimulate the flow of prāna in the nasal and sinus passages and alleviate sinus headaches and migraines. It regulates hyperactive udāna vāyu that results in vertigo. It also enhances the flow of vyāna vāyu, relieving congestion and pain in different parts of the body, including the liver and spleen. The marma on the right is affiliated with the liver and that on the left with the spleen. Hence, it is associated with rañjaka pitta, which is present in both organs. Angushtha Mūla benefits the hands and fingers locally and it treats pain, numbness, tingling and arthritis. In addition, it releases suppressed emotions that are vāta, pitta or kapha in nature. All these functions can be ascribed to the marma's powerful ability to circulate prāna and unblock stagnation. **During pregnancy this marma should not be pressed, because it may stimulate apāna vāyu and bring on uterine contractions.**

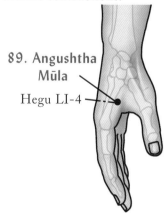

89. Angushtha Mūla

Hegu LI-4

Bāhya Manibandha

. . . .

Location
On the radial side of the wrist in a depression between the tendons extensor pollicis longus and brevis. In the "anatomical snuff box" when the thumb is extended.

Action
♦ Benefits the wrist and hand
♦ Detoxifies the liver
♦ Enhances immunity

Associated Doshic Subtypes
Prāna Vāyu, Vyāna Vāyu, Rañjaka Pitta, Shleshaka Kapha

Indications
♦ Pain or swelling in the wrist joint and thumb
♦ Arthritis of the hand
♦ Toxins in the liver

Treatment
Steady pressure for one minute or application of heat on this point helps to detoxify the liver. Massage **mahānārāyana oil** into the hand and wrist to relieve pain and stiffness.

For hepatitis A, an effective therapy is called *agni karma*. Holding a chunk of dry turmeric root with tongs or forceps, burn one end, blow out the flame, hold close to Bāhya Manibandha. Blow the heat and smoke toward the marma for 1–2 minutes. This action will stimulate the liver to release gamma globulin (ojas), acting to prevent and heal hepatitis A. In hepatitis B and C, this procedure may help to reduce the viral load by its anti-inflammatory property.

Corresponding Acupoint
LI 5, Yangxi (Yang Stream)

LI 5 also benefits the wrist joint and is mentioned for difficulty in raising the elbow. It is primarily indicated for clearing heat in the same regions as for LI 4: the eyes, ears, nose, teeth, head and throat. Unlike Bāhya Manibandha, LI 5 does not have an influence on the liver or on immunity. However, the acupoint does have an ability to calm the mind.

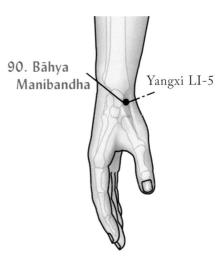

Arms
Hands

Commentary
Bāhya means external and manibandha is the point where a woman ties a watch or jewelry to her wrist. Bāhya Manibandha benefits the wrist joint and treats pain or weakness of the wrist. It also reduces swelling and arthritis in the wrist. The marma on the right is associated with the liver and gallbladder, and the one on the left with the spleen and pancreas. It stimulates bhūta agni, the fire component of the liver. Hence, it is effective for removing toxins in the liver, and is associated with rañjaka pitta. Steady pressure for one minute on this marma strengthens ojas and increases immunity.

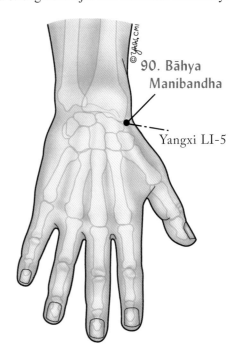

Manibandha

Location
At the midpoint of the wrist crease when the hand is in a supine position, between the tendons of the palmaris longus and flexor carpi radialis.

Arms Hands

Action
♦ Frees movement in the wrist joint
♦ Relieves localized pain
♦ Influences the reproductive organs
♦ Unfolds mental tranquility, balances emotions
♦ Strengthens the rectum and benefits sexual activity

Associated Doshic Subtypes
Apāna Vāyu, Vyāna Vāyu, Shleshaka Kapha

Indications
♦ Pain or swelling in the wrist joint
♦ Carpal tunnel syndrome
♦ Arthritis of hand
♦ Sexual dysfunction such as low libido, premature ejaculation
♦ Hemorrhoids
♦ Emotional disturbances

Treatment
Dashamūla oil or **nutmeg oil** can be applied to Manibandha to reduce vāta symptoms. **Jasmine oil** or **jatamāmsī oil** will soothe the mind and emotions. A yogic method for treating sexual dysfunction, the elevated lotus pose (ūrdhva padmāsana), stretches the wrist joint and places pressure on this marma. This yoga posture is beneficial for both shukra and ārtava dhātus (male and female reproductive tissues) and provides results similar to stimulating Manibandha. Other helpful yoga postures for sexual dysfunction include the peacock pose (mayūrāsana) and cobra pose (bhujangāsana).

Corresponding Acupoint
PC 7, Daling (Great Mound)

PC 7 possesses a broader range of action than Manibandha. Both act on the wrist joint and are used for the treatment of carpal tunnel syndrome and wrist pain. Both points address emotional imbalance, but PC 7 also influences heart disorders such as chest pain and palpitations, because it is a principal point on the Pericardium meridian. Unlike Manibandha, PC 7 does not affect the reproductive organs. Instead, it harmonizes the stomach and intestines and is used for treatment of pain and vomiting.

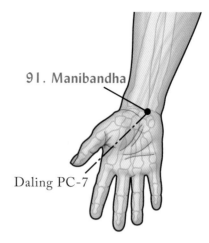

91. Manibandha

Daling PC-7

It is used to cool excess heat and related disorders such as red eyes, fever and blood in the urine. It also treats the breasts for local pain and abscesses. Locally, PC 7 relieves pain and contraction of the elbow, heat in the palms, contraction of the hand and swelling of the axilla.

Commentary
The Sanskrit word *mani* is interpreted as precious jewels and *bandha* means to lock. Accordingly, the marma is named for the point where a woman's bracelet is tied and touches her wrist. This marma is on the ventral surface of the hand, while Bāhya Manibandha is on the dorsal side. Both marmāni help to relieve pain, swelling and numbness in the wrist joint. Gentle pressure here stimulates shleshaka kapha (thus synovial fluid) to provide lubrication and facilitate easy movement of the joints.

Manibandha is functionally related to the reproductive organs, rectum, prostate and cervix. It directly corresponds to shukra dhātu in males and ārtava dhātu in females. It is indicated for sexual dysfunction, including low libido and premature ejaculation. In addition, Manibandha pacifies hemorrhoids. These disorders are linked to a disturbance of apāna vāyu. Treatment to Manibandha is also very effective for balancing many doshic emotional fluctuations.

Kūrcha Shira

Location
At the ulnar end of the wrist crease, in a depression between the ulnar styloid process and the triquetral bone.

Action
♦ Benefits the wrist joint
♦ Influences the reproductive organs

Associated Doshic Subtypes
Prāna Vāyu, Apāna Vāyu, Vyāna Vāyu, Sādhaka Pitta, Shleshaka Kapha

Indications
♦ Pain or swelling in the wrist joint
♦ Arthritis of the hand
♦ Ulnar neuropathy
♦ Pain during ovulation
♦ Rectal prolapse, hemorrhoids

Treatment
Use **vacha** or **nutmeg oils** to pacify vāta in the wrist joint. Massage with **mahānārāyana oil** or **Tiger Balm®** to relieve pain, numbness and stiffness of the finger joints.

Corresponding Acupoint
SI 5, Yanggu (Yang Valley)

SI 5 is indicated for pain of the arm and shoulder, along with a number of points on the Bladder channel. It also treats hemorrhoids, perhaps because of the paired connection between the Small Intestine and Bladder meridians. Unlike Kūrcha Shira, SI 5 is not considered to have an influence on the reproductive organs.

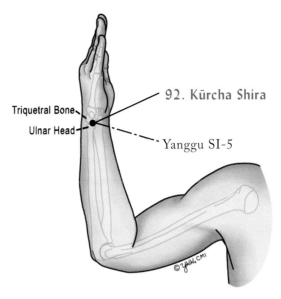

Triquetral Bone
Ulnar Head
92. Kūrcha Shira
Yanggu SI-5

Arms
Hands

Commentary
Kūrcha Shira is translated as head of the ligaments. Like other marmāni located on the wrist joint, it treats local dysfunctions, including ulnar neuropathy, numbness, and tingling due to repetitive stress affecting the ulnar nerve. Stimulation of Kūrcha Shira promotes shleshaka kapha to lubricate the joints and prevent friction.

Like Manibandha, the marma also benefits the reproductive organs, specifically the ovaries in women and spermatic cord in men. Hence, Kūrcha Shira is associated with shukra and ārtava dhātus. Stimulation of Kūrcha Shira benefits reproductive disturbance, rectal prolapse and hemorrhoids, all due to disturbance of apāna vāyu.

Tala Hrida

Location
On the palm of the hand, in the depression between the second and third metacarpals, at the point where the middle finger touches the palm when a fist is made.

Action
♦ Balances heart and mind
♦ Harmonizes emotions and relieves stress
♦ Regulates functions of the lungs and diaphragm
♦ Benefits the hand

Associated Doshic Subtypes
Prāna Vāyu, Vyāna Vāyu, Udāna Vāyu, Sādhaka Pitta, Avalambaka Kapha

Indications
♦ Attention Deficit Hyperactive Disorder (ADHD), poor concentration
♦ Cardiac arrhythmias, chest pain
♦ Pain or swelling in the wrist joint
♦ Arthritis of hand
♦ Carpal tunnel syndrome
♦ Sweating of the palms, heat in palms
♦ Emotional disturbance

Treatment
Vacha oil pacifies vāta conditions and **coconut oil** reduces high pitta. Both **jatamāmsī** and **brahmī oils** soothe the nervous system and help to alleviate emotional imbalances.

Corresponding Acupoint
PC 8, Laogong (Labor Palace)

PC 8, a significant point on the Pericardium meridian, is associated with the heart and emotions, as is Tala Hrida. Both treat cardiac or chest pain and calm disturbance of the mind. PC 8 is needled in acupuncture to treat more severe conditions that the marma does not address, such as mania. PC 8 is also indicated for depression, fear, sadness, anxiety, anger and restlessness. Locally, both the acupoint and marma benefit the hand for symptoms such as tremors, arthritis, pain and sweating of the palms. Unlike the marma, PC 8 clears heat manifesting as fever, hypertension and mouth ulcers. Heat also leads to Blood disturbances, such as vomiting blood, persistent nosebleed and blood in the stools.

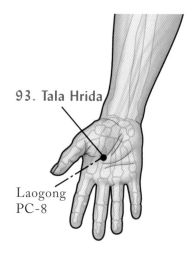

93. Tala Hrida

Laogong PC-8

Unlike Tala Hrida, the acupoint also can be used in treatment of epilepsy and wind-stroke (apoplexy).

Commentary
Tala Hrida is translated as the heart (*hrid*) or center of the palm. It is a highly effective marma to calm the mind, balance the emotions and relieve stress. When prāna does not flow smoothly through the prāna nādīs (channels), it tends to become hyperactive. This can result in hyperactivity of the mind and ADHD in children. Massaging Tala Hrida in conjunction with Mūrdhni very quickly settles the mind, whether of an adult or a child.

Massage to Tala Hrida pacifies many emotional disturbances. This is because of the marma's direct action on mano vaha srotas (channels of the mind) and majjā dhātu (nervous tissue), which are adversely affected in conditions such as emotional imbalance, mood swings and difficulty concentrating.

Tala Hrida is functionally related to the heart through vyāna vāyu, to the diaphragm through udāna vāyu, and to the lungs through prāna vāyu. It is indicated in the treatment of cardiac arrhythmias, especially anxiety tachycardia. This marma is considered the "solar plexus" of the hand, as the hand is thought to be a microcosm of the chakra system.

Kūrcha

. . . .

Location
At the midpoint of the belly of the abductor pollicis brevis muscle on the thenar eminence of the hand.

Action
♦ Benefits the hand and fingers
♦ Reduces stress
♦ Enhances the flow of prāna and benefits lungs
♦ Enhances immune response
♦ Influences the reproductive organs

Associated Doshic Subtypes
Apāna Vāyu, Prāna Vāyu, Sādhaka Pitta, Avalambaka Kapha

Indications
♦ Pain or swelling in the wrist joint
♦ Carpal tunnel syndrome
♦ Arthritis of the hand
♦ Emotional stress and tension
♦ Pulmonary congestion, difficulty breathing
♦ Poor immunity
♦ Testicular pain, pain during ovulation

Treatment
Using **nutmeg, castor** or **eucalyptus oil** at Kūrcha helps to pacify both vāta and kapha.

Corresponding Acupoint
LU 10, Yuji (Fish Border)

LU 10 is a key point on the Lung meridian for alleviating cough and disturbances of the throat. Like Kūrcha it effectively relieves difficulty breathing; unlike the marma, it is also helpful for chest pain. Where Kūrcha is indicated for general stress and tension, LU 10 pacifies more specific emotions such as anger, mania, sadness and fear. Locally, Kūrcha is used in treatment of the hand and wrist joint, but LU 10's action extends beyond the thumb to the palm, elbow and arm. LU 10 also treats impotence and genital itching.

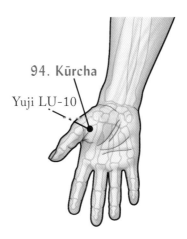

94. Kūrcha
Yuji LU-10

Arms Hands

Commentary
Kūrcha means ligament or fascia. Like other marmāni on the hand, it has a specific local action for pain reduction, but its influence is widespread. By enhancing the flow of prāna, pressure here relieves shortness of breath and pacifies emotional tension. By acting to enhance ojas, it improves immune response. Its influence on avalambaka kapha, a subtype of kapha dosha located in the lungs, relieves pulmonary congestion. Kūrcha also has an influence on the reproductive organs, especially the ovaries in females and testicles in males. The mount of Venus on the hand astrologically corresponds to shukra and ārtava dhātus, the reproductive tissues.

Hasta Kshipra

• •

Arms
Hands

Location
On the dorsal surface of the thumb, at the midpoint of the base of the nail.

Action
♦ Benefits the hand
♦ Relieves headaches
♦ Enhances flow of prāna to the lungs and brain

Associated Doshic Subtypes
Prāna Vāyu, Vyāna Vāyu, Tarpaka Kapha

Indications
♦ Headaches in any region, sinus headaches, migraines
♦ Vertigo
♦ Seizure disorder
♦ Excess heat
♦ Pain, swelling, arthritis of the thumb

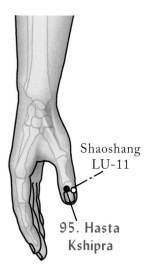

Shaoshang
LU-11

95. Hasta
Kshipra

Treatment
Vacha and **nutmeg oils** used on Hasta Kshipra will pacify vāta, while **sandalwood oil** will cool pitta. Traditionally, Ayurvedic physicians have bled a few drops at this marma to instantly relieve pain and soothe migraines.

Corresponding Acupoint
None

Close to LU 11, Shaoshang (Lesser Shang)

LU 11, the last point on the Lung meridian, is located on the thumb, 0.1 cun lateral to the base of the nail on the radial side. Some of the acupoint's functions match Hasta Kshipra's. LU 11 is also an important point for clearing heat. Locally it treats pain of the thumb and wrist, and sweaty palms. Unlike the marma, LU 11 helps relieve painful obstruction of the upper arms, where qi or blood is stagnant. LU 11 addresses loss of consciousness, while the marma is indicated for seizure disorder, vertigo and headache. Although Hasta Kshipra benefits the lungs, LU 11 does this more specifically by treating sore throat, cough and shortness of breath. LU 11 benefits the throat region because the internal pathway of the Lung meridian ascends to the throat.

Commentary
Hasta means hand, differentiating the marma from Pāda Kshipra located on the toe. *Kshipra* is translated as instantaneous or immediately acting. It acts without delay to relieve sinus, frontal, temporal or occipital headaches. Gentle pressure applied here enhances the flow of prāna, specifically to the lungs and brain. Thus, it is a principal marma in the treatment of headaches, migraines, vertigo and any seizure disorder where prāna is destabilized. Hasta Kshipra is located on the thumb, which is correlated to the brain, space element, and vāta dosha. Many of the conditions treated by this marma are disturbances of vāta, but it can also cool down heat that accumulates due to excess pitta.

Tarjani

Location
On the dorsal surface of the index finger, immediately lateral to the base of the nail on the radial side.

Action
♦ Benefits lungs and enhances the flow of prāna
♦ Regulates colon and apāna vāyu
♦ Balances udāna and apāna vāyu
♦ Acts on the hands and fingers

Associated Doshic Subtypes
Prāna Vāyu, Udāna Vāyu, Apāna Vāyu, Avalambaka Kapha

Indications
♦ Flatulence (gas in the colon)
♦ Constipation, diarrhea
♦ Asthma, chronic cough, shortness of breath
♦ Pain, swelling, arthritis of index finger

Treatment
Mahānārāyana oil relieves pain, numbness or stiffness of the finger joints.

Corresponding Acupoint
LI 1, Shangyang (Metal Yang)

There is a functional relationship between the paired meridians of the metal element, the Lung and Large Intestine. LI 1 shares similar lung indications as Tarjani for cough, asthma and shortness of breath. Unlike Tarjani, LI 1 has no influence on colon disorders. It clears heat and treats shoulder and back pain that radiates to the supraclavicular region which the Large Intestine meridian traverses.

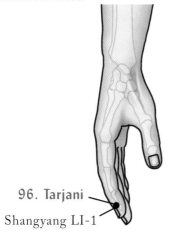

96. Tarjani
Shangyang LI-1

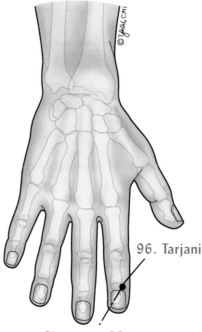

96. Tarjani
Shangyang LI-1

Commentary
Tarjani is derived etymologically from the root *tarja*, meaning to show, indicate or point out. The index finger, known as tarjani in Sanskrit, is used for this function. Each finger has a corresponding element: the thumb with ether, index finger with air, middle finger with fire, ring finger with water and the little finger with earth. Thus, Tarjani is connected to the air element and vāta dosha. It enhances lung capacity when used in conjunction with other marmāni on the chest.

Tarjani simultaneously regulates the functions of three vāyus: apāna vāyu in the colon, udāna vāyu in the diaphragm and prāna vāyu in the lungs. Therapeutically, it addresses imbalances of the organs associated with each vāyu. Udāna is the upward moving vāyu; its imbalance manifests as asthma, cough, and difficulty breathing. Apāna, the downward moving vāyu, tends to manifest as colon dysfunction, especially flatulence.

Kanīshthika

Location
On the dorsal surface of the little finger, immediately below the midpoint of the base of the nail.

Action
♦ Regulates heart functions
♦ Enhances coronary circulation
♦ Benefits the hands
♦ Balances emotions

Associated Doshic Subtypes
Prāna Vāyu, Vyāna Vāyu, Sādhaka Pitta, Avalambaka Kapha

Indications
♦ Angina pain that radiates down the arm to little finger, cardiac pain
♦ Anxiety, palpitations
♦ Pain, swelling, arthritis of the little finger

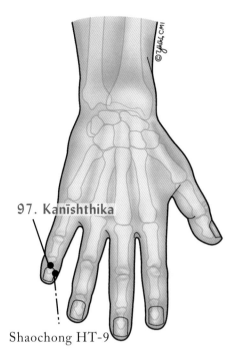

97. Kanīshthika

Shaochong HT-9

Treatment
Nutmeg and **nirgundi oils** pacify vāta and relieve cardiac pain. **Mahānārāyana oil** relieves pain, numbness or stiffness of the finger joints.

Corresponding Acupoint
None

Close to HT 9, Shaochong (Lesser Rushing)

HT 9 is also located on the little finger at the root of the nail, close to Kanīshthika. It is 0.1 cun lateral from the radial root of the nail. HT 9 is the terminal point on the Heart Meridian and has a similar influence as Kanīshthika on the heart. However, HT 9 has a broader range of action; it is indicated for loss of consciousness, epilepsy and for clearing heat conditions. It calms the mind in emotional disturbances such as mania, depression, fright, agitation and restlessness. HT 9 affects the tongue, throat and eyes. Locally, it relieves pain, stiffness and swelling of the fingers, extending its influence along the meridian to relieve pain in the palm, forearm and elbow.

Commentary
Kanīshthika is the name for the little finger, which represents the earth element. Kanīshthika marma is used primarily for treating cardiac dysfunction manifesting as pain, anxiety and palpitations. Angina pain can radiate from the heart down the arm to the little finger. Squeezing or biting Kanīshthika marma can relieve anginal pain to some extent, but Ayurvedic herbs or other medical treatment are suggested for this condition. Locally, Kanīshthika can relieve pain, stiffness or swelling of the little finger.

Marma Massage for the Arms and Hands

• •

If you are not very familiar with Ayurvedic marma therapy, before attempting the following procedure, please review chapter 8, especially "Guidelines for Touch and Pressure" on page 75 that offers information for massaging marmāni. Appendix C has the series of marma massage directions and illustrations starting on page 284.

The instructions here refer to the drawings on these pages. The numbers are for use with these massage drawings only; they are different from the numbering system for the marma points used throughout the book. To look up details on a particular marma point, refer to the beginning of this chapter, page 169, to the tables that reference all the marma points and their page numbers.

Apply a few drops of essential oil to the tips of the fingers. Start with gentle pressure on the marma points, and gradually increase according to the capacity of the individual. If you use too much pressure, the person will show discomfort by saying "ouch" or through facial expressions, such as wrinkling of the face. Pressure on all marmāni should be held for approximately one to two minutes. If you feel that stronger pressure is needed you can apply it when the patient exhales.

Have the patient lie in supine position (face up) with the practitioner at the head. Begin by stimulating Ūrdhva Skandha marma (1). Then apply gentle pressure on Kakshadhara marma (2) with the thumbs. Both of these marmāni are often tender and require deep stimulation if the patient can tolerate it. Then move to the patient's left side and pull the left arm slightly away from the body. Stimulate Kaksha marma (3) at the armpit with the thumb and hold for one minute. Then move to Amsa marma (4). Massage the deltoid muscle with a "squeezing" motion, giving special emphasis to Adhah Skandha (5), and then apply either a clockwise or a counterclockwise rotation. Clockwise pressure increases pitta and relieves kapha and vata, while counterclockwise pressure increases vata and kapha and relieves or pacifies pitta. So if the pain or discomfort is pitta type, massage with a counterclockwise motion, and if it is vata and kapha type, the motion should be clockwise.

With the elbow in a flexed position, slide downwards to Bāhu Ūrvī (6), followed by Ānī (7) and then Bāhū Indrabasta (8). Slide the thumb gently along the midline of the forearm from Ānī (7) to Manibandha (9) at the wrist crease. Use gentle circular rotation to relax the patient. Massage Kūrcha Shira (10), followed by Bāhya Manibandha (11). Continue towards Angushtha Mūla (12) and hold for one minute. Turn the hand over and apply pressure to Kūrcha (13). Next, firmly hold Tala Hrida (14) at the center of the palm. Massage each finger from the base to the tip, starting with the little finger. Give special emphasis to Kanīshthika (15), Tarjani (16) and Hasta Kshipra (17).

Repeat on the opposite side.

While standing again at the head, end the massage with both thumbs applying deep pressure on Kakshadhara marma (2).

Arms Hands

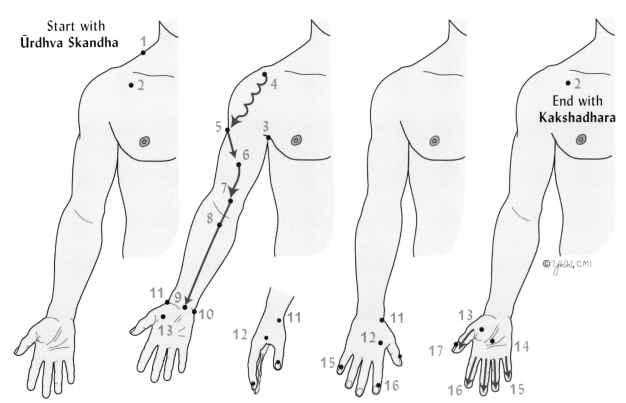

Start with **Ūrdhva Skandha**

End with **Kakshadhara**

©Yhshi, CMI

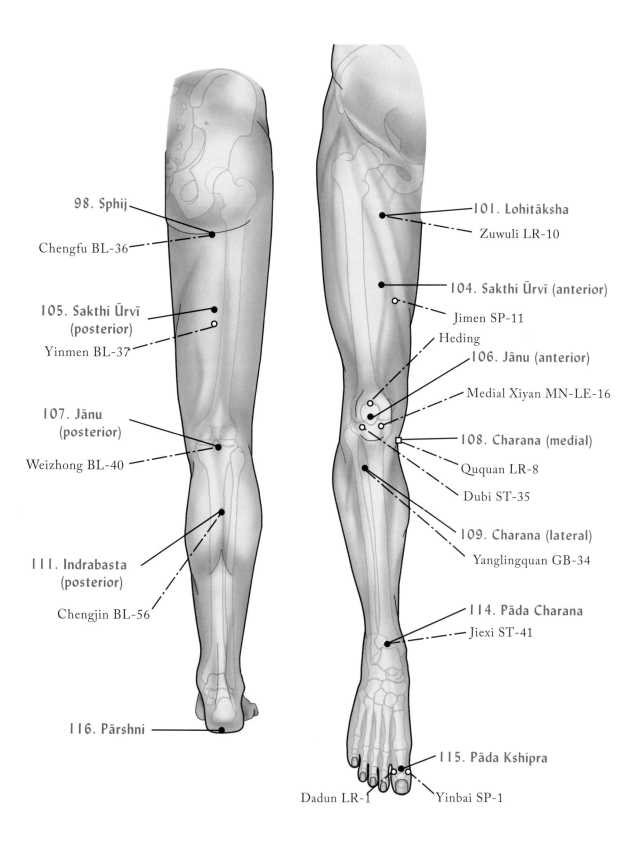

98. Sphij

Chengfu BL-36

101. Lohitāksha

Zuwuli LR-10

104. Sakthi Ūrvī (anterior)

Jimen SP-11

105. Sakthi Ūrvī (posterior)

Yinmen BL-37

Heding

106. Jānu (anterior)

Medial Xiyan MN-LE-16

107. Jānu (posterior)

108. Charana (medial)

Weizhong BL-40

Ququan LR-8

Dubi ST-35

109. Charana (lateral)

Yanglingquan GB-34

111. Indrabasta (posterior)

Chengjin BL-56

114. Pāda Charana

Jiexi ST-41

116. Pārshni

115. Pāda Kshipra

Dadun LR-1

Yinbai SP-1

190

Adha Shakha (Lower Extremities) Marmāni

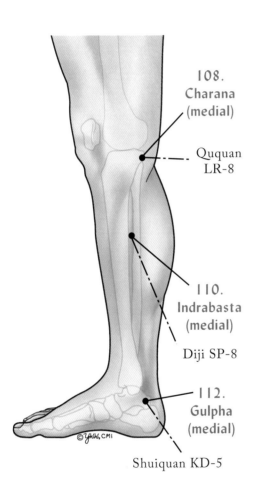

108.
Charana
(medial)

Ququan
LR-8

110.
Indrabasta
(medial)

Diji SP-8

112.
Gulpha
(medial)

Shuiquan KD-5

©Yuki, CMI

Sakthi (Thighs) Marmāni (14)

#	Marma Points	Page	Acupoints
98	Sphij	193	BL 36
99	Ūrū 1	194	----------
100	Ūrū 2	194	GB 31
101	Lohitāksha	195	LR 10
102	Medhra/Yoni Jihvā	196	-----------
103	Vrushana/ Yoni Oshtha	197	-----------
104	Sakthi Ūrvī (anterior)	198	≈SP 11
105	Sakthi Ūrvī (posterior)	198	≈BL 37
106	Jānu (anterior)	199	≈Heding, ≈medial Xiyan, ≈ST 35
107	Jānu (posterior)	199	BL 40
108	Charana (medial)	200	LR 8
109	Charana (lateral)	200	GB 34
110	Indrabasta (medial)	202	SP 8
111	Indrabasta (posterior)	202	BL 56
112	Gulpha (medial)[a]	203	KD 5

a. Part of the Foot Marmāni.

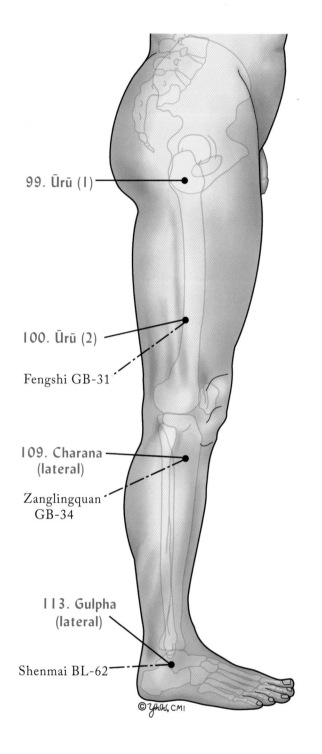

99. Ūrū (1)

100. Ūrū (2)

Fengshi GB-31

109. Charana
(lateral)

Zanglingquan
GB-34

113. Gulpha
(lateral)

Shenmai BL-62

© Yhshi, CMI

Pāda (Foot) Marmāni (6)

#	Marma Points	Page	Acupoint
99	Ūrū 1	194	----------
100	Ūrū 2[a]	194	GB 31
109	Charana (lateral)	200	GB 34
112	Gulpha (medial)	203	KD 5
113	Gulpha (lateral)	203	BL 62
114	Pāda Charana	204	ST 41
115	Pāda Kshipra	205	≈SP 1, LR 1
116	Pārshni	206	---------
117	Pāda Madhya	207	KD 1

a. Part of the Thigh Marmāni.

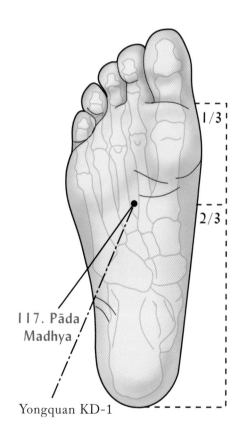

1/3

2/3

117. Pāda
Madhya

Yongquan KD-1

Sphij

• •

Location
At the midpoint of the transverse gluteal crease that lies below each buttock.

Action
♦ Enhances circulation in the lower extremities
♦ Relieves pain
♦ Benefits the colon

Associated Doshic Subtypes
Vyāna Vāyu, Apāna Vāyu

Indications
♦ Pain, neuropathy of lower extremities
♦ Pain in gluteal and coccygeal regions
♦ Low back pain
♦ Lumbosacral radiculopathy (sciatica)
♦ Colon dysfunction: constipation

Treatment
Mahānārāyana oil relieves pain and stiffness locally and soothes muscles. **Nirgundi oil** pacifies vāta, **sandalwood oil** reduces pitta and vacha oil treats excess kapha.

Corresponding Acupoint
BL 36 Chengfu (Hold and Support)

Both BL 36 and Sphij are used for treating localized pain and are especially effective for sciatic pain. They also address apāna vāyu dysfunction; Sphij for constipation and BL 36 for difficult urination, genital pain and hemorrhoids.

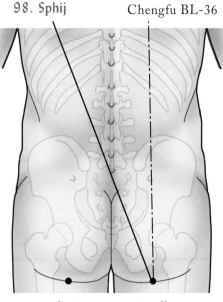

98. Sphij   Chengfu BL-36

Legs
Feet

(points are paired)

Commentary
Sphij translates as gluteal fold. Pressure applied to this marma relieves pain locally in the lumbar region, sacrum, coccyx and buttock. Low back and gluteal pain may be due to lumbar strain, lumbosacral radiculopathy and sacroiliac joint dysfunction. Sphij is especially effective for treatment of sciatic pain that descends along the posterior aspect of the leg along the track of the sciatic nerve. These conditions result from impaired vyāna vāyu, which reduces circulation. Sphij addresses colon dysfunction and is particularly associated with the sigmoid colon and rectum. The marma on the right side of the body is functionally related to the ascending colon and on the left side with the descending colon.

Ūrū (2)

* * * * * * * * * * * * * * * * * * * *

Legs
Feet

Location

Two points on the lateral aspect of the thigh.
Ūrū 1 – on the prominence of the greater trochanter.
Ūrū 2 – when a patient stands with the arms held comfortably at the side, the point is located where the tip of the middle finger touches the thigh, 8.5 to 9 anguli superior to the popliteal crease.

Action

♦ Balances apāna vāyu
♦ Benefits lower extremities
♦ Enhances circulation
♦ Relieves pain

Associated Doshic Subtypes

Apāna Vāyu, Vyāna Vāyu, Shleshaka Kapha

Indications

♦ Pain, neuropathy of lower extremities
♦ Lumbosacral radiculopathy (sciatica)
♦ Hip pain, knee pain, arthritis of hip and knee
♦ Edema in lower extremities
♦ Constipation
♦ Low libido, genital disorders

Treatment

Mahānārāyana oil relieves thigh pain and stiffness and soothes the muscles.

Corresponding Acupoint

Ūrū 1 – None

Ūrū 2 – GB 31, Fengshi

GB 31 is located below the greater trochanter and 7 cun (or 8.5-9 angula) superior to the popliteal crease. These points benefit the hips, thighs and knees when there is pain, numbness, weakness or stiffness. Unlike Ūrū 2, GB 31 is also indicated for heaviness of the legs. In TCM GB 31 is considered one of the primary acupoints for expelling Wind from the body that manifests as pain, numbness, tingling and weakness. The acupoint does not share the marma's ability to benefit the pelvic area and genital organs.

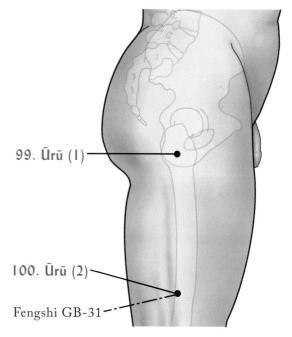

99. Ūrū (1)

100. Ūrū (2)

Fengshi GB-31

Commentary

Ūrū literally means the origin of the thighs. Both Ūrū marmāni are located on the lateral aspect of the thighs, along the same line and sharing similar actions. Locally, they relieve numbness and tingling by promoting circulation to the lower extremities via vyāna vāyu. They also relieve lumbosacral radiculopathy, commonly referred to as sciatica. These points benefit arthritis by stimulating shleshaka kapha, enhancing lubrication of the joint and relieving dryness and inflammation. Ūrū 1 provides relief for arthritis of the hip joint and Ūrū 2 for arthritis of the knee joint.

Ūrū marmāni also benefit the pelvic area and genital organs by balancing apāna vāyu. They are functionally related to the ovaries and testicles. Bhaga marma, located on the pubic bone (see page 153) has a more direct action on these organs and on low libido. Ūrū marmāni on the right thigh are related to the ileocecal valve and cecum, while those on the left thigh are related to the sigmoid colon. They relieve constipation by regulating apāna vāyu.

Lohitāksha

● ●

Location
Inferior to the midpoint of the inguinal ligament on the anterior aspect of the thigh.

Action
♦ Promotes circulation in lower extremities
♦ Balances apāna vāyu
♦ Relieves pain locally
♦ Regulates blood flow to the legs
♦ Benefits the heart and colon

Associated Doshic Subtypes
Vyāna Vāyu, Apāna Vāyu, Shleshaka Kapha, Rañjaka Pitta

Indications
♦ Peripheral vascular disease (PVD), poor circulation
♦ Lumbar radiculopathy (sciatica)
♦ Pain, neuropathy of lower extremities
♦ Arthritis of the hip
♦ Edema of lower extremities
♦ High blood pressure
♦ Cardiac dysfunction
♦ Flatulence
♦ Testing cremasteric reflex in paralyzed male patients[a]

a. If this reflex is gone, chances for recovery are poor.

Treatment
Refer to Ūrū Treatment section, page 194. **Dashamūla oil** pacifies vāta dosha, **sandalwood oil** is used for pitta and **vacha oil** for kapha.

Corresponding Acupoint
LR 10, Zuwuli (Leg Five Miles)

LR 10 does not share the same sphere of action as the marma. It is primarily used for urinary disorders and abdominal pain and fullness.

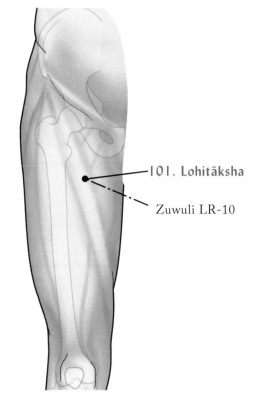

101. Lohitāksha

Zuwuli LR-10

Legs
Feet

Commentary
Lohita translates as blood and *aksha* as eyes. The most literal translation, "vision of the blood," is strikingly appropriate, as Lohitāksha is an excellent diagnostic tool for detecting cardiovascular disorders. Lohitāksha is located close to the femoral nerve, artery and vein. The femoral nerve is involved in conditions such as radiculopathy and neuropathy. The femoral artery is affected in valvular heart disease, while the femoral vein is affected in diminished venous return leading to edema. The marma treats lymph edema and venous congestion of the lower extremities. Lohitāksha is functionally related to the heart and colon. It is also associated with the testicles and ovaries through the function of apāna vāyu. Lohitāksha on the left corresponds to the descending colon and on the right with the ascending colon.

Medhra and Yoni Jihvā

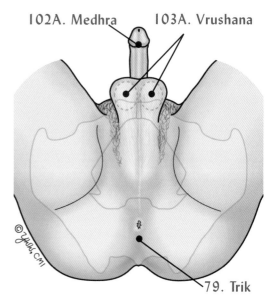

102A. Medhra   103A. Vrushana

79. Trik

Location
Medhra is on the dorsal surface of the midpoint of the glans penis.
Yoni Jihvā is the tip of the clitoris.

Action
♦ Acts on shukra or ārtava dhātu
♦ Stimulates ojas

Associated Doshic Subtypes
Apāna Vāyu, Vyāna Vāyu, Rañjaka Pitta

Indications
♦ Dysmenorrhea
♦ Low libido
♦ Premature ejaculation and premature orgasm

Treatment

Ashvagandha (*withania somnifera*) and **bala** (*sida cordifolia*) **oils**[6] are tonifying and strengthen the reproductive system. For stronger therapeutic results when shukra or ārtava dhātu is affected, the patient should take the herbs ashvagandha and bala herbs internally. *Ashvini mudrā,* a practice in Yoga that involves contracting the anus inwards, creates pressure at this marma and is useful for treating sexual dysfunction.

Note: It is not recommended that the practitioner touch the patient at these locations. If you feel that using them is beneficial for treatment, you can verbally instruct the client.

Corresponding Acupoint
None

Commentary

These marmāni are not used in clinical treatment but are good for self-healing. Medhra is the Sanskrit term for penis. The marma is associated with shukra dhātu, the male reproductive tissue, and male sex energy. Yoni Jihvā is the term for clitoris and is related to ārtava dhātu, the female reproductive tissue, and female sex energy. Both stimulate awakened sex energy and the production of ojas, the superfine essence that is released in the form of orgasmic fluid. Āyurveda gives a great deal of importance to controlling sexual desires and regulat-

ing the ejaculation of orgasmic fluid in accordance with one's constitution. Excessive or frequent ejaculation (which varies according to constitutional type as well as overall health and vitality) may deplete ojas, weaken immune function and adversely affect the health and harmony of the entire being. These delicate marmāni are considered vital points; a kick to the genitals can lead to severe pain and cardiac arrest and the person may collapse or die.

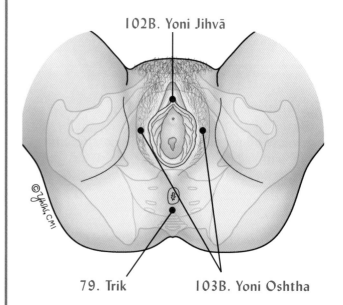

102B. Yoni Jihvā

79. Trik   103B. Yoni Oshtha

---

6. These are medicated oils, different from the essential oils usually recommended for marma chikitsā. Medicated oils are decoctions and are less volatile and milder for this sensitive area. For more on decoctions, see *The Complete Book of Ayurvedic Home Remedies,* appendix 2, page 287.

Vrushana and Yoni Oshtha

· ·

Location
Vrushana is at the central point of each testicle, which is anatomically related to the junction between the epididymis and the testicle.
 Yoni Oshtha is at the midpoint of the labia majora, on each side.

Action
♦ Acts on shukra or ārtava dhātu
♦ Stimulates ojas
♦ Relieves pain locally
♦ Awakens sexual energy

Associated Doshic Subtypes
Apāna Vāyu, Vyāna Vāyu

Indications
♦ Epididymitis
♦ Inflammation of penis, testicles
♦ Hydrocele
♦ Reduced tissue elasticity during pregnancy

Treatment
Refer to Medhra and Yoni Jihvā Treatment section, page 196.

Corresponding Acupoint
None

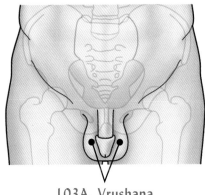

103A. Vrushana

Commentary
Vrushana and *Yoni Oshtha* correspond to the male and female reproductive tissues respectively. Refer to the Commentary section of Medhra and Yoni Jihvā for more information (see page 196). The name vrushana means testicle, while yoni describes the marma's location as part of the female genitalia and oshtha means lips. Vrushana is used for cooling epididymitis, inflammation of the penis as well as inflammation of the testicles. Hydrocele is the pathological accumulation of fluid in the membrane covering the testes; self-pressure applied to Vrushana helps to reduce hydrocele. Yoni Oshtha may be used during pregnancy to enhance tissue elasticity and in childbirth to relax the birth canal.

Legs
Feet

Sakthi Ūrvī (2)

Legs
Feet

Location
Two points located on the anterior and posterior aspect of the thigh.
Anterior Sakthi Ūrvī is located at the level of the mid thigh on the anterior surface of the quadriceps muscle. Posterior Sakthi Ūrvī is 1-2 anguli superior to the midpoint of a line drawn from Sphij (midpoint of gluteal fold) to Posterior Jānu (center of popliteal crease).

Action
♦ Promotes circulation in lower extremities, especially the thighs
♦ Benefits bladder, colon, and kidneys
♦ Benefits ovaries and testicles

Associated Doshic Subtypes
Vyāna Vāyu. Udāna Vāyu, Apāna Vāyu

Indications
♦ Peripheral vascular disease (poor circulation)
♦ Pain, neuropathy of lower extremities
♦ Edema of lower extremities
♦ Low back pain
♦ Arthritis of hip and knee
♦ Renal colic, cystitis, urinary incontinence
♦ Sexual dysfunction: low libido, impotence
♦ Pain in ovaries, testicles, epididymis

For posterior Sakthi Ūrvī
♦ Lumbosacral radiculopathy (sciatica)

Treatment
Refer to Ūrū Treatment section, page 194. **Neem or brahmī oil** can be used to treat cystitis.

Corresponding Acupoint
None

Anterior Sakthi Ūrvī: Close to SP 11, Jimen (Winnowing Gate)

Posterior Sakthi Ūrvī: Close to BL 37, Yinmen (Gate of Abundance)

Anterior Sakthi Ūrvī is slightly superior and lateral to SP 11. Both help to regulate urination and are helpful in treating urinary disturbances. SP 11 drains Damp-heat that can lead to urinary conditions, eczema, genital itching, inguinal swelling and abdominal pain.

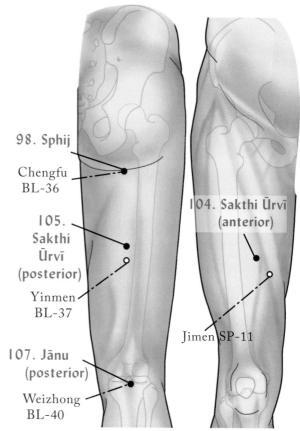

98. Sphij
Chengfu BL-36
105. Sakthi Ūrvī (posterior)
Yinmen BL-37
107. Jānu (posterior)
Weizhong BL-40
104. Sakthi Ūrvī (anterior)
Jimen SP-11

BL 37 corresponds to Posterior Sakthi Ūrvī and is located on a line drawn from Chengfu BL 36 (Sphij marma) to Weizhong BL 40 (Posterior Jānu). Like the marma, the acupoint treats pain and swelling of the thighs, as well as sciatica. Unlike Posterior Sakthi Ūrvī, it helps to relieve pain of the lumbar spine.

Both Sakthi Ūrvī marmāni promote circulation in the lower extremities and benefit the reproductive organs, unlike the corresponding acupoints.

Commentary
Sakthi ūrvī translates as power or energy of the thighs; *ūrvī* is derived from the Sanskrit term *ūrū*, which means thighs. Both marmāni (posterior and anterior) revitalize and boost energy by stimulating udāna vāyu. Udāna is responsible for upward moving energy and strength. Massaging these marmāni provides strength for the lower limbs, promotes circulation and helps to alleviate pain, weakness, numbness and tingling. Sakthi Ūrvī marmāni address vāta-type fluctuating pain as well as pitta-type sharp radiating pain such as sciatica.

Both marmāni are functionally related to the kidneys and bladder and are used in the treatment of renal colic, urinary incontinence and cystitis. They also benefit the ovaries and testicles and are used to treat pain and low libido. Sakthi Ūrvī reduces inflammation due to elevated pitta. The marmāni on the right thigh are associated with the ascending colon and the ones on the left with the descending colon.

Jānu (2)

• •

Location
Two points located on the anterior and posterior aspect of the knee joint.
Anterior Jānu – at the center of the patella.
Posterior Jānu – at the midpoint of the popliteal crease.

Action
♦ Benefits the knees
♦ Promotes circulation in lower extremities
♦ Relieves pain locally

Posterior Jānu only
♦ Enhances the flow of prāna
♦ Improves cerebral circulation
♦ Relieves respiratory distress

Associated Doshic Subtypes
Vyāna Vāyu, Prāna Vāyu, Apāna Vāyu, Udāna Vāyu, Shleshaka Kapha, Kledaka Kapha, Avalambaka Kapha

Indications
♦ Arthritis of the knee joint
♦ Limited range of motion of the knee
♦ Peripheral vascular disease (PVD), poor circulation
♦ Pain, neuropathy or edema of lower extremities

Posterior Jānu only
♦ Lumbosacral radiculopathy (sciatica)
♦ Low back pain
♦ Vertigo
♦ Asthma, pulmonary congestion

Treatment
Mahānārāyana oil relieves vāta pain in cases of degenerative arthritis. **Nirgundi oil** pacifies vāta dosha, **sandalwood oil** is used for pitta, and **vacha oil** for kapha. **Garlic oil** also pacifies vāta-type pain and **ginger oil** increases movement and circulation locally.

Corresponding Acupoint
Anterior Jānu – None. Close to extra points medial and lateral Xiyan (Eye of the Knee) and Heding

Posterior Jānu – BL 40, Weizhong (Middle of the Creek)

Anterior Jānu has no corresponding acupoint. It is in close proximity to two points in the medial and lateral hollow that are immediately below the patella when the knee is flexed. Lateral Xiyan is also known as Dubi or ST 35, located on the Stomach meridian. Anterior Jānu is also slightly inferior to extra point Heding at the mid-

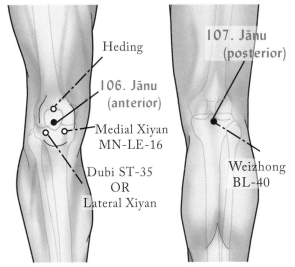

point of the superior border of the patella. All these points benefit the knee joint locally.

BL 40 is an influential and frequently used point on the Bladder meridian. It is similar to Posterior Jānu in its local action and for treatment of sciatic pain. Both also treat pain and stiffness of the lumbar region, including the sacrum and coccyx. Unlike the marma, BL 40 is not indicated for dizziness or respiratory conditions. In TCM theory, BL 40 is known to clear heat, cool the blood, and treat vomiting and diarrhea. It also strengthens the bladder in cases of enuresis (bed wetting) and difficult urination.

Commentary
Jānu means knee. These marmāni address pain, tenderness, swelling and weakness of the knee. Applying gentle repetitive pressure (stopping and starting) can alleviate stiffness and arthritis of the knee joint. In degenerative arthritis, shleshaka kapha is diminished and fails to lubricate the joints, resulting in dryness and degenerative changes in the articular tissue of the joints. On the other hand, systemic pitta may go into the joint via the circulatory system, causing inflammation, resulting in accumulation of inflammatory exudates and leading to edema, swelling of the joint. Posterior Jānu is an excellent point for treating sciatic pain, while anterior Jānu is excellent for inflammatory disorders.

Stimulation of Jānu marmāni increases blood flow to the brain, and is effective for relieving vertigo or dizziness. Medial Charana corresponds to LR 8, an acupoint known to "invigorate the blood". The Liver meridian travels through the genital region, hence it benefits the genital area and the uterus. It is used for swelling, itching, and pain of the genitals. LR 8 also treats impotence, seminal emission, difficult urination, retention of urine and enuresis. In women, the acupoint treats uterine prolapse, abdominal masses, amenorrhea and umbilical pain. It can also address headache, dizziness, mania, nosebleeds and shortness of breath.

199

Charana (2)

Location
Two points on the medial and lateral aspect of the knee joint.

Lateral Charana is in a depression anterior and inferior to the head of the fibula.

Medial Charana is located, when the knee is flexed, 1.5 anguli superior to the medial end of the popliteal crease.

Action
♦ Promotes circulation in lower extremities
♦ Acts locally to relieve knee pain
♦ Supports the kidneys, bladder and adrenals

Associated Doshic Subtypes
Apāna Vāyu, Vyāna Vāyu, Shleshaka Kapha

Indications
♦ Arthritis of the knee joint
♦ Limited range of motion of the knee
♦ Peripheral vascular disease (PVD), poor circulation
♦ Pain, neuropathy or edema of lower extremities

Treatment
Refer to Jānu Treatment section, page 199.

Corresponding Acupoint
Lateral Charana – GB 34, Yanglingquan (Yang Mound Spring)

Medial Charana – LR 8, Ququan (Spring at the Crook)

Both marmani have a strong local action to benefit the knee joint and lower extremities. The acupoints have a wider range of influence in addition to their local action. Lateral Charana corresponds to GB 34, a commonly used acupoint. It is an influential point to benefit the sinews, providing pain relief in all the muscles and joints. It is also a major point to harmonize "shaoyang" conditions such as excess damp-heat by benefiting the shaoyang meridians: Liver and Gallbladder. GB 34 relieves shaoyang symptoms such as vomiting, constipation, hypertension, and chills and fever.

Medial Charana corresponds to LR 8, an acupoint known to "invigorate the blood". The Liver meridian travels through the genital region, hence it benefits the genital area and the uterus. It is used for swelling, itching, and pain of the genitals. LR 8 also treats impotence,

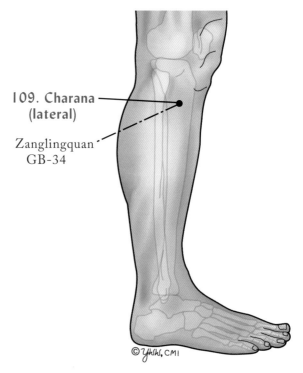

109. Charana (lateral)

Zanglingquan GB-34

© Yhīhī, CMI

seminal emission, difficult urination, retention of urine and enuresis. In women, the acupoint treats uterine prolapse, abdominal masses, amenorrhea and umbilical pain. It can also address headache, dizziness, mania, nosebleeds and shortness of breath.

Commentary
Charana is translated as movement. These marmāni are related to the functioning of the lower extremities and are responsible for their movement. They regulate circulation through vyāna vāyu. Similar to Jānu marmāni, they influence the knees and legs for relief of pain, tingling, numbness and edema. Medial Charana is related to the bladder and Lateral Charana to the kidneys. Tenderness on palpation of these marmāni may reveal toxins in the colon. The marma on the right is connected to the ascending colon and on the left with the descending colon.

Legs Feet

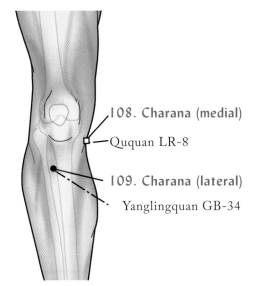

108. Charana (medial)

Ququan LR-8

109. Charana (lateral)

Yanglingquan GB-34

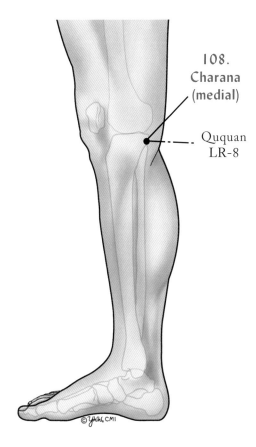

108. Charana (medial)

Ququan LR-8

Indrabasta (2)

**Legs
Feet**

Location

Two points on the medial and posterior aspect of the calf muscle.

Medial Indrabasta is 4 to 5 anguli inferior to the medial condyle of the tibia in a depression just posterior to the medial crest of the tibia.

Posterior Indrabasta is in the center of the belly of the gastrocnemius muscle, at the line that connects posterior Jānu to Pārshni.

Action

◆ Promotes circulation in the lower extremities
◆ Benefits the legs and relaxes the muscles
◆ Regulates menses (medial Indrabasta)
◆ Regulates functions of the colon (posterior Indrabasta)
◆ Stabilizes mind (posterior Indrabasta)

Associated Doshic Subtypes

Apāna Vāyu, Vyāna Vāyu, Rañjaka Pitta, Sādhaka Pitta

Indications

◆ Peripheral vascular disease (poor circulation)
◆ Pain, neuropathy or edema of lower extremities
◆ Muscle cramps
◆ Colon dysfunction: constipation, diarrhea, flatulence
◆ Hemorrhoids, irritable bowel syndrome (IBS)
◆ Inflammatory bowel disease: Crohn's disease, ulcerative colitis
◆ Emotional disturbance

Medial Indrabasta
◆ PMS, dysmenorrhea (painful menses), menstrual cramps

Posterior Indrabasta
◆ Lumbosacral radiculopathy (sciatica)

Treatment

Use these points in conjunction with other local marmāni to enhance the desired therapeutic effect. Refer to Jānu Treatment section, page 199.

Corresponding Acupoint

Medial Indrabasta – SP 8, Diji (Earth Pivot)

Posterior Indrabasta – BL 56, Chengjin (Support of the Sinews)

SP 8 has similar functions as the marma to regulate blood and menstruation. As a Xi-cleft point, it specifically addresses blood stagnation manifesting as irregular

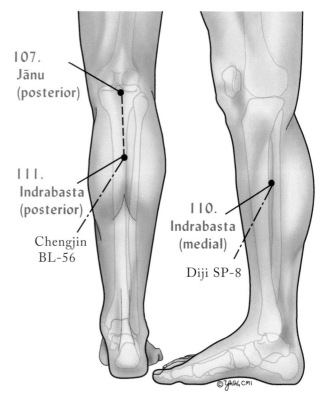

107. Jānu (posterior)

111. Indrabasta (posterior)

Chengjin BL-56

110. Indrabasta (medial)

Diji SP-8

menses, dysmenorrhea, abdominal masses, distention or pain. It does not share the marma's ability to treat colon dysfunction.

Posterior Indrabasta corresponds to Chengjin BL 56. Both locally benefit the legs, feet, heels and soles as well as relieving cramps in the calf muscle. Both share the ability to treat hemorrhoids and constipation. The acupoint also relieves incontinence.

Commentary

Basta can be translated as colon and the term *basti* as bladder. Indrabasta is considered the inner door of the colon. A corresponding point on the arm, Bāhū Indrabasta, has similar energetics (see page 176). Indrabasta marmāni on the legs relieve pain of the lower extremities, while Bāhū Indrabasta affects the upper extremities.

All Indrabasta marmāni affect the colon and the mind. According to Āyurvedic psychology, the colon is the seat of vāta and all vāta-related emotions, such as anxiety, fear and nervousness. These can be relieved by treating Indrabasta marma. Indrabasta on the right leg is affiliated with the ascending colon; the marma on the left leg relates to the descending colon. It is recommended to treat the marmāni related to the descending colon first, followed by those associated with the ascending colon. Indrabasta marmāni address colon dysfunction and pacify vāta-type emotions. Refer to the Bāhū Indrabasta Commentary additional information, page 176.

Medial Indrabasta is known for regulating the blood, relieving menstrual cramps and treating PMS. Posterior Indrabasta is effective for reducing sciatic pain and muscle cramps.

Gulpha (2)

Location
Two points located on the medial and lateral aspects of the ankle joint.
Medial Gulpha is one angula inferior and one angula posterior to the tip of the medial malleolus.
Lateral Gulpha is in a depression below the lateral malleolus.

Action
♦ Benefits the ankles
♦ Improves circulation in the feet
♦ Relieves pain locally
♦ Regulates kidney function and water filtration
♦ Pacifies kapha dosha

Associated Doshic Subtypes
Prāna Vāyu, Apāna Vāyu, Vyāna Vāyu, Shleshaka Kapha

Indications
♦ Ankle pain
♦ Edema, swelling due to arthritis
♦ Cold feet
♦ Kidney dysfunction: renal colic
♦ Urinary incontinence, dribbling urine, retention of urine, difficulty of urination
♦ Emotional disturbance

Contraindications
♦ Pregnancy

Treatment
Refer to Jānu Treatment section, page 199.

Corresponding Acupoint
Medial Gulpha – KD 5, Shuiquan (Water Spring)

Lateral Gulpha – BL 62, Shenmai (Extending Vessel)

Similar to medial Gulpha, KD 5 improves circulation locally and relieves ankle pain or swelling. It also regulates kidney function and benefits difficult urination or dribbling urination. However, KD 5's primary influence is to regulate menstruation and treat menstrual disorders such as irregularity, amenorrhea and dysmenorrhea. TCM describes a close connection between the Kidneys, the uterus, blood and menstruation.

BL 62 acts on the ankle as Lateral Gulpha does. However, it has a broader range of action than Gulpha,

because it is the master point of the *Yangqiao,* one of the Eight Extraordinary Vessels. These vessels are meridians that run much deeper in the body than the 14 primary meridians located on the body's surface. They affect qi, blood, yin and yang more profoundly. Hence, BL 62 is used to treat headaches, vertigo, epilepsy and hemiplegia. It is indicated for Bell's palsy, stiff neck and back pain in the lumbar region. BL 62 also addresses insomnia, palpitations, fright or mania.

Commentary
The Sanskrit translation of *gulpha* is dimple or ditch. A ditch is a place where water collects. Edema, a swelling due to build-up of fluids, often becomes noticeable under the loose skin of both the ankle and lower eyelid. If the puffiness is evident under the eyelid in the morning, it is renal edema. If it becomes more pronounced in the evening along with swollen ankles, it is likely due to poor venous return and is called cardiac edema. Edema is due to disturbance of ambu vaha srotas, the channels that transport water, and mūtra vaha srotas, the channels of the urinary system. Gulpha is functionally related to both these systems.

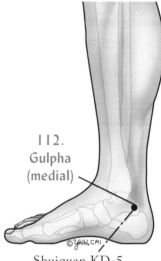

Legs Feet

112. Gulpha (medial)

Shuiquan KD-5

With gentle pressure, Gulpha alleviates local pain, sprain and swelling of the ankle joint. When shleshaka kapha is diminished, the joints are not properly lubricated, resulting in dryness, inflammation and arthritis. Gulpha also influences the kidneys. Lateral Gulpha is associated with the ovaries in women

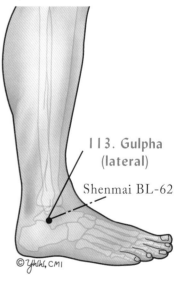

113. Gulpha (lateral)

Shenmai BL-62

and prostate and testicles in men. Gulpha marmāni pacify kapha dosha and kapha-type emotions. It also influences the kidneys and treats dysfunction such as renal colic.

Pāda Charana

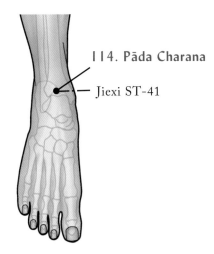

114. Pāda Charana

Jiexi ST-41

Legs
Feet

Location
On the anterior aspect of the ankle joint. In a depression between the tendons of extensor hallucis longus and extensor digitorum longus.

Action
♦ Benefits the ankles
♦ Improves circulation in the feet
♦ Relieves pain locally
♦ Regulates functions of the colon and bladder

Associated Doshic Subtypes
Apāna Vāyu, Prāna Vāyu, Vyāna Vāyu, Shleshaka Kapha, Ālochaka Pitta

Indications
♦ Ankle pain
♦ Edema, swelling due to arthritis
♦ Cold feet, poor circulation
♦ Pain, swelling, or tenderness of the feet
♦ Colon dysfunction, constipation, flatulence
♦ Cystitis, bladder pain

Treatment
Refer to Jānu Treatment section, page 199.

Corresponding Acupoint
ST 41, Jiexi (Stream Divide)

ST 41 benefits the foot and ankle. Similar to Pāda Charana, it also treats constipation. However, ST 41 has a broader action that encompasses treating hypertension and vertigo. It relieves sciatic pain, headaches, and abdominal pain and distention. The acupoint also addresses emotional disturbances such as mania, agitation, sadness and fear.

Commentary
Pāda translates as foot and *charan* as movement. The marma is connected to the movement of the foot. Locally, it helps the foot and ankle, like the Gulpha marmāni. Pāda Charana benefits the colon and bladder as well. The marma located on the right foot corresponds to the ascending colon, while the one on the left foot is related to the descending colon. The marma has some affiliation with the eyes, via prāna vāyu and ālochaka pitta; the prāna nādī that originates between the second and third toes travels from Pāda Charana towards the eyes.

Pāda Kshipra

Location
Midpoint of the base of the nail on the big toe.

Action
♦ Relieves headaches
♦ Activates prāna
♦ Regulates kundalinī
♦ Benefits shukra and ārtava dhātus

Associated Doshic Subtypes
Prāna Vāyu, Udāna Vāyu, Apāna Vāyu, Vyāna Vāyu, Tarpaka Kapha, Shleshaka Kapha

Indications
♦ Vertex headaches, migraines
♦ Insomnia
♦ Shortness of breath
♦ Hormonal imbalance, pituitary dysfunction

Treatment
A silver ring can be worn on the big toe to pacify pitta and to control migraines. **Nirgundi oil** applied here pacifies vāta dosha, **sandalwood oil** reduces pitta, while **vacha oil** is used for kapha.

Corresponding Acupoint
None

Midway between SP 1, Yinbai (Hidden White) and LR 1, Dadun (Big Mound)

Pāda Kshipra is located midway between SP 1 and LR 1, the first points on the Spleen and Liver meridians, respectively. Both are located at the base of the nail on the big toe; SP 1 is 0.1 cun from the medial corner, while LR 1 is 0.1 cun from the lateral corner.
Both regulate the Blood and stop excessive menstrual bleeding. SP 1 also treats blood in the urine, stools or vomit, and is used for nosebleeds. Locally, both points alleviate cold feet and cold sensations in the lower leg. Both points restore consciousness and influence the emotions. SP 1 also addresses digestive disturbances, such as vomiting, diarrhea, loss of appetite and abdominal distention. LR 1 has an effect on the genital area and

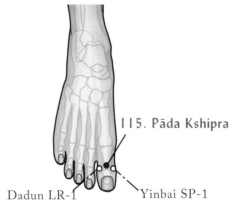

115. Pāda Kshipra

Legs
Feet

Dadun LR-1   Yinbai SP-1

treats urinary dysfunction. Unlike Pāda Kshipra, neither of them treat insomnia or hormonal imbalance.

Commentary
Pāda means foot and *kshipra* is instantaneous or immediately acting. Its location on the big toe mirrors that of Hasta Kshipra on the thumb. Both are at the midpoint of the base of the nail. Each of these marmāni activates prāna, because of a prāna nādī (energy channel) that runs from the marma to the brain. Hence, they instantaneously begin to relieve headaches. Pāda Kshipra is functionally related to the heart, lungs and pituitary. This marma addresses pituitary dysfunction and hormonal imbalance. Pāda Kshipra on the right foot stimulates pitta, while left Pāda Kshipra stimulates Kapha. To enliven vāta, press both simultaneously.

Via apāna vāyu, Pāda Kshipra acts on the ovaries in women and testicles in men. Yogis influence this vāyu by sitting in half-lotus pose, so that the left heel presses against mūlādhāra chakra at the perineum. This pressure activates Pāda Kshipra marma, regulates kundalinī energy and decreases libido. When sitting in this posture, yogis also suck in the anus, performing ashvini mudrā. It is important to keep kundalinī energy moving upward rather than downward. Upward flowing kundalinī brings spiritual awakening, while downward flow of kundalinī makes the person materialistic and lost in worldly affairs. One way to channel kundalinī energy is to wear a copper ring on the left big toe. This helps to direct the kundalinī flow to the right brain hemisphere, awakening intuition, poetry and spirituality.

Pāda Kshipra marma can be pressed or the big toe pulled to bring a person to a normal state of consciousness if kundalini becomes hyperactive. Kundalini is said to arise from the mūlādhāra chakra, which is governed by Lord Ganesha. He is known as Kshipra Prasāda because he offers his devotees immediate prasāda or fulfillment.

Pārshni

Location
One angula inferior to the calcaneal tubercle on the posterior aspect of the heel.

Action
♦ Benefits the heels
♦ Promotes circulation in the feet
♦ Relieves pain locally
♦ Balances prāna and apāna in the pelvic cavity

Associated Doshic Subtypes
Apāna Vāyu, Vyāna Vāyu, Shleshaka Kapha

Indications
♦ Pain in the heel or foot
♦ Local swelling due to arthritis, tendonitis, plantar fasciitis
♦ Lumbar radiculopathy (sciatica)
♦ Pain in ovaries or prostate

Treatment
Agni karma, the application of heat, can be used to treat sciatic pain via this marma and all the marmāni that run down the posterior aspect of the leg. Stimulating the marma with a shalākā effectively reduces pain locally. (See "Agni Karma (Application of Heat)" on page 73.) **Nirgundi oil** pacifies vāta dosha, **sandalwood oil** pacifies pitta and **vacha oil** is used for kapha.

Corresponding Acupoint
None

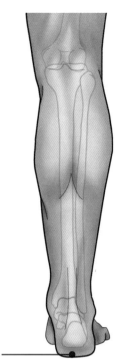

116. Pārshni

Commentary
Parshni means heel. Locally, it relieves pain, as do Gulpha and Pāda Charana. Deep pressure here relieves sciatic pain and lumbosacral pain. The marma is used in conjunction with Sphij, Posterior Sakthi Ūrvī, Posterior Jānu and Posterior Indrabasta to effectively reduce sciatic pain. Pārshni has a connection to the pelvic cavity and organs. In men, it treats problems with the testicles and prostate by balancing apāna vāyu. In women, it addresses disorders of the ovaries and cervix. As described above (page 205) under Pāda Kshipra marma, yogis press the heel against the perineum and mūlādhāra chakra while sitting in the half-lotus pose, stimulating Pārshni marma. This helps to moderate sexual desire, traditionally considered to be an obstacle to spiritual development.

Pāda Madhya

Location
On the sole of the foot, between the second and third metatarsals. If a line is drawn from the base of the second toe to the heel, the point is one-third of the distance from the toe.

Action
♦ Benefits the feet and lower extremities
♦ Relieves pain locally
♦ Relieves headaches
♦ Maintains equilibrium
♦ Calms the mind and relieves stress

Associated Doshic Subtypes
Prāna Vāyu, Vyāna Vāyu, Pāchaka Pitta

Indications
♦ Pain in the feet, cold feet
♦ Pain, neuropathy of lower extremities
♦ Headaches, migraines
♦ Hyperglycemia
♦ Vertigo, light-headedness
♦ Insomnia, stress, hyperactivity

Treatment
Castor oil or **coconut oil** can be used to relieve pain or soreness, especially for flat feet. For insomnia, it is recommended to massage the soles of the feet with **bhringarāja oil** before bedtime, giving special emphasis to Pāda Madhya.

Corresponding Acupoint
KD 1, Yongquan (Bubbling Spring)

Like Pāda Madhya, KD 1 benefits the lower extremities. It is especially indicated for lower limb paralysis, pain and swelling of the leg. It also treats cold or heat sensations, chronic pain and numbness of the feet. KD 1 similarly descends excessive energy from above that manifests as ungroundedness, insomnia, vertigo, headaches and migraines. Thus, it stabilizes the mind. In addition, KD 1 treats epilepsy, loss of consciousness and hypertension. It strengthens the mind in cases of poor memory, agitation, fear and rage. It alleviates respiratory conditions, such as cough and shortness of breath. KD 1 also addresses constipation, difficult urination or defecation, abdominal pain, infertility and impotence.

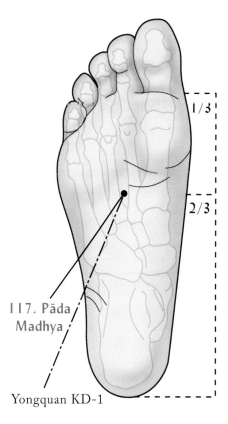

Legs Feet

117. Pāda Madhya

Yongquan KD-1

Commentary
Pāda translates as foot and *madhya* as middle, describing the marma's location precisely in the middle of the foot. Sushruta calls this point Tala Hridaya. In addition to benefiting the lower extremities, Pāda Madhya calms the mind and helps to reduce stress, insomnia and hyperactivity by effectively descending excess energy in the head and bringing it down to the feet—hence its effectiveness in pacifying headaches and migraines. It maintains equilibrium and grounds individuals who feel dizzy, spacey and light-headed due to disturbance of vāta dosha. Pāda Madhya is functionally related to the pancreas and diaphragm.

The foot can be seen as a map of the body; this marma in the center of the foot corresponds to the center of the body, the solar plexus. Treatment here pacifies pāchaka pitta, which works in the stomach and pancreas to digest, absorb and assimilate food. It is also helpful for hyperglycemia and peptic ulcer.

To balance the body's polarity, Pāda Madhya at the sole of the foot and Mūrdhni at the top of the head can be stimulated together. Nābhi marma, at the center of the navel, is the central pole that harmonizes both forces, positive and negative.

Marma Massage for the Legs And Feet

Before using the following procedure please review chapter 8, especially "Guidelines for Touch and Pressure" on page 75 that offers instructions about massaging marmāni. Appendix C has the series of marma massage directions and illustrations starting on page 284.

Legs
Feet

The instructions here refer to the drawings on these pages. The numbers are for use with these massage drawings only; they are different from the numbering system for the marma points used throughout the book. To look up details on a particular marma point, refer to the beginning of this chapter, page 191, to the tables that reference all the marma points and their page numbers.

Apply a few drops of essential oil to the tips of the fingers. Start with gentle pressure on the marma points, and gradually increase according to the capacity of the individual. If you use too much pressure, the person will show discomfort by saying, "ouch!" or through facial expressions, such as wrinkling of the face. Pressure on all marmāni should be held for approximately one to two minutes. If you feel that stronger pressure is needed, you can apply it when the patient exhales.

It's possible to perform the Prone Position series on both legs simultaneously but you can do one leg at a time as well. The Supine Position series should be done on one leg at a time.

Prone Position. Ask the patient to lie in prone position to massage the posterior aspect of the legs. These large muscles require greater pressure to be exerted with the thumbs. Begin at Sphij marma (1) and hold for one minute. Slide down the midline from Sphij to Posterior Sakthi Ūrvī (2), and then Posterior Jānu (3). Repeat this sequence three times. Slide down the midline again from Posterior Jānu (3) to Posterior Indrabasta (4) and hold. Repeat this sequence two or three times as well.

From Posterior Jānu (3), move to Medial Charana (5) and slide down the medial aspect of the calf with a "squeezing" motion. Next, move from Posterior Jānu (3) to Lateral Charana (6) and repeat the "squeezing" technique down the lateral aspect of the calf. Massage Lateral and Medial Gulpha (7, 8) together at the ankle. Apply pressure on Pārshni (9), followed by Pāda Madhya (10).

Supine Position. Next, ask the patient to lie in supine position so the anterior aspect of the legs can be massaged. Begin by stimulating Ūrū 1 (11) and sliding the thumb towards Lohitāksha (12). Next apply pressure on Ūrū 2 (13), followed by Anterior Sakthi Ūrvī (14). Slide down the midline from Lohitāksha (12), to Anterior Sakthi Ūrvī (14), and then Anterior Jānu (15). Repeat this procedure three times.

From Lateral Charana (16), apply the squeezing technique down the lateral aspect of the calf. Repeat the squeezing technique down the medial aspect of the calf. Give emphasis to Medial Indrabasta followed by Medial Charana (5). Continue towards the ankles and massage both Gulpha marmāni (7, 8) simultaneously, followed by Pāda Charana (18) and Pāda Kshipra (19).

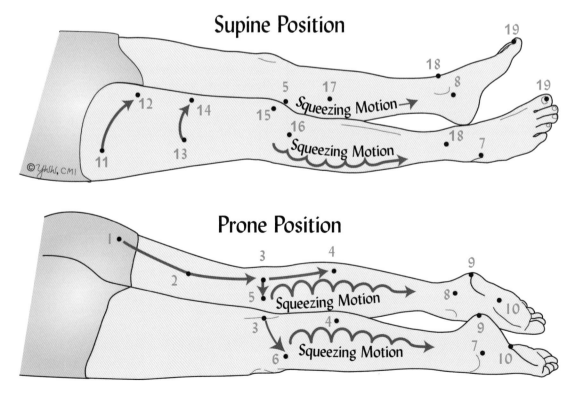

Supine Position

Prone Position

Introduction to Part Three

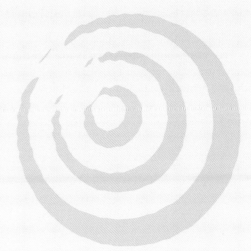

In Parts 1 and 2, we have explored the marmāni of Āyurveda from numerous perspectives, including their anatomy, physiological functions, relation to subdoshas, therapeutic effects, influence on the mind and emotions, and their significance for spiritual unfoldment. Part 3 focuses on the practical application of marma therapy in the management of numerous disorders, including aggravation and disturbance of the bodily channels known as srotāmsi. We also discuss the use of several other types of therapy, including aromatherapy and yoga, in the context of marma chikitsā.

Marma chikitsā is a vast subject that illustrates interconnectedness, a view of life central to both TCM and Āyurveda. Effective practice of marma chikitsā entails an extensive background understanding of etiology, pathogenesis, pathways of disease, channel disturbance and vikruti (current imbalance). Equally important is the integration of marma chikitsā with various other branches of therapy as well as a mastery of specific techniques to stimulate the energy points.

In short, marma chikitsā is an art and science that requires dedication, cultivation and clinical acumen. While it is true that simply pressing here and there on the body at appropriate marma points can bring immediate relief for conditions such as headaches or nausea,[1] we urge our readers, especially those responsible for the health of others, not to be tempted to practice marma chikitsā without expert guidance and without first gaining at least some understanding of the broad framework in which these energy points are utilized. Like the other aspects of Āyurveda, marma therapy is especially effective when it is practiced in the context of the entire medical system and not in isolation.

Throughout this book, we emphasize the therapeutic value of the marmāni but it is important to remember that these energy points can also be utilized as diagnostic tools. Marmāni are a language of the body that a sensitive practitioner can learn to read in daily clinical life. The internal organs speak through the marmāni, and a tender marma is a call for prompt, proper attention. For example, if Jānu marma is tender, this is a sign of toxins in the colon. If Gulpha marma is sensitive, this indicates a disturbance of kidney energy. Then the very same marma can be used for treatment.

If you are a medical practitioner, a massage therapist, chiropractor, physician, nurse, acupuncturist, naturopath and so on, study this material; get some training and guidance from an experienced practitioner of marma chikitsā, and incorporate this knowledge for the benefit of your patients. And everyone, whether a health care provider or not, can learn enough from these pages to promote healing and balance in their lives and the lives of their families and friends.

As this book goes to press, there is much talk of Western medicine moving into the age of the "empowered patient," capable of substantial self-care and of discerning and demanding the most appropriate treatment. This trend is welcomed by Ayurvedic practitioners, as self-care and empowerment have always been at the core of this ancient knowledge. Indeed, the heart of Āyurveda is self-care and prevention in conjunction with a disciplined and self-managed lifestyle. A primary task of Ayurvedic practitioners is education to help their

---

1. We list a number of these points and conditions in the section on First Aid at the beginning of chapter 17.

patients live long and healthy lives. Thus, we encourage everyone to put the knowledge in this book to use.

From our long experience using marma therapy in clinical practice, we don't hesitate to say that if you are a medical professional and put this knowledge to use, a miracle will happen in your clinical life. Patients who come to your clinic or your office with pain and tears will leave with a smiling face.

Aromatherapy, Essential Oils and Attars in Āyurveda

In chapter 7 we discussed the various types of therapy or chikitsā employed in Āyurveda. One category is called Tanmātrā Chikitsā, or Five Element Therapy, which promotes health and treats illness using the five senses. Among these, aromatherapy, known as *gandha chikitsā* or therapy based on the sense of smell, is the venerable art of using fragrant essential oils for therapeutic purposes.

Essential oils may be derived from the roots, leaves, bark, seeds, stems, fruits or flowers of an herb, plant or tree and carry its concentrated healing properties. These potent fragrances affect mind, body and spirit in numerous ways. They may elevate or pacify the doshas, excite or calm the mind, relieve pain, stimulate circulation, work as an antibiotic and antiseptic, enliven kundalinī, act as an aphrodisiac and much more.

The oils have an affinity to various structures of the body. When they are applied to specific marmāni, the sensory perceptions of smell and touch are engaged. Essential oils alter the body's neurochemistry and trigger the release of neurotransmitters and neuropeptides through the olfactory bulb and chemoreceptors under the skin. (These are the same neuropeptides released in the central nervous system that govern psycho-neuro-immunological response.) The influence of the oils comes through three fields of action:

* *Rasa* (taste)
* *Vīrya* (heating or cooling energy)
* *Vipāka* (post-digestive effect[1])

Specific properties of essential oils influence the doshas and their associated organs. For example, applying sandalwood oil to Ājñā marma (the third eye) and Shankha marma (the temple) has a cooling effect on the entire body. In general, oils that are heating and ground-

ing in nature are best to pacify vāta dosha. Hina, cinnamon, chamomile, eucalyptus, ginger, clove and nirgundi may be used for vāta conditions. Cooling oils soothe pitta dosha, as they are anti-inflammatory. These include sandalwood, khus, lavender, jasmine, peppermint and rose. Kapha is calmed by heating and energizing essential oils, such as saffron, vacha, camphor, ginger, hina, clove, nutmeg and eucalyptus. A therapist chooses which oils to use according to the patient's constitution and the condition being treated. Table 26 on page 212 shows the vīrya of the 27 oils we discuss in this chapter.

Both essential oils and attars are used in Ayurvedic treatments. Essential oils are highly concentrated, complex chemicals extracted from whole plant matter. Attars are extracted through distillation and blended in a base of sandalwood essential oil. This chapter includes a brief description of 27 of the most commonly used oils and attars and summarizes their therapeutic properties. For each oil, a few marmāni are listed as examples of where the healing qualities of the oil may be most effectively used. At the end of this chapter is a detailed chart summarizing the properties and actions of these oils and attars.

Brahmī, *centella asiatica,* medicated oil takes on brahmī's qualities, which are sweet, astringent and bitter in taste, with a sweet vipāka. Its vīrya is cooling if the herb is fresh, but heating if older than a year. It balances all three doshas. Brahmī oil is a rejuvenative for memory, intelligence and concentration. It improves the clarity of perception and is a rasāyana for the brain and majjā dhātu, the nervous system. It calms the mind, especially when applied to Mūrdhni, Brahmarandhra, Shivarandhra or Ājñā marmāni.

Camphor, *cinnamomum camphora,* essential oil is sweet, slightly pungent and astringent to the taste. Its vīrya is heating and vipāka is pungent. It pacifies vāta and kapha doshas because of its heating properties. As a bronchodilator, decongestant and expectorant, its action is primarily on the lungs, so it can be applied to Apast-

---

1. Bhrājaka agni promotes digestion through the medium of the skin. Substances applied on the skin can influence sweating and cellular metabolism via their vipāka.

ambha, Amsa Phalaka, Prushtha and Bruhatī marmāni. Its action is calming because it is a nervine sedative. Camphor is said to unfold divine love in one's consciousness and compassion in the heart; it also enhances devotion. Thus, it can be applied to marmāni associated with the heart: Hrid and Hridayam.

Chamomile, *anthemis nobilis,* essential oil is sweet and astringent in taste. It is cooling with a sweet vipāka. It pacifies pitta and can provoke kapha because of its sweet nature. The chamomile flower has a lovely fragrance. With an affinity for the brain, nervous system, heart and muscles, it enhances tranquility and relaxation, and is a frequent ingredient in sleep inducing tea. For insomnia, apply chamomile to Ājñā marma. Chamomile is antispasmodic, analgesic and a muscle relaxant.

Champa, *michelia champaca* or *magnolia champaca,* attar is bitter, slightly sweet and astringent. It has a heating vīrya and pungent vipāka. The green form of champa is cooling; snakes like it, and thus it is known as the "cobra" type. The yellow type is heating and is good for vāta and kapha, but may be too strong for pitta individuals. Acting to improve circulation and release deep-seated emotions, it also serves as a mood elevator and relieves feelings of heaviness. It is a decongestant. This oil can be applied to Nābhi marmāni for stagnant pitta that may manifest as gallstones. Application on Ganda marmāni is effective for sinus congestion.

Cinnamon, *cinnamomum zeylanicum,* essential oil is sweet, pungent and slightly astringent in taste, with a pungent vipāka. Its vīrya is heating and thus not recommended for high pitta. It pacifies vāta and kapha doshas. Similar to camphor, cinnamon oil has an affinity for the lungs and is classified as a decongestant and expectorant. It acts to improve lymphatic circulation. Influential especially on the heart, in cardiac conditions the oil can be applied directly to the pericardial area, including Apastambha, Hrid and Hridayam marmāni. Cinnamon reduces cholesterol and triglycerides, induces vasodilatation, and thins the blood; do not use it when there is bleeding disorder. Cinnamon is a mild aphrodisiac; the oil may be applied, carefully, onto the pubic bone at Bhaga marma. But if the oil touches the mucous membrane, it causes burning, so be careful!

Clove, *syzygium aromaticum,* essential oil has a sweet and pungent rasa, heating vīrya and sweet vipāka. It pacifies vāta and kapha because of its heating nature, but can easily stimulate pitta. It has a sharp, penetrating action. This essential oil is analgesic and can instantaneously relieve pain. It is effective for headaches and toothaches if applied to Shankha, Hanu, Oshtha or Chibuka marmāni. Clove applied to Apastambha and Agra Patra marmāni acts on the lungs as an expectorant and decongestant. Applied to the stomach it can improve

digestion, especially via Nābhi marma. Clove oil also has an affinity for the nervous system.

Table 26: Heating or Cooling Properties of Oils

Essential Oil	Cooling Vīrya	Essential Oil	Heating Vīrya
Chamomile	Cooling	Camphor	Heating
Jasmine	Cooling	Cinnamon	Heating
Jatamāmsī	Cooling	Clove	Heating
Kadamba	Cooling	Deodara	Heating
Khus	Cooling	Hina	Heating
Lavender	Cooling	Kewrā	Heating
Mitti	Cooling	Musta	Heating
Patchouli	Cooling	Champa	Heating
Peppermint	Cooling[c]	Nirgundi	Heating
Rose	Cooling	Nutmeg	Heating
Sandalwood (Chandan)	Cooling	Tulsi (Holy Basil)	Heating
Eucalyptus	Cooling/heating[a]	Vacha	Heating
Brahmī	Cooling/heating[b]	Tea Tree[c]	Heating/cooling[d]
		Saffron	Warming

a. In moderate doses, eucalyptus is cooling but it is heating in large quantity. Externally, it is cooling, internally it is heating.
b. Brahmī medicated oil made from fresh herbs is cooling; made from dried herbs it is heating.
c. All essential oils should be applied only to unbroken skin; avoid getting into the eyes or mucous membranes unless otherwise stated.
d. Tea tree oil is internally heating; externally this oil is cooling. It has a heating effect on mucous membranes – it will burn!

Deodara, *cedrus deodara,* essential oil has a pungent rasa and vipāka. Its heating nature pacifies vāta and kapha doshas. Grounding and a muscle relaxant, it is a strong nervine sedative and has an affinity for the nervous system. When used in conjunction with sandalwood, deodara oil can open blocked chakras. It can be applied to all chakras for meditation and chakra attunement.

Eucalyptus, *eucalyptus globulus,* essential oil has a pungent rasa and vipāka. In moderate doses it is cooling, but it is heating in large quantity. Pacifying to vāta and kapha doshas, it primarily acts on the lungs and sinuses as a decongestant and bronchodilator, and can be applied to Apastambha, Ājñā, Kapola Nāsā or Nāsā Puta marmāni. Eucalyptus oil is also a stimulant that effectively acts on kapha dosha. It is a diaphoretic, that is, it induces sweating. Eucalyptus has a cooling effect on the surface of the skin, but is heating on the mucous lining.

Hina, an Indian attar blend of various herbs, spices, roots and seeds in a base of mehendi (*lawsonia inermis*), saffron and sandalwood, has a bitter, slightly pungent and sweet taste. It is heating, with a pungent vipāka. It is balancing to all three doshas in small amounts, but may increase pitta in higher doses or in summertime, because of its strong scent. Due to its divinely pleasing smell, it is considered sacred and it is commonly used in pūja (Hindu rituals). It strengthens the mind and body, enhancing clarity, intuition and psychic abilities. A rejuvenative and alterative nervine tonic with a tranquilizing effect, hina improves circulation, especially coronary circulation. It treats cardiac pain and vāta and kapha type of pain. Hina is said to have a mystical ability to open the heart chakra (Hridayam) and third eye (Ājñā), and to awaken kundalinī shakti. It unfolds bhakti (devotion).

Jasmine, *jasminum sambac,* essential oil or attar is sweet, astringent and slightly bitter to the taste. It is cooling with a sweet vipāka. Although it balances all three doshas, it elevates kapha with long-term use. It is an effective rasāyana for majjā dhātu (the nervous system), especially the memory. This oil has an affinity for the heart and the brain. It unfolds love in the heart and acts as an antidepressant. It can be applied to Hrid and Hridayam marmāni. A few drops applied to Bhaga marma (pubic bone) can act as an aphrodisiac.

Jatamāmsī, *nardostachys jatamansi,* essential oil is sweet, astringent and bitter to the taste with a sweet vipāka. It balances the three doshas, but elevates kapha through long-term use, because it is cooling. A nutritive tonic that soothes the nervous system, it is a sedative and tranquilizer, but overuse can make a person slow and sluggish. It has expectorant and demulcent qualities. Jatamāmsī works on majjā dhātu, including the sympathetic and parasympathetic nervous systems. Apply to Mūrdhni, Brahmarandhra, Shivarandhra, Ājñā and Nābhi marmāni. It is grounding and can be used to enhance clarity of perception.

Kadamba, *neolamarckia cadamba,* essential oil is sweet, astringent and bitter to the taste. It is cooling and has a sweet vipāka. Its heavy nature increases kapha and balances vāta and pitta, which are both light. It is grounding and can be applied to Mūrdhni and Ājñā marmāni to calm hyperactivity. It is a decongestant, diuretic and a sedative. Kadamba promotes ojas and helps unfold love in the heart. It awakens kundalinī energy. Kadamba has an affinity to the spleen and can be applied to Plīhā marma for spleen disorders.

Kewrā,[2] *pandanus odoratissimus,* attar is a flower essence derived from a bush. It is sweet and bitter to the taste, and has a sweet vipāka. It is calming and tridosha balancing, but increases pitta if used in excess, because of its heating nature. However, compared to Hina, this oil is better for pitta individuals. It is a blood tonic, nervine stimulant and improves circulation. It has an affinity for the heart and liver and can be used on Hrid, Hridayam and Yakrut marmāni. The sweet aroma of kewrā makes it an excellent choice for pūja (rituals) and worship. This plant is used for worship of Durga, a form of the Divine Mother, and Lord Ganesha. It is a mystical oil that is said to enhance bhakti (devotion) and promotes ojas and immunity.

Khus, *vetiveria zizanioides,* essential oil or attar is sweet and bitter in taste with a sweet vipāka. Its cooling vīrya and grounding properties are good for pitta, but may increase vāta and kapha doshas with long usage. By applying Khus to Ājñā and Shankha marmāni and the carotid and radial arteries, the aura is calmed and anger cooled. It also calms the solar plexus, especially when applied to Sūrya marma. Khus oil is a strengthening tonic and relaxant, and it has an affinity for the nervous system. It improves concentration and purifies the mind. It is antiseptic, a blood purifier and can be used on the skin. Khus balances female hormones and is used as an aphrodisiac oil.

Lavender, *lavandula augustifolia* or *vera,* essential oil is sweet and astringent in taste, with a cooling vīrya and sweet vipāka. Tridosha balancing, tranquilizing and sedative, it calms the mind and induces a deep sense of relaxation. Its properties are similar to rose, but it is sweeter. It also has an affinity for the lungs and bronchi, acting as a bronchodilator. Lavender is an antidepressant and treats anxiety and insomnia. It can be used on Apastambha, Agra Patra and Mūrdhni marmāni.

Mitti, a "baked earth" attar, is a combination of sandalwood and clay. Its rasa is sweet, vīrya cooling and vipāka sweet. It is grounding, calming and centering for vāta, while sweet and cooling for pitta. Excessive use may elevate kapha. Many of its properties are similar to khus oil, particularly its grounding ability.

Musta, *cyperus rotundus,* essential oil is sweet and astringent in taste and pungent in vipāka. Many pitta individuals cannot tolerate musta because of its heating nature. It is an analgesic and a muscle relaxant, often used in the treatment of fibromyalgia. A nervine sedative and tranquilizer, it can relieve vāta and kapha headaches if applied to Shankha, Ājñā, Kapāla and Kapola Nāsā marmāni. Musta is also a mood elevator for those suffering from kapha-type depression.

Nirgundi, *vitex nirgundo,* essential oil is pungent, bitter and slightly astringent. Due to its heating vīrya and pungent vipāka, it may stimulate pitta dosha. Because of its sharp penetrating qualities, nirgundi oil relaxes the muscles and improves circulation. It is a strong analgesic

---

2. Also known as kevrā.

213

and nervine sedative with an affinity for the nervous system.

Nutmeg, *myristica fragrans,* essential oil tastes pungent, bitter, astringent or slightly sweet. Its heating vīrya and pungent vipāka can stimulate pitta dosha. It pacifies vāta and kapha dosha. Nutmeg is a strong analgesic with narcotic properties. It is effective in marma chikitsā for sinus and joint pain, as well as muscle spasms and sprains. It is a tranquilizer and sedative for inducing sound sleep. A drop can be applied to Ājñā marma for insomnia, or to Shankha marma for headaches and migraines. Nutmeg has an affinity to the colon. Because of its astringent action, it helps to bind the stools.

Patchouli, *pogostemon cablin,* essential oil is sweet and astringent to the taste, with a cooling vīrya and a sweet vipāka. It has a pleasant aroma and is pacifying to all three doshas. This oil is grounding, calming and has a soothing effect on the mind. It effectively quiets anxiety, agitation and irritation. Patchouli can be applied to Mūrdhni, Brahmarandhra, Shivarandhra and Ājñā marmāni. Antibacterial and antiseptic, it is also an antidepressant and a memory stimulant. A mild aphrodisiac, it can be applied to Bhaga marma to treat impotence.

Peppermint, *mentha piperita,* essential oil has a sweet, pungent and astringent rasa, cooling vīrya and sweet vipāka. It is tridosha balancing. With an affinity for the lymphatic system and lungs, it is a decongestant. Peppermint oil also acts on the stomach and relieves burning gastric sensations, especially when a few drops are ingested with a small portion of sugar. Peppermint can be used to treat bad breath and indigestion. In marma chikitsā, it can be applied to Apastambha, Sūrya and Nābhi marmāni.

Rose, *rosa damascena,* essential oil or attar has a bitter, sweet or astringent rasa. It has a cooling vīrya, sweet vipāka and is tridosha balancing. Due to its fragrant, pleasing essence, it is used for pūja (ritual and worship). It promotes love and compassion and is a romantic stimulant. Because rose has an affinity for the heart and genitals, it is an aphrodisiac that unfolds sensual love and it can help to open the heart chakra. Rose oil is also a mild laxative, antidepressant and rejuvenates the cells. It can be used for anxiety and insomnia. Rose promotes ojas (immunity). Apply rose oil to Mūrdhni, Ājñā and Hridayam marmāni for depression.

Saffron, *crocus sattivus,* attar is called *keshara* in Sanskrit. It is pungent, bitter and sweet in rasa, slightly heating, with a pungent vipāka. It pacifies vāta and kapha doshas, but may stimulate pitta. This oil is extremely sattvic and beneficial for yoga and spiritual practices. It can bring clarity of perception to the mind and open the heart chakra. It improves the color of complexion, cleanses the blood, and acts as a decongestant. Saffron has an affinity for the spleen and cerebrovascular system. It is an aphrodisiac and acts on the reproductive tissue (shukra and ārtava), balancing male and female hormones. A drop of saffron oil in milk decreases kapha and minimizes the mucus-forming properties of milk.

Sandalwood, *santalum album,* essential oil is called *chandana* in Sanskrit. It is the basis for almost all attars, and can be called the mother of all attars. Its rasa is sweet, bitter and astringent, the vīrya is cooling and its vipāka is sweet. It is tridosha balancing and also balances ojas, tejas and prāna. Sandalwood is calming, with a celestially tranquilizing effect. An antidepressant and nervine sedative, it improves concentration and meditation and has an affinity to the brain, mind, crown chakra and majjā dhātu (nervous tissue). It can be helpful for anxiety, depression and insomnia. Sandalwood is also antispasmodic, anti-inflammatory, antibacterial and antipyretic. It has an affinity for the bladder and can be used to relieve bladder irritation. It acts as a diuretic when applied to Bhaga and Basti marmāni. Sandalwood applied to the skin soothes itching and eczema. It is used in pūja, especially in worshipping Lord Shiva.

Tea Tree, *melaleuca alternifolia,* essential oil is bitter, astringent and pungent to the taste, cooling, and has a pungent vipāka. Tea tree pacifies vāta and kapha, and may stimulate pitta in excess. It has affinity for the skin and rasa and rakta dhātus. It can be used for skin conditions such as athlete's foot or fungal infections. It is antibacterial, antiviral, antifungal, antibiotic and a disinfectant. It is contraindicated for inflammatory conditions or the mucous membranes of the eyes, mouth and genitalia because it creates burning sensations. Tea tree combined with neem oil is a powerful antiseptic for topical use.

Tulsi (Holy Basil), *ocinum sanctum,* essential oil is tridosha balancing and made from the seed of the tulsi plant. The rasa of green tulsi is sweet, while that of purple tulsi is pungent, and its aftertaste is bitter. Due to its heating vīrya and pungent vipāka, tulsi oil stimulates pitta dosha, but pacifies vāta and kapha. It is diaphoretic, decongestant, eliminates toxins and its bitter aftertaste makes it antipyretic. It can be used for generalized body ache and flu-like symptoms. It is antispasmodic and reduces muscle spasms and sprains. It enhances circulation and metabolism. Tulsi benefits the complexion and purifies the body, mind and spirit. It soothes the nervous system. It also has an affinity for the heart and lymphatic system and unfolds love in the heart chakra. It can be applied to Hrid, Hridayam and Apastambha marmāni. Tulsi stands for prosperity, purity, love and devotion and is traditionally considered a favorite of Lord Krishna and Lord Vishnu.

Vacha or calamus root, *acorus calamus,* essential oil is pungent and astringent, and its aftertaste is bitter. Because of its heating vīrya and pungent vipāka, it may stimulate pitta dosha, but it pacifies vāta and kapha. Vacha has a quick-acting effect to enhance clarity of perception. It acts primarily on the brain. It is anticonvulsant, decongestant and analgesic for kapha-type pain. To induce vomiting, vacha oil can be used, as it has emetic action. Vacha oil relieves numbness and is a strong stimulant. It has an affinity for the nervous system, sinuses, lungs and lymphatic system. Vacha oil can be applied to Mūrdhni, Brahmarandhra, Shivarandhra, Ājñā and Apastambha marmāni. Vacha can enhance cellular intelligence.

Table 27: Properties and Actions of Essential Oils

Essential Oil	Rasa	Vīrya	Vipāka	Doshic Influence	Organs / Systems Affected	Action[a]
Brahmī	Sweet, astringent, bitter	Cooling/ heating[b]	Sweet	V↓ P↓ K↓	Nervous system, brain	Nervine tonic, enhances clarity, concentration, memory, and intelligence
Camphor	Sweet, slightly pungent, astringent	Heating	Pungent	V↓ P↑ K↓	Lungs	Decongestant, bronchodilator, expectorant, nervine sedative, unfolds divine love
Chamomile	Sweet, astringent	Cooling	Sweet	V↓ P↓ K↑	Brain, nervous system, heart, muscles	Muscle relaxant, antispasmodic, analgesic, sedative, tranquilizing, antidepressant
Cinnamon	Sweet, pungent, slightly astringent	Heating	Pungent	V↓ P↑ K↓	Heart, lungs, lymphatics	Decongestant, expectorant, enhances circulation, mild aphrodisiac, heart stimulant
Clove	Pungent, sweet	Heating	Sweet	V↓ P↑ K↓	Stomach, lungs, throat, nervous system	Analgesic, decongestant, expectorant, enhances digestion
Deodara	Pungent	Heating	Pungent	V↓ P↑ K↓	Joints, skeleto-muscular system	Analgesic, muscle relaxant, nervine sedative, balances chakras
Eucalyptus	Pungent	Cooling externally / heating internally	Pungent	V↓ P↑ K↓	Lungs, sinuses	Decongestant, diaphoretic, bronchodilator
Hina	Bitter, slightly pungent, sweet	Heating	Pungent	V↓ P↑ K↓	Heart, brain, mental channels	Strengthens mind and body, rejuvenative, alterative nervine tonic, tranquilizer, enhances circulation
Jasmine	Sweet, astringent, slightly bitter	Cooling	Sweet	V↓ P↓ K↓	Heart, brain, nervous system	Antidepressant, antibacterial, enhances memory, aphrodisiac
Jatamāmsī	Sweet, astringent, bitter	Cooling	Sweet	V↓ P↓ K↓	Brain, nervous system	Tranquilizer, sedative, expectorant, demulcent, nutritive tonic, enhances clarity, grounding
Kadamba	Sweet, astringent, bitter	Cooling	Sweet	V↓ P↓ K↑	Spleen, lymphatics, heart	Grounding, calms hyperactivity, decongestant, sedative, enhances ojas, awakens kundalinī

Table 27: Properties and Actions of Essential Oils

Essential Oil	Rasa	Vīrya	Vipāka	Doshic Influence	Organs / Systems Affected	Action[a]
Kewrā	Sweet, bitter	Heating	Sweet	V↓ P↓ K↓	Liver, heart	Blood tonic, nervine stimulant, enhances circulation, increases bhakti and ojas
Khus	Sweet, bitter	Cooling	Sweet	V↑ P↓ K↑	Central nervous system, mind	Tonic, relaxant, purifies mind, blood and skin, antiseptic, enhances concentration, balances female hormones, aphrodisiac
Lavender	Sweet, astringent	Cooling	Sweet	V↓ P↓ K↓	Lungs, mind	Relaxant, tranquilizer, sedative, calms mind, antidepressant, bronchodilator
Mitti	Sweet	Cooling	Sweet	V↓ P↓ K↑	Heart, brain, blood, circulation, muscular system	Calming, cooling, grounding effect
Musta	Sweet, astringent	Heating	Pungent	V↓ P↑ K↓	Skeleto-muscular system	Analgesic, muscle relaxant, nervine sedative, tranquilizer, mood elevator, relieves headaches
Champa	Bitter, slightly Sweet, slightly astringent	Heating	Pungent	V↓ P↑ K↓	Blood, heart, circulation, mind	Promotes circulation, mood elevator, releases emotions, decongestant, enhances romantic feelings
Nirgundi	Pungent, bitter, slightly astringent	Heating	Pungent	V↓ P↑ K↓	Muscle, nervous system	Analgesic, muscle relaxant, nervine sedative, enhances circulation
Nutmeg	Pungent, bitter, astringent or slightly sweet	Heating	Pungent	V↓ P↑ K↓	Colon, central nervous system (CNS)	Analgesic, muscle relaxant, sedative, tranquilizer, binds stools
Patchouli	Sweet, astringent	Cooling	Sweet	V↓ P↓ K↓	Brain, heart, mind, urinary system	Calms mind, antidepressant, antibacterial, antiseptic, mild aphrodisiac, memory stimulant, grounding
Peppermint	Sweet, pungent, astringent	Cooling	Sweet	V↓ P↓ K↓	Lymphatics, lungs, stomach	Decongestant, relieves burning, relieves gastric irritation
Rose	Bitter, sweet or astringent	Cooling	Sweet	V↓ P↓ K↓	Heart, genitals, mind	Romantic, aphrodisiac, mild laxative, antidepressant, promotes immunity
Saffron	Pungent, bitter, sweet	Warming	Pungent	V↓ P↑ K↓	Cerebrovascular system, spleen, reproductive system, heart, mind	Blood cleanser, improves color of complexion, enhances clarity of perception, decongestant, aphrodisiac, balances hormones

Table 27: Properties and Actions of Essential Oils

Essential Oil	Rasa	Vīrya	Vipāka	Doshic Influence	Organs / Systems Affected	Action[a]
Sandalwood (chandan)	Sweet, bitter, astringent	Cooling	Sweet	V↓ P↓ K↓	Brain, heart, bladder, mind, nervous system	Antidepressant, nervine sedative, tranquilizer, enhances concentration, antispasmodic, anti-inflammatory, antibacterial, antipyretic, diuretic, relieves burning and itching of urinary tract
Tea Tree[c]	Bitter, pungent, astringent	Heating internally / cooling externally	Pungent	V↓ P↑ K↓	Skin, rasa and rakta dhatus	Antibacterial, antifungal, antiviral, antibiotic, antiseptic, disinfectant
Tulsi/Holy Basil	Sweet, pungent, bitter	Heating	Pungent	V↓ P↑ K↓	Heart, mind, lungs, lymphatic system	Decongestant, antipyretic, diaphoretic, antispasmodic, enhances circulation and metabolism, benefits complexion, decreases toxins, purifies body, mind, spirit
Vacha	Pungent, astringent, bitter	Heating	Pungent	V↓ P↑ K↓	Brain, nervous system, sinuses, lungs, lymphatics	Anticonvulsant, emetic, stimulant, analgesic, relieves numbness, enhances clarity, decongestant

a. All oils act on the mind.

b. Brahmī essential oils made from fresh herbs are cooling and those from dried herbs are heating.

c. Care must be taken to keep this oil from entering the eyes or mucous membranes.

Marmāni that Treat Channel Disturbance

Introduction to Srotāmsi

As we briefly discussed in chapter 4, comparing various aspects of Āyurveda and Traditional Chinese Medicine, srotāmsi are the channels and channel networks in the body.[1] The channels resemble rivers with various tributaries and branches, each with its own origin, pathways and openings. Srotāmsi are related to organs and other anatomical structures via the seven dhātus (tissues) and to physiological functions, such as the transportation of air, blood, nutrients and fluids.

Srotāmsi are the pathways that facilitate the flow of bodily substances, including glandular secretions, nutrients, hormones and biochemical mucus secretions at the cellular level. All biological secretions originate at the *sroto mūla* (root, origin), flow through the *sroto mārga* (passage) and are excreted via the *sroto mukha* (opening). These are the three components of all srotāmsi.

Part of the vast interlinked communication network that pervades the mind-body, which includes the neurological pathways that allow information to leap and flow from cell to cell, srotāmsi are minute openings or porosities in the cell walls of the tissues that allow communication and exchange of materials in the body. The cell is termed *anusrotas* in Sanskrit, because it is considered a type of channel. Srotāmsi process and regulate the body's biochemistry and metabolism.

Some srotāmsi are physical structures that are comparable to Western anatomical systems, such as the respiratory or digestive systems. Srotāmsi also exist on subtle, biochemical and neurological levels as circuits for communication. There are innumerable srotāmsi. There is an Ayurvedic sūtra that says, *"Man is nothing but a bundle of srotāmsi."* Every thought, feeling and emotion has its own srotas, unique pathway; implying an origin, movement along a pathway and a flowering or opening. There are srotāmsi for the manas (mind), buddhi (intellect), chitta (subconscious faculty that stores vast experience as images) and ahamkāra (ego). These are called *antahkarana,* the inner equipment of experience.

Among the virtually innumerable channels, for practical, clinical purposes Āyurveda highlights sixteen principal srotāmsi, differentiating them into the following categories:

* Receiving channels for food, water and air

* Eliminating channels for urine, feces and sweat

* Tissue channels, corresponding to the seven bodily dhātus

* Channel for the mind, including intellect, memory and emotions

* Additional channels in women for lactation and menstruation

There is a close relationship between the dhātus (tissues), which govern the *structural* aspect of the body, and the srotāmsi (channels), which govern the *functional* aspects. Each srotas is viewed as a physiological and functional unit of a particular dhātu (tissue). The srotas is the container or space within which the dhātu functions, while the dhātu is comparable to the content or substance within the container. The srotāmsi facilitate communication between the tissues and the rest of the body by transporting neural messages and nutrients. Agni (digestive fire) is the fuel that enables the dhātu or srotas to perform its functions. For example, māmsa agni enables māmsa dhātu (muscle tissue) to move through its associated srotāmsi, in order to provide strength and support and give form to the muscles.

Each dhātu has an *upadhātu* (by-product) that is formed when the tissue is nourished. For example, teeth are a by-product of asthi dhātu (bone tissue). An excess or insufficiency of a particular upadhātu reflects the state of agni that leads to the under- or over-nourishment of

---

1. Srotas is the singular form and srotāmsi the plural.

the particular tissue. For instance, lactation is a by-product of rasa dhātu (plasma/lymph); thus, disturbances of rasa dhātu agni can lead to insufficient or excessive lactation. Each upadhātu in turn is associated with its corresponding srotas, which regulates its function. Lactation disturbance is related to rasa vaha srotas.

See table 47 on page 255 in appendix A for detailed information on the srotāmsi, including their functions, roots, pathways and openings.

Disturbance and Treatment of Srotāmsi

Several kinds of etiological factors can aggravate the srotāmsi and lead to disease. These include genetic disposition, poor diet, unhealthy lifestyle choices, aggravation of the doshas and disturbance of the dhātus. Repressed emotions, unresolved tensions in relationships and seasonal factors are also influential. When a srotas is disturbed, it may overflow, stagnate, dilate, constrict or create a false passage. Channels may also experience hypertrophy, atrophy, stagnation, distention, consolidation, inflammation or irritation. For example, stagnation may manifest as blood clots or constipation, hypertrophy as overgrowth or tumor formation, consolidation as calcification, dilation as aneurism or tumors, and false passage as fistulae or diverticula. Disturbances may range from mild to severe. For example, mild overflow can result in diarrhea, whereas severe overflow may cause vomiting. Understanding channel disturbances and the forms they may take is essential for an Ayurvedic clinician to diagnose and treat a patient appropriately.

Treatment of channel disturbances is known as *srotas chikitsā*. Because marmāni communicate internally with the channels and their corresponding tissues, part of the treatment can involve marma chikitsā. Marmāni also influence the upadhātu, mūla, mārga and mukha of each srotas; thus, each marma can help address the pathology and disturbances of its related srotāmsi. Marma treatment can help to rebalance the channel by unblocking stagnation, dispelling accumulation, and so on.

This chapter briefly elucidates the functions, components and disturbances of each srotas, and includes a list of marmāni associated with each channel. The list contains marmāni affecting a particular dhātu (tissue), upadhātu, sroto mūla, sroto mārga or sroto mukha. In the list for each srotāmsi, *the principal marmāni for treatment are italicized.* Refer to part 2 for information on how specific marmāni are related to srotas disturbance and can be used in their treatment.

At the level of sroto mūla, each srotas has its own agni, and ojas, tejas and prāna. Agni maintains the nutritional aspect; prāna governs the communication aspect of the srotas, tejas the intelligence aspect and ojas the immune mechanism. The sroto mūla governs the activity of the srotas through ojas, tejas and prāna and re-establishes normal physiological functioning.

The reason marma chikitsā is so effective, is that it directly stimulates the agni of the srotas which brings functional integration between ojas, tejas and prāna.

Table 28: Srotāmsi, Their Functions and Marmāni

Srotāmsi	Essential Substance
Prāna Vaha Srotas	Prāna
Ambu/Udaka Vaha Srotas	Water
Anna Vaha Srotas	Food
Rasa Vaha Srotas	Plasma
Rakta Vaha Srotas	Blood
Māmsa Vaha Srotas	Muscle
Meda Vaha Srotas	Fat
Asthi Vaha Srotas	Bones
Majjā Vaha Srotas	Marrow, Nervous Tissue
Shukra Vaha Srotas	Semen
Ārtava Vaha Srotas	Female Eggs
Purīsha Vaha Srotas	Feces
Mūtra Vaha Srotas	Urine
Sveda Vaha Srotas	Sweat
Stanya Vaha Srotas	Lactation
Mano Vaha Srotas	Mind

Prāna Vaha Srotas

Prāna is the vital energy of life. As cellular intelligence, the flow of information that facilitates communication to every part of the body, including each cell, it is the bridge between body and mind. It regulates the flow of emotions and sensory perception. Prāna is also responsible for gaseous exchange and respiration. Thus, prāna vaha srotas is the channel that distributes life energy to all bodily tissues and cells.

The sroto mūla (roots) of prāna vaha srotas are the left chamber of the heart and the entire GI tract (mahā srotas). Its sroto mārga (pathway) corresponds to the respiratory tract, including the bronchial tree and alveoli. The sroto mukha (opening) is the nose.

Diseases of prāna vaha srotas may be caused by smoking, over-exercise, exposure to cold and damp or dry weather. Respiratory allergies and infections weaken this channel system. Dry food, choking or entry of food particles into the trachea, deep-seated grief and repression of the natural urge to sneeze, cough or yawn can all aggravate prāna vaha srotas, resulting in colds, congestion, cough, asthma and wheezing. Other symptoms may include hoarseness of voice, difficulty breathing, sleep

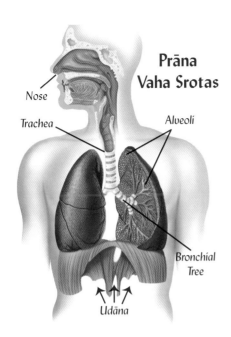

Prāna Vaha Srotas

Nose

Trachea

Alveoli

Bronchial Tree

Udāna

apnea and dyspnea. Bronchitis, pharyngitis, laryngitis or pneumonia are also disturbances of prāna vaha srotas.

The following marmāni benefit prāna vaha srotas. Of these, Mūrdhni is the principal marma to regularize prāna function.

Marmāni (36). Agra Patra, Ājñā, Akshaka, Amsa, Amsa Phalaka, Angushtha Mūla, Antara Vartma, Apastambha, Bruhatī, Brahmarandhra, Bhrūh, Ūrdhva Ganda, Adhah Ganda, Grīvā, Hridayam, *Hrid,* Jatrū, Kakshadhara, Kanīnaka, Kantha, *Kanthanādī,* Kapāla, Kapola Nāsā, Krikātikā, *Mūrdhni,* Nābhi, Nāsā Agra, Nāsā Madhya, Nāsā Mūla, Nāsā Puta, Pārshva Sandhi, Prushtha, Adhah Skandha, Ūrdhva Skandha, Tarjani, Vidhuram.

Ambu/Udaka Vaha Srotas

Ambu or *udaka* is translated as water. This system comprises the water-carrying channels of the body. Its agni is responsible for electrolyte balance, body temperature regulation and maintaining optimum pH. Ambu vaha srotas performs lubrication, hydration and elimination of wastes, providing energy to the body. It is functionally related to mūtra vaha srotas (urinary channels) and to sveda vaha srotas (channels of sweat). The sroto mūla (roots) of ambu vaha srotas are the soft palate, called *tālu* in Sanskrit, the arachnoid villi in the brain, and the pancreas, known as *kloma.* Its sroto mārga (pathway) is the GI mucous membrane and its sroto mukha (openings) are the tongue (jihva), kidneys (*vrukka*) and sweat glands (*roma kūpa*).

Ambu vaha srotas can be disturbed by too much dry, hot or spicy food, insufficient or excessive water intake, and excessive sugar and salt. Extreme physical exercise, profuse sweating, intense fear and exposure to extreme heat and dryness also can disturb this channel system. In addition, alcohol, tobacco, or nicotine use can damage ambu vaha srotas. These disturbances may manifest as dehydration, extreme thirst, dry skin, low blood pressure and impaired electrolyte balance. Hypotension, renal failure, scanty urination, edema or kidney stones are other disturbances of ambu vaha srotas.

The following marmāni may be used as an adjunctive therapy for treatment of these conditions:

Marmāni (32). Ānī, Agra Patra, Ājñā, Amsa, Amsa Phalaka, *Apastambha,* Basti, Bhaga, Bruhatī, Charana, *Chibuka,* Gulpha, Hanu, Indrabasta, Jānu, Kaksha, *Kapola Madhya,* Kati, Kukundara, Lohita, Manyāmūla, Nābhi, Pāda Madhya, Sakthi Ūrvī, Shivarandhra, Sūrya, Trik, Ūrū, Vankri, Vartma, Vrukka, Vrushana.

Ambu / Udaka Vaha Srotas

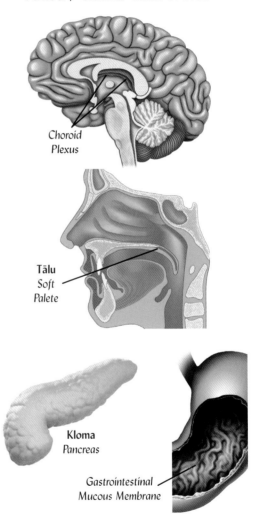

Choroid Plexus

Tālu Soft Palete

Kloma Pancreas

Gastrointestinal Mucous Membrane

Anna Vaha Srotas

Annam is the Sanskrit term for food. Anna vaha srotas is the channel system responsible for digestion, absorption and assimilation of nutrients from food. It corresponds to the GI or gastrointestinal tract. It governs the transformation of food into āhāra rasa, which directly

Anna Vaha Srotas

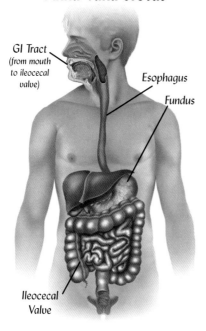

GI Tract
(from mouth
to ileocecal
valve)

Esophagus

Fundus

Ileocecal
Valve

nourishes the dhātus. The GI tract is also termed *mahā srotas,* "the great or major channel," because of its pre-eminent importance in the health and functioning of the body. According to Āyurveda, eighty percent of all diseases originate in the GI tract.

The sroto mūla (roots) of anna vaha srotas are the esophagus and the upper fundus of the stomach. The sroto mārga (pathway) is the GI tract, beginning from the lips and ending at the ileocecal valve. The sroto mukha (openings) are the ileocecal valve and the mouth.

Disturbances of the anna vaha srotas originate in dietary and eating habits. Eating too quickly, under stress or at an improper time adversely affects this srotas. Overeating, undereating, emotional eating, improper or unwholesome diet, and poor food combining also disturb this channel. Signs of distress are diminished ability to taste, loss of appetite, nausea, vomiting and burping. Other symptoms may include heartburn, acid reflux, constipation, bloating, distention and abdominal pain.

Marmāni to treat digestive imbalances are listed below.

Marmāni (31). Ānī, *Agra Patra,* Akshaka, Apastambha, Basti, Chibuka, Ūrdhva Ganda, Adhah Ganda, Grīvā, Hanu, Indrabasta, Kaksha, Kantha, Kapola Madhya, Kukundara, Lohita, Mantha, Manyāmūla, *Nābhi,* Oshtha, Pāda Madhya, Pāda Charana, Plīhā, Sakthi Ūrvī, Shankha, Stanya Mūla, *Sūrya,* Vankri, Vankshana, Vartma (Bāhya and Madhya), Yakrut.

Rasa Vaha Srotas

Rasa vaha srotas is the channel system responsible for nutrition, nourishment and immunity. It governs the flow of nutrients in the body and circulates rasa dhātu (lymph and plasma) via the lymphatic, venous and capillary circulation. The upadhātus (by-products) of rasa dhātu are the top layer of the skin and *stanya* (breasts and breast milk) and *rajah* (menstrual fluid) in females. These two additional channels in women are functionally related to ārtava vaha srotas and are discussed in that section, below.

In the Āyurvedic view, rasa and rakta dhātu circulate together through the cardiovascular system. The liquid component of the blood, plasma, is rasa dhātu, while the cellular component, white blood cells and red blood cells, are a part of rakta dhātu. The secretions of the lymph glands are also rasa dhātu. Venous blood and the venous system primarily come under rasa vaha srotas, and the arterial system, which carries oxygenated blood, is functionally related to rakta vaha srotas. In reality, both the venous and arterial systems belong to rakta vaha srotas. All venous blood comes to the right chamber of the heart, hence that is considered the root of rasa vaha srotas. On the other hand, the left chamber of the heart receives fresh oxygenated blood and is responsible for arterial circulation, which circulates prāna (oxygen) throughout the body via the blood. So, the left chamber of the heart is the root of prāna vaha srotas.

In addition to the right chamber of the heart, the other sroto mūla (roots) of rasa vaha srotas are the *ten great pathways.* These are subtle energy pathways of sensory perception connected to the heart chakra. There are two for each sense: two optical pathways, two olfactory pathways, two auditory pathways, two tactile path-

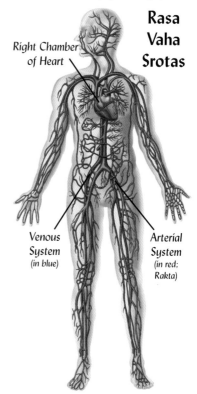

Rasa
Vaha
Srotas

Right Chamber
of Heart

Venous
System
(in blue)

Arterial
System
(in red;
Rakta)

Lymphatic System

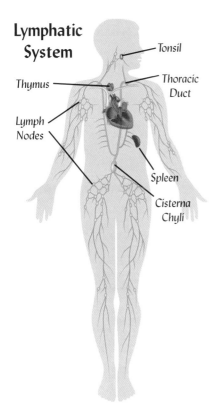

- Tonsil
- Thymus
- Thoracic Duct
- Lymph Nodes
- Spleen
- Cisterna Chyli

ways and two gustatory pathways. These five pairs of prānic pathways influence the sensory motor sympathetic and parasympathetic nerve pathways, affecting cardiac activities due to their connection to the cardiac plexus, which regulates the activities of the pacemaker sino-auricular node and the atrial ventricular node. That is why, if we suddenly hear somebody screaming, or we smell a terrible smell or see a terrible sight, it affects the heart.

The mārga (pathway) of rasa vaha srotas is the venous system and lymphatic system. The mukha (mouth) is the arteriovenous junction in the capillaries.

Rasa dhātu and rasa vaha srotas are affected adversely by a diet that is predominantly cold, heavy, oily, fatty or fried. Incompatible food combinations, leftovers, excessive dairy and hydrophilic substances (yogurt, watermelon and salty foods) are disturbing to rasa vaha srotas. A sedentary lifestyle, too much exposure to heat, anxiety, worry and bacteria all affect this channel system as well. Signs of disturbance include diminished sense of taste, desire for inappropriate or unhealthy foods, nausea and food allergies. Generalized body ache, fatigue, hypersensitivity to sound, and lack of faith and clarity are indicators of imbalance within rasa vaha srotas.

Marmāni used to treat both rasa channel and rasa tissue are listed below.

Marmāni (31). Agra Patra, Akshaka, Angushtha Mūla, Bāhu Ūrvī, Bruhatī, Charana, Grīvā, Gulpha, *Hrid, Indrabasta,* Jānu (posterior), Jatrū, *Kaksha,* Kakshad-

hara, Karnapāla, Karnapālī, Lohita, Lohitāksha, Mantha, Manyāmūla, Nābhi, Pāda Madhya, Pāda Charana, Plīhā, Sakthi Ūrvī, *Sīrāmantha,* Sphij, Stanya Pārshva, *Stanya Mūla,* Sūrya, Vidhuram.

Rakta Vaha Srotas

This srotas is the same as the hematopoietic system of Western medicine, which produces and develops blood cells. The srotas transports rakta (blood) throughout the body. Its function is *jīvana,* which means to oxygenate and to promote life. Rakta vaha srotas transports respiratory gases, nutrients, hormones, minerals, vitamins and enzymes with the aid of rasa dhātu. It is responsible for the drainage of metabolic waste products, maintenance of water-electrolyte balance, and regulation of body temperature. Rakta vaha srotas maintains blood volume and blood pressure. Rakta dhātu has two upadhātus (by-products): *sirā* (blood vessels, especially capillaries) and *kandara* (tendons/ligaments).

The sroto mūla (root) of rakta vaha srotas is the liver and spleen. Its mārga is the arterial circulatory system and the sroto mukha (opening) is the arteriocapillary junction. This srotas is principally connected to rañjaka pitta, which is also associated with the liver, to prāna vāyu, and to kledaka and avalambaka kapha.

Dietary factors that disturb this srotas include excess sugar and salt consumption, food that is hot, spicy, fatty, fried, fermented or incompatibly combined. Alcohol, tobacco, marijuana, excess exposure to sun or radiation, and liver and spleen disorders all weaken rakta vaha srotas. Symptoms may include skin disorders, such as acne, discoloration, eczema, dermatitis, boils or scabies. Other consequences may be varicose veins, glossitis, stomatitis, splenitis, hepatitis and thrombophlebitis. Additional symptoms may include herpes, hepatosplenomegaly, appendicitis or blood-borne disorders. Marma chikitsā administered along with medicine can alleviate many of these conditions.

Rakta Vaha Srotas

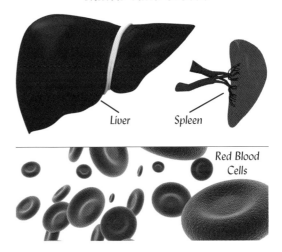

- Liver
- Spleen
- Red Blood Cells

The marmāni below affect the functioning of rakta vaha srotas, which as mentioned above is closely connected with rasa vaha srotas, as both rasa and rakta function together. Marmāni related to the heart, and therefore rakta dhātu, can be referenced in chapter 11.

Marmāni (29). Akshaka, Amsa Phalaka, Angushtha Mūla, Apastambha, Bāhya Manibandha, Bāhū Indrabasta, Basti, Bhaga, Bruhatī, *Hridayam,* Hrid, Jānu (posterior), Lohita, *Lohitāksha,* Mantha, Mūrdhni, *Nābhi,* Nāsā Agra, Nāsā Madhya, Nāsā Mūla, Nāsā Puta, Oshtha, Pārshva Sandhi, *Plīhā, Sīrāmantha,* Stanya Mūla, Vankri, Vidhuram, *Yakrut.*

Māmsa Vaha Srotas

Māmsa is muscle, which gives the body strength, form and coordination, and permits locomotion. Without muscle, the body cannot move. Māmsa dhātu covers the vital organs and skeletal system and forms the walls of body cavities. Māmsa facilitates speech, communication and facial expression. It also maintains body temperature.

The sroto mūla (roots) of māmsa vaha srotas are the *snāyu* (fascia), *tvak* (six layers of skin), mesoderm and small tendons. Its mārga (pathway) is the entire muscular system, including the heart and involuntary muscles like the uterus and diaphragm. The mukha (opening) for the srotas is the superficial layer of the skin. The upadhātus (by-products) of māmsa dhātu are the skin and subcutaneous fat while the inferior by-products are earwax, smegma and nasal crust. These are known as *khamala.*

A diet rich in meat and protein, or lacking in electrolytes, calcium or potassium, may adversely affect māmsa vaha srotas. Insufficient or excessive exercise, heavy weight lifting, inadequate rest, emotional stress and trauma may also deplete māmsa vaha srotas. The result can be muscle aches, pain, sprain, cramps or fatigue. Tremors, tics, spasms or twitching may occur.

Muscular pain is due to lack of prāna or lack of awareness in a particular area. Activating marmāni locally will enhance the flow of prāna directly to that area and allow the pain to subside. All marmāni located on the muscle system are connected to māmsa vaha srotas. Thus, all marmāni treat māmsa vaha srotas.

Marmāni. Marmāni for māmsa dhātu and māmsa vaha srotas vary according to the affected muscle. For example, if there is pain in the pectoralis major muscle, then we can use Apastambha marma and Kakshadhara marma. If there is pain in the neck muscle, Manyāmūla marmāni can be used. For shoulder pain or pain in the muscles of the shoulder, we can use Skandha marma. And in case of pain in the calf muscle, Indrabasta marma is effective.

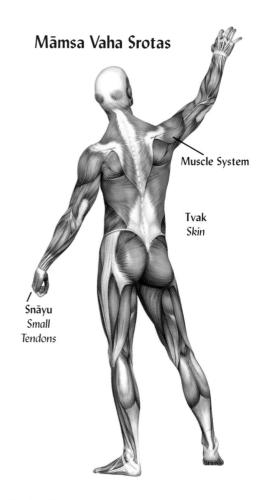

Māmsa Vaha Srotas

Muscle System

Tvak
Skin

Snāyu
Small Tendons

Meda Vaha Srotas

Meda vaha srotas is the channel system for meda dhātu (fat or adipose tissue). The important functions of fat are lubrication, protection, and, as an insulating material, retention of heat. That is why skinny people are always cold, and chubby people are hot. Meda adds sweetness to the voice and gives the physical body beauty, bulk and energy. The upadhātu (by-product) of meda dhātu is snāyu, the flat muscles, sinews, tendons and ligaments. Snāyu is also a sroto mūla of māmsa vaha srotas.

The sroto mūla (root) of meda vaha srotas is the omentum of the abdomen and the adrenals (*vrukka granthi*). Subcutaneous fatty tissue is the sroto mārga (pathway). The sroto mukha (opening) of meda vaha srotas is the sweat glands (roma kūpa).

This srotas is aggravated by dietary factors, such as high protein levels and oily, fatty, fried foods as well as excess sugar and dairy products. Emotional eating, steroid therapy, stress and unresolved emotions are also contributing factors to disturbances of meda vaha srotas. A sedentary lifestyle, eating, sitting and doing nothing, with insufficient exercise and lack of stimulation also negatively affects meda vaha srotas. Disturbance manifests as obesity, fluctuations of weight, underactive thyroid and excessive hunger and thirst. Increased meda dhātu may also result in steatorrhea and low libido. All marmāni that address the digestive system also treat meda vaha srotas. Those that increase jāthara agni (digestive fire of the stomach) or the dhātu agni (digestive fire of the tissues), may be effectively used to reduce excess meda. Nābhi and Sūrya have the most powerful influence on agni.

Meda Vaha Srotas

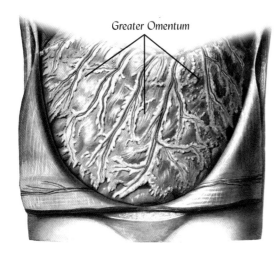

Greater Omentum

Marmāni (20). Agra Patra, Bāhu Ūrvī, *Chibuka,* Grīvā, Jatrū, Kantha, *Kanthanādī,* Kapola Madhya, Kūrpara, Manyāmūla, *Nābhi,* Oshtha, Plīhā, Shankha, Stanya Mūla, *Sūrya,* Vankri, Vartma, Vrukka, Yakrut.

Asthi Vaha Srotas

Asthi means bone or osseous tissue. Asthi vaha srotas comprises the entire skeletal system that provides the framework to support the body. It protects the vital organs, such as the brain, spinal cord and lungs. The sense of hearing and sense of vibration are important functions of asthi vaha srotas; we hear through the bones. Asthi vaha srotas includes the joints where muscles attach to enable leverage and movement. The sroto mūla (root) of asthi vaha srotas is the pelvic girdle and sacrum, the sroto mārga (pathway) is the entire skeletal system, and the sroto mukha (opening) the hair and nails. The hair and nails help to eliminate toxic substances from the body. The upadhātu (by-product) of asthi dhātu is the teeth and cartilage.

Asthi vaha srotas can be weakened by excess consumption of vāta-provoking foods, lack of minerals, excessive traveling or trauma. Other factors include over-exercise, overexcitement, anxiety or feeling unsupported. This results in spinal misalignment, joint pain, impaired movement, stiffness, arthritis, and cracking and popping of the joints. It can also lead to cavities in the teeth, receding gums, swollen or inflamed gums, and disorders of the hair and nails.

The following marmāni can be stimulated for treatment of asthi vaha srotas.

Marmāni (30). Agra Patra, Amsa, Bāhya Kūrpara, Basti, *Bhaga, Brahmarandhra,* Grīvā, Hanu, Hasta Kshipra, Jānu, Karnapāla, Kati, Krikātikā, Kukundara, Kūrpara, Lohita, *Manyāmani,* Manyāmūla, Nāsā Madhya, Nāsā Mūla, Oshtha, Pāda Madhya, Shivarandhra, Adhah Skandha, Ūrdhva Skandha, *Trik,* Ūrdhva Ganda, Ūrū, Vankshana, Vidhuram.

Asthi Vaha Srotas

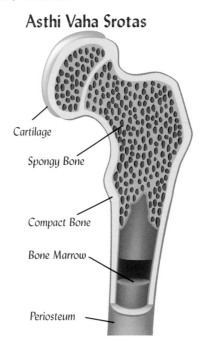

Cartilage

Spongy Bone

Compact Bone

Bone Marrow

Periosteum

Majjā Vaha Srotas

Majjā can be translated as intelligence, motivation, inner core or essence of perception. The root *majjan* means "to merge," "to immerse" or "to sink." Therefore, majjā vaha srotas is the flow of intelligence that allows one to sink deep into the ocean of knowledge, or to become immersed in the ocean of emotion.

Majjā dhātu includes the bone marrow and nervous tissue, while majjā vaha srotas is the channel through which the nervous system operates. Majjā as bone marrow produces red blood cells, and also fills up the space within the bone. As nervous tissue, Majjā has the important function of communication. Majjā vaha srotas facilitates the higher functions of the mind: intelligence, communication, comprehension, recognition, understanding, and memory storage. Through the functioning of sādhaka pitta, it promotes the transformation of sensory perception into knowledge. Majjā vaha srotas transmits neuro-electrical impulses via prāna vāyu. Tarpaka kapha has the important function of retaining knowledge, information and memory. It is the storehouse of memories. Out of memory, majjā vaha srotas reacts to the present situation in the form of thoughts, feelings,

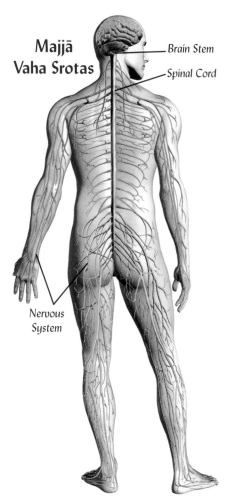

Majjā
Vaha Srotas

Brain Stem

Spinal Cord

Nervous
System

All marmāni stimulate majjā dhātu because they are a part of the nervous tissue. Particular marmāni that treat majjā vaha srotas are listed below. Marmāni that treat emotional disturbance, stress, poor memory, poor concentration and insomnia are referenced in chapter 17.

Marmāni (33). Adhah Skandha, *Ājñā, Angushtha Mūla,* Apānga, Ashrū, *Brahmarandhra,* Bhrūh, Hasta Kshipra, Hridayam, Hrid, Kanīnaka, Kantha, Kapāla, Karnamūla, Karnapāla, Karnapālī, Mantha, Manyāmani, Manyāmūla, Mūrdhni, Nāsā Agra, Nāsā Madhya, Nāsā Mūla, Oshtha, Pāda Madhya, Pāda Kshipra, Prushtha, *Shankha,* Shivarandhra, Sphij, Tala Hridayam, Ūrdhva Skandha, Vidhuram.

Shukra/Ārtava Vaha Srotas

Shukra and ārtava are the tissues that constitute the male and female reproductive systems. These channels produce ojas, the upadhātu of shukra and ārtava dhātus, which is transformed into supreme intelligence. Ojas is cellular immunity, but it is also the fluid that is vital for reproduction, orgasm and emotional release.

In males, shukra vaha srotas has its mūla (root) in the nipples and testicles. Its sroto mārga (pathways) are the vas deferens, epididymis, prostate, urethra and genitourinary tract. The urethral opening is the sroto mukha (opening).

Ārtava vaha srotas is the female reproductive system. It includes the ovaries, fallopian tubes and uterus. The ovaries and the areolae of the nipples are its sroto mūla (roots). The sroto mārga (pathway) includes the fallopian tubes, uterus, cervical

Shukra Vaha Srotas

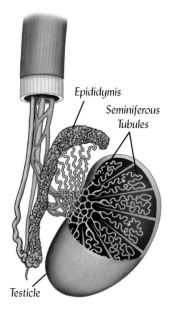

Epididymis

Seminiferous
Tubules

Testicle

canal and vaginal passage. The *yoni oshtha,* or vagina, labia minor and major are the sroto mukha (openings) for ārtava vaha srotas.

The function of both channels can be impaired by a poor quality diet, sexual promiscuity, over-exercise, stress, intense emotions or trauma. These factors may result in excessive or low libido, painful coitus or sexually transmitted diseases. For women, disturbance may manifest in numerous ways, including irregular menses, endometriosis, ectopic pregnancy, or spontaneous miscarriage.

and emotions. Majjā vaha srotas maintains equilibrium and governs coordination and the development of nerves. It conveys the tactile sensations of touch, pain, temperature and pressure.

Majjā vaha srotas has its mūla (roots) in the brain stem, spinal cord and bone marrow. The mārga (passage) is the central nervous system, including sympathetic and parasympathetic systems. The sroto mukha (opening) is the synaptic space and neuromuscular cleft within each nerve cell. Thus, majjā vaha srotas is an integral component of the mental and emotional bodies. The upadhātu (by-product) of majjā dhātu is tears, which are the expressions of emotion. Excessive lacrimation is one sign of impairment of this srotas.

Majjā vaha srotas can be disturbed by a vāta-aggravating diet, incompatible food combinations, drug addiction, trauma or extreme temperatures. It is also adversely affected by stress, lack of sleep, a hectic lifestyle and repressed emotions. These can lead to misunderstanding, poor communication, loss of memory and sleep disorders. Majjā vaha srotas disorders include lack of coordination and complex neurological problems, such as epilepsy or stroke.

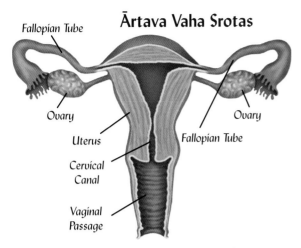

Ārtava Vaha Srotas

Fallopian Tube
Ovary
Ovary
Uterus
Fallopian Tube
Cervical Canal
Vaginal Passage

In females, two additional channels, for menstruation and lactation, are related to ārtava vaha srotas. Rajah vaha srotas is the channel responsible for menstrual cleansing. The endometrial lining is shed, regenerating a new lining after each ovulation. Rajah vaha srotas includes the uterus, endometrium, cervical canal and vaginal passage. Stanya vaha srotas is the channel that transports the mother's milk. Its mūla (roots) are the lactiferous glands, the mārga (passage) is the lactiferous ducts and the mukha (openings) are the nipples.

Marmāni that benefit these channels are listed below. Chapter 17 references marmāni that treat specific reproductive and genitourinary disorders.

Stanya Vaha Srotas

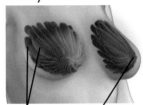

Lobules   Lactiferous Duct

Marmāni (36). Ānī, Angushtha Mūla, Bāhū Indrabasta, Basti, *Bhaga, Chibuka,* Gulpha, Hanu, Indrabasta, Kaksha, Kakshadhara, Kati, Kūrcha, Kūrcha Shira, Lohita, Manibandha, *Medhra,* Mūrdhni, *Nābhi 3 and 4,* Nāsā Agra, Nāsā Mūla, Pāda Kshipra, Pārshni, Sakthi Ūrvī, Stanya, Stanya Mūla, Stanya Pārshva, Ājñā, Stanya, Trik, Ūrū, Vankshana, Vrushana, *Yoni Jihvā, Yoni Oshtha.*

Marmāni for Stanya Vaha Srotas (4). Ājñā, Stanya, Stanya Mūla, Stanya Pārshva.

Purīsha Vaha Srotas

This channel system is responsible for the formation of feces and the absorption of minerals in the colon. Purīsha vaha srotas gives strength, support and vitality to the body. The sroto mūla (root) includes the colon, rectum and sigmoid colon. Its sroto mārga (passageway) is the entire pathway of the colon, opening into the anal orifice, which is its mukha (opening).

Purīsha vaha srotas is adversely affected by a diet lacking sufficient fiber or over-consumption of meat,

and by improper food combining. Polluted water or insufficient water intake also disturbs purīsha vaha srotas. Excess consumption of beans or chickpea flour can result in dryness of the feces. The srotas is aggravated by poor bowel habits, such as postponing the natural call of defecation, suppressing the urge to pass gas or sitting on hard and rough surfaces. Insufficient exercise can also be a cause of constipation. Chronic indigestion can lead to the formation of āma (toxins) that clog the colon, leading to further disturbances of the srotas, such as foul breath or gases.

Purīsha Vaha Srotas

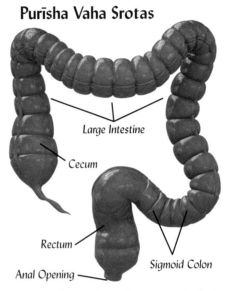

Large Intestine
Cecum
Rectum
Anal Opening
Sigmoid Colon

Symptoms of purīsha vaha srotas imbalance can therefore include constipation, flatulence, bloating and distention. Another symptom is tenesmus, painful straining during defecation with a sense of incomplete evacuation. Other symptoms include fissures, fistulae, hemorrhoids, diverticulosis and rectal prolapse, rectal polyps, and cancerous growths. These symptoms all primarily reflect vāta imbalance. If pitta dosha is affected, it may result in diarrhea, dysentery, ulcerative colitis and Crohn's disease. Kapha imbalance leads to amebiasis, giardiasis, amoeboma, mucus dysfunction or parasites (krumi).

The following marmāni benefit purīsha vaha srotas. Of these, Indrabasta marmāni have the strongest influence on the colon.

Marmāni (25). *Bāhū Indrabasta, Basti,* Charana, Grīvā, Hanu, *Indrabasta,* Jānu, Kapola Madhya, Karnamūla, Kūrcha Shira, Kukundara, Manibandha, Mūrdhni, *Nābhi,* Nāsā Agra, Pāda Charana, Plīhā, Shankha, Shivarandhra, Sphij, Sūrya, Tarjani, *Trik,* Ūrdhva Ganda, Yakrut.

Mūtra Vaha Srotas

Mūtra vaha srotas governs the elimination of *mūtra* (urine) from the body. In addition, it regulates blood

227

Mūtra Vaha Srotas

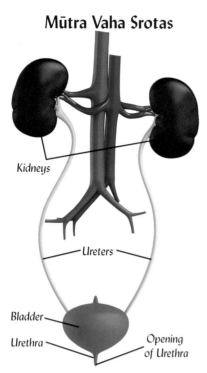

Kidneys

Ureters

Bladder

Urethra

Opening
of Urethra

Sveda Vaha Srotas

Sveda vaha srotas governs perspiration and the elimination of liquid waste. It maintains body temperature, blood pressure, water regulation and lubrication. *Kleda,* the liquid component present in all bodily tissues, is filtered through the kidneys and then eliminated by the bladder. One of the important functions of sveda is to retain the kleda (water component) in order to maintain lubrication of the skin. Both mūtra (urine) and sveda (sweat) help to regulate the water-electrolyte balance and the liquid component of kleda. That is why a person experiences more profuse sweating and decreased urination in the summer, and the opposite effect in winter.

Sveda Vaha Srotas

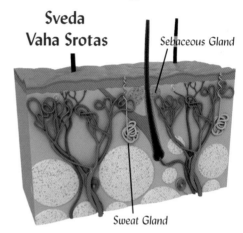

Sebaceous Gland

Sweat Gland

The sebaceous glands are the mūla (roots) of sveda vaha srotas and the sebaceous ducts are its mārga (pathway). The pores of the skin and the sweat glands (roma kūpa) constitute the sroto mukha (openings). Sveda (sweat) is the mala (waste product) of meda dhātu (adipose tissue) and it is also functionally related to ambu vaha srotas, the water-carrying channels. Marmāni that release heat, a form of excess pitta in the body, help in the elimination of sweat. Several marmāni of ambu vaha srotas, mūtra vaha srotas and meda vaha srotas are also applicable, because they are functionally connected to sveda.

The following marmāni activate sveda vaha srotas, ambu vaha srotas, mūtra vaha srotas and meda vaha srotas. Kaksha is the most influential marma for this srotas.

Marmāni (10). Agra Patra, Ājñā, Apastambha, Basti, Gulpha, *Hrid,* Jatrū, *Kaksha,* Mūrdhni, *Nābhi.*

Mano Vaha Srotas

Mano vaha srotas is the pathway of the mind. It encompasses the entire body. This understanding is unique to Āyurveda, in which mind and body are not perceived as two separate entities, but as one entity functioning through two interconnected media. Since this srotas incorporates the entire body, all srotāmsi belong to mano vaha srotas.

pressure and the water-electrolyte balance. The kidney is the organ of filtration and it is the sroto mūla (root) of this srotas. The urethra and bladder constitute the mārga (passages), and the opening of the urethra is the mukha (opening) of mūtra vaha srotas.

Mūtra vaha srotas can be aggravated by excess or insufficient intake of water, and over-consumption of alcohol. It is adversely affected by excess caffeine, sugar, salt, and foods rich in oxalic acid, such as tomatoes, spinach and eggplant. Other causes of disturbance include trauma, intense labor under the hot sun, and intense emotions, such as fear, anxiety and nervousness and suppression of the natural call of urination or micturition. Pathogens such as bacteria, which may cause kidney or bladder infections, also imbalance this srotas.

Disturbances of mūtra vaha srotas result in urinary dysfunction, such as polyuria (excessive urination) and dysuria (painful urination). Retention of urine, increased frequency of urination and bladder atony are mūtra vaha srotas ailments of vāta dosha. Albumin urea, polycystic kidneys, benign prostatic hypertrophy and kidney stones are all kapha disturbances of mūtra vaha srotas. High pitta in mūtra vaha srotas may manifest as blood in the urine (hematuria), or as infections of the bladder (cystitis), kidney (nephritis) or prostate (prostatitis).

Marmāni that address disturbance of mūtra vaha srotas are listed below.

Marmāni (18). Ānī, Basti, Bhaga, Charana, Gulpha, Jānu, Karnamūla, Kati, Kukundara, Lohita, Medhra, *Nābhi 3* and *4,* Sakthi Ūrvī, Trik, Vankshana, Vartma, *Vrukka.*

The sroto mūla (root) of mano vaha srotas consists of the heart, cardiac plexus, brain and chakra system. The chakra system is a network of seven principal neuroplexuses that have functional integration with one another and with the body. They are aligned along the central axis of the body. The sroto mārga (passage) is the entire body. This communication system includes all the nerve pathways and the five koshas (sheaths or bodies).

As we briefly discussed in chapter 3, "The Spiritual Dimension of Marmāni," the koshas represent an understanding of the human body that views it as much more than the physical form. These five levels of existence range from the gross to the subtle: annamaya kosha (physical or food body), prānamaya kosha (breath body), manomaya kosha (mental body), vijñānamaya kosha (knowledge body) and ānandamaya kosha (bliss body). Each level has its corresponding mode of consciousness and depends on nourishment from food, breath, experience, knowledge and bliss respectively. Mano vaha srotas opens (mukha) into the sense organs (doors of perception), the synaptic spaces between neurons, and the marmāni. Therefore, the marmāni link perception, mental function, and physical and mental experience.

The functions of mano vaha srotas integrate with the functions of majjā vaha srotas. These include the higher cognitive functions, such as memory, concentration, judgment, reasoning and communication. *Mano agni,* the fire component of the mind, is the fuel for this srotas. It enlivens the capacity for concentration, perception, one-pointed attention and understanding. Mano vaha srotas also involves the harmonious interaction between prāna vāyu, sādhaka pitta and tarpaka kapha.

Mano vaha srotas is adversely affected by a *tamasic* diet that is dull, heavy, stale and contains processed foods. Rajasic foods that are hot, spicy and fermented, or substances such as alcohol and marijuana also negatively affect this srotas. Sattvic fresh fruits, grains and vegetables support the healthy functioning of mano vaha srotas. Troubled relationships, undigested emotions, emotional extremes and unhealthy habitual lifestyle patterns are factors that can upset the mind. Psychological trauma and emotional imbalance may also be contributing factors. In the Ayurvedic paradigm, stress is said to be the product of a mind that is unable to digest thoughts, feelings, emotions or experiences.

The qualities of sattva, rajas and tamas can clearly be seen in mano vaha srotas. The natural expression of mind is a sattvic quality of consciousness, awareness and meditative potential. Rajas guna represents the movement of thought and the constant activity of the mind. Tamas guna yields sensory perception into mano vaha srotas. Tamas, the quality of inertia and darkness, allows the mind to rest and the body to sleep. In daily operating consciousness, the perceiver is sattva; the object of perception is tamas; and the flow of perception is rajas. Overall, sattva is the mūla (root of mano vaha srotas), rajas is its mārga (path) and tamas is the mukha (opening) of mano vaha srotas.

Since marmāni are the openings of mano vaha srotas and its related doors of perception, they directly affect the mind. Other marmāni that treat disorders of this srotas, such as emotional disturbances, stress, poor memory, poor concentration and insomnia, can be referenced in chapter 17.

Marmāni (9). *Ājñā, Brahmarandhra,* Hasta Kshipra, Hrid, Jānu, Jatrū, *Mūrdhni,* Nābhi and *Shivarandhra.*

There is no disease without disturbed srotas. And there is no perfect health without balanced srotas. So one can prevent potential or even incipient ailments by massaging specific marmāni to affect specific srotāmsi. The marmāni listed in this chapter can not only prevent disease, they can also act as a rasāyana or rejuvenation. Thus, the knowledge in this chapter can help to bring healthy, long life.

Management of Specific Disorders with Marma Chikitsā

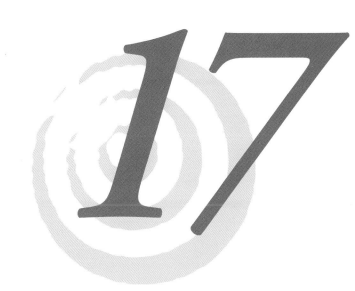

We have emphasized throughout that marma chikitsā is rarely used alone, but is most often utilized as part of a comprehensive, multi-faceted treatment program. This approach requires of the practitioner a broad and in-depth understanding of etiology, symptomatology and the stages of pathogenesis as well as sensitivity and skill in diagnosis and the ability to design an integrated treatment protocol according to the patient's prakruti (constitution) and vikruti (current state). However, in addition to its role as a team player in a general management program, marma chikitsā can be used alone effectively for immediate pain relief, long-term pain management and for first aid.

Sadyah Phaladai Chikitsā – Āyurvedic First Aid

First aid therapy in Āyurveda is called *sadyah phaladai chikitsā,* or "that which is instantly fruit-giving." Like Western-style first aid management, marma chikitsā can be useful for acute, emergency conditions such as nosebleed, convulsions, tremors, fever and pain. Though using marma therapy in these conditions may not eradicate the pathogenesis completely, it can give temporary symptomatic relief and may prevent serious complications from arising. A quick reference chart for using marma chikitsā for first aid is in table 29 on page 232.

The experience of many years of clinical practice has shown that very often, the patient comes to the Ayurvedic physician with pain, and after marma therapy he or she leaves with a smiling face! For treatment of pain, marmāni may be selected according to the body region affected or by the doshic nature of pain (whether it is primarily vāta, pitta, or kapha) and the severity of symptoms. In general, stimulating a marma enhances the flow of prāna locally and thereby reduces pain. For mild and short-term conditions, marma therapy alone can be quite effective. As the complexity of a disease increases,

other therapies become essential. These may include herbal or dietary recommendations, exercise, pañcha-karma and lifestyle changes.

This chapter enumerates dozens of disorders and the marmāni that can be used to treat them, either by a therapist/clinician or by an individual for self-healing. For instance, an individual with recurrent headaches can self-massage specific marmāni as a preventative measure, or to mitigate an existing headache. The most beneficial points for each condition are highlighted in italic type. Additionally, the marmāni are listed in order of treatment, from top of head to bottom of foot.

An initial knowledge of which marmāni are relevant for a condition is vital, but then this must be tailored to the specific situation. A good example is the treatment of headaches: occipital, temporal and frontal pain each involves different marmāni. Then appropriate stimulation techniques must be chosen and other therapies such as the use of medicated paste or oils can be incorporated. Additionally, essential oil that is analgesic and reduces the aggravated dosha may be selected.

For complete information on the marmāni in the tables below—including their precise locations, indications, actions, and methods of use—please refer to part 2 of this book.

Please note: Marma chikitsā is not a substitute for medical treatment or consultation with a physician.

Table 29: Marma Chikitsā for First Aid

Symptom/Condition	Marmāni Used for Relief of Symptom
Abdominal Pain	Sūrya, Nābhi, Basti
Acute Asthma	Jatrū, Kanthanādī, Prushtha
Arm Pain	Adhah Skandha, Ānī, Indrabasta
Bell's Palsy	Karnamūla, Kapāla, Shankha
Cardiac Pain	Hrid, Apastambha, Agra Patra, Pārshva Sandhi
Convulsions	Oshtha, Mūrdhni
Diarrhea	Nābhi 3 and 4, Vankshana
Dizziness	Oshtha, Ājñā
Dry Cough	Kantha, Jatrū, Kanthanādī
Elbow Pain	Kūrpara, Ānī
Epigastric Pain	Sūrya, Agra Patra, Vankri
Excess Urination	Vrukka, Nābhi 1 and 2
Headache, General	Mūrdhni
Headache, Frontal	Ājñā
Headache, Occipital	Manyāmūla
Headache, Ophthalmic	Kanīnaka, Bhrūh Antara
Headache, Sinus	Adhah Ganda
Headache, Temporal	Shankha
High Fever	Ājñā, Shankha, Nābhi (all)
Hip Pain	Lohitāksha, Sakthi Ūrvī, Ūrū
Hoarseness Of Voice	Kantha, Jatrū
Knee Pain	Jānu, Sakthi Ūrvī, Charana
Leg Pain	Sakthi Ūrvī, Indrabasta, Charana
Lower Backache	Kati, Vankshana, Trik
Neck Pain	Manyāmūla, Karnapāla, Sīrāmantha
Nosebleed	Nāsā Puta, Oshtha
Palpitations	Hrid, Agra Patra, Kanīshthika
Pelvic Pain	Bhaga, Vankshana, Lohitāksha
Pleuritic Pain	Apastambha, Agra Patra, Kakshadhara
Sciatica	Trik, Sphij, Indrabasta
Shoulder Pain	Adhah Skandha, Ūrdhva Skandha, Amsa Phalaka
Stroke Paralysis	Adhipati (Mūrdhni), Brahmarandhra, Shivarandhra, Kshipra
TMJ Pain	Shankha, Karnapāla, Kapola Madhya
Toothache	Oshtha, Adhah Ganda, Kapola Madhya
Wrist Pain	Manibandha, Kūrcha Shira, Tala Hrida

Table 30: Pain

Region	General Marmāni
Headache, Migraine	Adhah Ganda, Ājñā, *Angushtha Mūla*, Apānga, Ashrū, Brahmarandhra, Bhrūh, Grīvā, Hanu, Hasta Kshipra, Kanīnaka, Kapāla, Karnamūla, Karnapālī, Krikātikā, Manyāmūla, *Mūrdhni*, Nāsā Mūla, Pāda Kshipra, Pāda Madhya, *Shankha*, Shivarandhra, Ūrdhva Ganda, Ūrdhva Skandha, Vidhuram
TMJ Pain	Chibuka, Hanu, *Kapola Madhya*, Karnapāla, *Karnamūla, Shankha*
Toothache	Adhah Ganda, *Chibuka, Hanu*, Kapola Madhya, Karnamūla, *Oshtha*, Shankha
Neck Pain	Ājñā, Amsa Phalaka, *Grīvā*, Karnapāla, *Krikātikā*, Mantha, *Manyāmani*, Manyāmūla, Shivarandhra, Sīrāmantha, Ūrdhva Skandha, Vidhuram
Shoulder Pain	Adhah Skandha, *Amsa*, Amsa Phalaka, Kaksha, Kakshadhara, Prushtha, *Ūrdhva Skandha*
Upper Back Pain	*Amsa Phalaka*, Bruhatī, *Prushtha*, Ūrdhva Skandha
Low Back Pain	Jānu (posterior), Karnapāla, *Kati, Kukundara*, Sakthi Ūrvī (posterior), Sphij, Trik, Vrukka
Abdominal Pain	Basti, Bhaga, Lohita, *Nābhi*, Pārshva Sandhi, Plīhā, Sūrya, Vankri, Vankshana, Yakrut
Pelvic Pain	Basti, *Bhaga*, Lohita, Trik, *Vankshana*
Hip Pain	Lohitāksha, Sakthi Ūrvī, *Ūrū*
Arm Pain	Ānī, Adhah Skandha, *Amsa*, Bāhya Kūrpara, Bāhū Indrabasta, *Bāhu Ūrvī*, Kaksha, Kakshadhara
Elbow Pain	*Ānī*, Bāhya Kūrpara, Kūrpara
Wrist Pain	Bāhya Manibandha, Hasta Kshipra, Kūrcha Shira, *Manibandha*, Tala Hrida
Leg Pain	Charana, Indrabasta, Lohitāksha, *Sakthi Urvi, Sphij*, Ūrū
Knee Pain	Charana, *Jānu*, Sakthi Ūrvī, Ūrū
Foot Pain	Gulpha, Pāda Charana, *Pāda Madhya*, Pārshni
Cardiac Pain	Agra Patra, Apastambha, *Hridayam, Hrid*, Kakshadhara, Kanīshthika, Pārshva Sandhi, Prushtha, Tala Hrida
Pleuritic Pain	Agra Patra, *Apastambha, Kakshadhara*, Hrid, Hridayam, Stanya Mūla, Vankri
Epigastric Pain	Plīhā, *Sūrya,* Vankri, Yakrut

Table 31: Neurological Disorders

Condition	General Marmāni
Stroke	Brahmarandhra, Karnapālī, Manyāmūla, *Mūrdhni, Oshtha*, Shivarandhra
Epilepsy	Mūrdhni, Oshtha
Syncope	Mantha, Manyāmūla, *Mūrdhni*, Nāsā Agra, *Oshtha*
Bell's Palsy (facial paralysis)	Chibuka, Hanu, *Kapola Madhya*, Karnamūla, Oshtha, Shankha
Trigeminal Neuralgia	Chibuka, Hanu, *Kapola Madhya*, Karnamūla, Oshtha, Shankha
Sciatica	*Indrabasta (posterior), Jānu (posterior)*, Pārshni, Sakthi Ūrvī (posterior), Sphij

Table 32: Eye, Ear, Nose, Throat and Speech Disorders

Condition	General Marmāni
Eye Disorders	Ājñā, Akshaka, *Apānga*, Bhrūh, *Kanīnaka*, Kapāla, Karnapālī, Nāsā Mūla, Shankha, Vartma, Vidhuram, Yakrut
Ear Disorders	Amsa, Kapola Madhya, *Karnamūla*, Karnapāla, Karnapālī, Krikātikā, Shankha, Shivarandhra
Nasal Disorders	*Adhah Ganda*, Ājñā, Angushtha Mūla, Apānga, Kanīnaka, Kapāla, Kapola Nāsā, Mūrdhni, Nāsā Agra, Nāsā Madhya, Nāsā Puta, *Ūrdhva Ganda*, Vartma, Vidhuram
Throat Disorders	*Jatrū, Kantha*, Akshaka, Grīvā, Kanthanādī, Mantha, Sīrāmantha
Speech Disorders	*Kantha, Kanthanādī*, Mantha, Oshtha, Shankha

233

Table 33: Organ or Glandular Disturbances

Organ	General Marmāni
Pituitary	Ājñā, Brahmarandhra, Kapāla, Manyāmani, *Mūrdhni*
Thyroid	Grīvā, *Jatrū*, Kantha, *Kanthanādī*, Mantha, Manyāmani, Sīrāmantha
Lung	Adhah Ganda, Adhah Skandha, Agra Patra, Akshaka, Amsa, Amsa Phalaka, *Apastambha*, Bruhatī, Hasta Kshipra, Hridayam, Hrid, Jatrū, Kakshadhara, Kantha, Kanthanādī, Kapola Nāsā, Krikātikā, Nāsā Agra, Nāsā Puta, Pārshva Sandhi, Prushtha, Tala Hrida, Tarjani, Ūrdhva Ganda, Ūrdhva Skandha
Heart	*Agra Patra*, Akshaka, Amsa Phalaka, Apastambha, *Hridayam, Hrid*, Kanīshthika, Kanthanādī, Lohita, Lohitāksha, Mantha, Prushtha, Sīrāmantha, Tala Hrida
Stomach	Adhah Skandha, Bāhu Ūrvī, Manyāmūla, *Nābhi*, Shankha, *Sūrya*
Spleen	Akshaka, Angushtha Mūla, Bruhatī, Jatrū, Nābhi 1 and 2, Pārshva Sandhi, *Plīhā*, Stanya Pārshva, Vankri, Vidhuram
Liver	Akshaka, Angushtha Mūla, Bāhya Manibandha, Bruhatī, Nābhi 1, Pārshva Sandhi, Vankri, Vidhuram, *Yakrut*
Gallbladder	Akshaka, Bruhatī, Nābhi 1, Pārshva Sandhi, Shankha, Vankri, *Yakrut*
Colon	*Bāhū Indrabasta*, Bāhu Ūrvī, *Indrabasta*, Kapola Madhya, Kukundara, *Nābhi 3 and 4*, Pāda Charana, Plīhā, Sakthi Ūrvī, Shankha, Sphij, Tarjani, Ūrdhva Ganda, Yakrut
Small Intestine	*Nābhi 1 and 2*, Plīhā, Yakrut
Kidneys, Adrenals	Ānī, Charana, *Gulpha*, Karnamūla, Kati, Kukundara, Nābhi 1–4, Pārshva Sandhi, Sakthi Ūrvī, Vartma, *Vrukka*
Pancreas	Ānī, Amsa, Bāhu Ūrvī, Manyāmūla, *Nābhi 2*, Sūrya, Vankri
Bladder	*Ānī, Basti*, Bhaga, Jānu (posterior), Kati, Kukundara, Pāda Charana, Sakthi Ūrvī, Vrukka

Table 34: Systemic Disorders

Condition	General Marmāni
Blood Pressure (high/low)	Apastambha, Lohita, Lohitāksha, Mantha, Manyāmūla, Mūrdhni, *Sīrāmantha*, Vidhuram
Chronic Fatigue Syndrome	Bāhu Ūrvī, Jatrū, *Nābhi*, Plīhā, Vrukka
Low Immunity and Immune Disorders	*Jatrū*, Kūrcha, Nābhi, Plīhā
Vertigo (Dizziness)	Angushtha Mūla, Brahmarandhra, Hasta Kshipra, Karnamūla, Karnapāla, Karnapālī, Mantha, Manyāmūla, *Mūrdhni, Oshtha*, Pāda Madhya, Shankha, Sīrāmantha, Vidhuram
High Fever	Ājñā, Mūrdhni, Oshtha, Shankha

Table 35: Circulatory Conditions

Condition	General Marmāni
Arterial/ Venous Circulation	Bāhu Ūrvī, Charana, Gulpha, Hridayam, *Hrid*, Indrabasta, Jānu (posterior), Kaksha, Lohita, Lohitāksha, Pāda Charana, Pāda Madhya, Sakthi Ūrvī, Sphij
Lymphatic Circulation	Akshaka, Angushtha Mūla, Bruhatī, Grīvā, Hrid, Jatrū, Kaksha, *Kakshadhara*, Lohita, Mantha, Manyāmūla, Plīhā, Sīrāmantha, Stanya Mūla, Stanya Pārshva
Cerebral Circulation	Ājñā, Brahmarandhra, Karnapālī, Manyāmūla, *Mūrdhni, Oshtha*, Shivarandhra

Table 36: Cardiac And Respiratory Disorders

Condition	General Marmāni
Coronary Artery Disease	*Hrid*, Hridayam, Kanīshthika and all heart marmāni
Palpitations, Arrhythmias	Agra Patra, Amsa, Amsa Phalaka, Apastambha, *Hridayam, Hrid*, Kanīshthika, Kanthanādī, Mantha, Mūrdhni, Prushtha
Chronic Asthma, Obstructive Pulmonary Disease (COPD)	Agra Patra, Amsa, Amsa Phalaka, *Apastambha*, Hrid, *Jatrū*, Kakshadhara, Kantha, Kanthanādī, Kapola Nāsā, Krikātikā, Mantha, Mūrdhni, Nāsā Agra, Nāsā Puta, Pārshva Sandhi, Prushtha, Tarjani, Ūrdhva Ganda, Ūrdhva Skandha

Table 37: Gastrointestinal Disturbances

Condition	General Marmāni
Weak Digestion	Agra Patra, Bāhu Ūrvī, Chibuka, Kapola Madhya, Madhya Vartma, Manyāmūla, *Nābhi*, Oshtha, Shankha, *Sūrya*, Vankri, Yakrut
Anorexia	Agra Patra, Nābhi, *Sūrya*, Vankri
Nausea, Vomiting	Agra Patra, Akshaka, Bāhu Ūrvī, Mantha, Mūrdhni, Stanya Mūla, *Sūrya*, Yakrut
Gastroesophageal Reflux Disease (GERD)	Agra Patra, Hridayam, Jatrū, Kanīnaka, Kantha, Kanthanādī, *Shankha*, Sūrya, Vankri
Peptic Ulcer	Agra Patra, Bāhu Ūrvī, Hridayam, Kanīnaka, Nābhi 1, *Shankha*, Sūrya, Vankri
Gastritis	Agra Patra, Bāhu Ūrvī, Hridayam, Kanīnaka, Nābhi 1, *Shankha*, Sūrya, Vankri
Abdominal Distension	*Bhaga*, Lohita, *Nābhi*, Plīhā, Sūrya, Vankshana, Yakrut
Constipation, Diarrhea	Bāhū Indrabasta, *Indrabasta (posterior),* Kapola Madhya, Kukundara, *Nābhi 3 and 4*, Plīhā, *Sūrya*, Tarjani, Yakrut
Diverticulosis	Bāhū Indrabasta, *Indrabasta (posterior), Kukundara, Nābhi 3 and 4*, Sphij, Tarjani
Irritable Bowel Syndrome (IBS)	Bāhū Indrabasta, *Indrabasta (posterior),* Nābhi 3 and 4
Inflammatory Bowel Disease	Bāhū Indrabasta, Bāhu Ūrvī, *Indrabasta (posterior),* Kapola Madhya, Nābhi 3 and 4
Hemorrhoids	Hanu, *Indrabasta (posterior),* Kūrcha Shira, Manibandha, Nāsā Agra, Trik

Table 38: Reproductive and Genitourinary Disorders

Condition	General Marmāni
Breast Disorders	Kaksha, Kakshadhara, Stanya, *Stanya Mūla, Stanya Pārshva*
Cervical and Ovarian Disorders	Ānī, *Bhaga*, Hanu, Kati, Kūrcha, Kūrcha Shira, Nāsā Agra, Nāsā Mūla, Pārshni, Sakthi Ūrvī, Trik, *Vankshana*
Menstrual Disorders	Bāhū Indrabasta, Basti, Bhaga, Indrabasta (medial), Lohita, *Nābhi 3 and 4,* Ūrū, Vankshana
Sexual Dysfunction	*Bhaga*, Chibuka, Hanu, Kati, Kūrcha, Kūrcha Shira, Manibandha, Medhra, Nābhi 3 and 4, Sakthi Ūrvī, Trik, Ūrū, Vrushana
Hormonal Imbalance	Ājñā, Hanu, Jatrū, Kapāla, *Mūrdhni*, Pāda Kshipra
Prostate/ Testicle Disorders	Ānī, *Bhaga*, Hanu, Medhra, Nāsā Agra, Nāsā Mūla, Pāda Kshipra, Pārshni, Sakthi Ūrvī, Trik, Vankshana, *Vrushana*
Urinary Tract Disorders	Ānī, *Basti, Bhaga*, Gulpha, Jānu (posterior), Kati, Kukundara, Medhra, Nābhi 3 and 4, Sakthi Ūrvī, Trik, Vankshana, Vrukka
Pelvic Disorders	Basti, *Bhaga*, Kshipra, Lohita, Pārshni, Trik, Ūrū

Table 39: Disorders of Extremities

Condition	General Marmāni
Lower Extremity Neuropathy	Charana, *Indrabasta (posterior)*, *Jānu (posterior)*, Lohita, Lohitāksha, Pāda Madhya, Pāda Charana, Sakthi Ūrvī, Sphij, Ūrū
Upper Extremity Neuropathy	Ānī, Adhah Skandha, Amsa, Bāhya Kūrpara, Bāhū Indrabasta, Bāhu Ūrvī, Kakshadhara, *Kūrcha, Kūrcha Shira*, Kūrpara, *Manibandha, Tala Hrida*
Arthritis of Hand	Angushtha Mūla, Bāhya Manibandha, Hasta Kshipra, Kanīshthika, Kūrcha, Kūrcha Shira, Manibandha, *Tala Hrida*, Tarjani
Carpal Tunnel Syndrome	Ānī, Bāhū Indrabasta, Kūrcha, *Manibandha*, Tala Hrida
Edema of Upper Extremities	Ānī, Adhah Skandha, Bāhū Indrabasta, Bāhu Ūrvī, Kaksha
Edema in Lower Extremities	Charana, Indrabasta, Jānu, Lohita, Lohitāksha, Sakthi Ūrvī, Ūrū, Vrukka

Table 40: Marmāni to Balance Prāna, Tejas and Ojas

Prāna[a]	Mūrdhni or Adhipati, Brahmarandhra, Shivarandhra, Ājñā or Sthapanī, Kapola Nāsā, Oshtha, Hanu, Jatrū, Hrid (3), Agra Patra, Nābhi (5), Basti, Bhaga, Vrushana, Yoni Oshtha, Medhra, Yoni Jihvā, (Guda), Jānu (Anterior), Pāda Kshipra
Tejas	Ājñā or Sthapanī, Nāsā Mūla, Oshtha, Sīrāmantha, Hrid (3), Sūrya or Āmāshaya, Yakrut, Plīhā, Nābhi (5), Stanya, Yoni Oshtha, Vrushana, Jānu (Posterior), Pārshni, Tala Hrida, Pāda Madhya
Ojas	Mūrdhni or Adhipati, Ājñā or Sthapanī, Kapola Nāsā, Karnamūla (2), Hanu, Jatrū, Hrid (3), Agra Patra, Nābhi (5), Angushtha Mūla, Ūrū 1, Ūrū 2, Indrabasta (Medial), Indrabasta (Posterior), Manibandha, Gulpha (Lateral), Gulpha (Medial), Pāda Kshipra

a. These marmāni are in order of treatment, from top of head to bottom of foot.

Table 41: Balancing Emotional Disturbances through Marmāni

Vāta Conditions	Balancing Marmāni
Loneliness	Ājñā or Sthapanī, Pāda Kshipra, Mūrdhni or Adhipati
Fear	Hrid (3), Nābhi (5), Vrukka
Anxiety	Agra Patra, Nābhi (5), Vrukka
Nervousness	Basti, Gulpha (Lateral), Gulpha (Medial), Jānu (Anterior), Nābhi (5), Sūrya or Āmāshaya
Insomnia	Ājñā or Sthapanī, Brahmarandhra, Pāda Kshipra, Mūrdhni or Adhipati, Nābhi (5)
Pitta Conditions	**Balancing Marmāni**
Judgment	Jatrū, Plīhā, Yakrut
Perfectionism	Jatrū, Nābhi (5), Sūrya or Āmāshaya, Yakrut
Anger	Nābhi (5), Plīhā, Tala Hrida, Yakrut
Hatred	Hrid (3), Jatrū, Sūrya or Āmāshaya, Yakrut
Envy	Jatrū, Nābhi (5), Sūrya or Āmāshaya, Yakrut
Jealousy	Nābhi (5), Plīhā, Tala Hrida, Yakrut
Kapha Conditions	**Balancing Marmāni**
Attachment	Agra Patra, Hrid (3), Plīhā
Greed	Hrid (3), Jānu (Posterior), Jatrū
Possessiveness	Hanu, Jānu (Anterior), Jānu (Posterior), Oshtha, Plīhā
Depression	Ājñā or Sthapanī, Hanu, Mūrdhni or Adhipati, Plīhā, Vrukka
Lethargy	Agra Patra, Hrid (3), Jatrū, Pāda Kshipra, Plīhā, Sūrya or Āmāshaya

Table 42: Marmāni for Disturbance of Dhātus

Dhātu	Marmāni Affected
Rasa	Ānī, Adhah Ganda, Adhah Skandha, Agra Patra, Akshaka, Amsa, Amsa Phalaka, Angushtha Mūla, Apastambha, Bāhu Ūrvī, Basti, Bhaga, Charana (Lateral), Charana (Medial), Chibuka, Gulpha (Lateral), Gulpha (Medial), Hanu, Hridayam, Hrid (3), Indrabasta (Medial), Indrabasta (Posterior), Jānu (Anterior), Jatrū, Kaksha, Kakshadhara or Skandadhara, Kanīshthika, Kantha, Kanthanādī, Kapola Madhya, Kapola Nāsā, Karnamūla (2), Karnapāla or Karna Ūrdhva, Karnapālī, Kati, Kūrcha, Kūrcha Shira, Lohita, Lohitāksha, Mantha, Nābhi (5), Nāsā Puta, Pāda Charana, Pārshni, Sakthi Ūrvī (Anterior), Sakthi Ūrvī (Posterior), Sīrāmantha, Sphij, Stanya, Stanya Mūla, Stanya Pārshva, Sūrya or Āmāshaya, Tala Hrida, Tarjani, Trik, Ūrdhva Ganda, Ūrū 1, Ūrū 2, Vankri, Vrukka, Yakrut
Rakta	Agra Patra, Akshaka, Amsa, Amsa Phalaka, Angushtha Mūla, Bāhya Manibandha, Bāhu Ūrvī, Basti, Bhaga, Bruhatī, Charana (Lateral), Charana (Medial), Gulpha (Lateral), Gulpha (Medial), Hanu, Hridayam, Hrid (3), Indrabasta (Medial), Indrabasta (Posterior), Jānu (Anterior), Jānu (Posterior), Jatrū, Kapola Madhya, Karnamūla (2), Karnapāla or Karna Ūrdhva, Karnapālī, Kūrcha Shira, Kukundara, Lohita, Lohitāksha, Manibandha, Mantha, Nābhi (5), Nāsā Puta, Oshtha, Pāda Charana, Pārshni, Pārshva Sandhi, Sakthi Ūrvī (Anterior), Sakthi Ūrvī (Posterior), Sīrāmantha, Sphij, Stanya, Stanya Mūla, Stanya Pārshva, Sūrya or Āmāshaya, Tala Hrida, Trik, Ūrdhva Skandha, Vankri, Vrukka, Yakrut
Māmsa	Ānī, Adhah Skandha, Agra Patra, Amsa, Amsa Phalaka, Angushtha Mūla, Apastambha, Bāhya Manibandha, Bāhū Indrabasta, Bāhu Ūrvī, Bruhatī, Charana (Lateral), Charana (Medial), Hridayam, Hrid (3), Indrabasta (Medial), Indrabasta (Posterior), Jānu (Anterior), Jānu (Posterior), Kaksha, Kakshadhara or Skandadhara, Kanīshthika, Kantha, Kanthanādī, Kati, Kūrcha Shira, Kukundara, Kūrpara, Lohitāksha, Mantha, Pāda Madhya, Pāda Charana, Pārshva Sandhi, Plīhā, Prushtha (3), Sakthi Ūrvī (Anterior), Sakthi Ūrvī (Posterior), Sphij, Stanya, Stanya Mūla, Stanya Pārshva, Tala Hrida, Tarjani, Trik, Ūrdhva Skandha, Ūrū 1, Ūrū 2, Vankri, Vankshana
Meda	Ānī, Bāhū Indrabasta, Kaksha, Kati, Kukundara, Pārshva Sandhi, Sūrya or Āmāshaya, Vankshana, Vrukka
Asthi	Bāhya Kūrpara, Bāhya Manibandha, Charana (Lateral), Charana (Medial), Gulpha (Lateral), Gulpha (Medial), Hasta Kshipra, Jānu (Anterior), Jānu (Posterior), Kūrcha, Lohitāksha, Manibandha, Pāda Charana, Pāda Kshipra, Pārshni, Tarjani, Ūrū 1, Ūrū 2
Majjā	Adhah Ganda, Adhah Skandha, Agra Patra, Ājñā or Sthapanī, Akshaka, Amsa, Amsa Phalaka, Angushtha Mūla, Antara Vartma, Apānga, Apastambha, Ashrū (3), Bāhya Kūrpara, Bāhya Manibandha, Bāhya Vartma, Bāhū Indrabasta, Bruhatī, Brahmarandhra, Bhrūh Agra, Bhrūh Antara, Bhrūh Madhya, Charana (Lateral), Charana (Medial), Chibuka, Grīvā (4), Gulpha (Lateral), Gulpha (Medial), Hanu, Hasta Kshipra, Hridayam, Hrid (3), Indrabasta (Posterior), Jānu (Anterior), Jānu (Posterior), Jatrū, Kaksha, Kakshadhara or Skandadhara, Kanīnaka, Kanīshthika, Kantha, Kanthanādī, Kapāla, Kapola Madhya, Kapola Nāsā, Karnamūla (2), Karnapāla or Karna Ūrdhva, Karnapālī, Kati, Kūrcha, Kūrcha Shira, Krikātikā, Kukundara, Kūrpara, Lohitāksha, Madhya Vartma, Manibandha, Mantha, Manyāmani, Manyāmūla, Medhra, Mūrdhni or Adhipati, Nāsā Agra, Nāsā Madhya, Nāsā Mūla, Oshtha, Pāda Madhya, Pāda Charana, Pāda Kshipra, Pārshni, Pārshva Sandhi, Plīhā, Prushtha (3), Sakthi Ūrvī (Posterior), Shankha, Shivarandhra, Sīrāmantha, Sūrya or Āmāshaya, Tala Hrida, Tarjani, Trik, Ūrdhva Ganda, Ūrdhva Skandha, Ūrū 1, Ūrū 2, Vankri, Vankshana, Vidhuram, Vrushana, Yakrut, Yoni Jihvā, Yoni Oshtha
Shukra/ Ārtava	Basti, Bhaga, Chibuka, Hanu, Hridayam, Indrabasta (Medial), Kati, Kūrcha, Lohita, Manibandha, Medhra, Nābhi (5), Nāsā Agra, Nāsā Puta, Pāda Kshipra, Pārshni, Sakthi Ūrvī (Anterior), Sakthi Ūrvī (Posterior), Sphij, Stanya, Stanya Mūla, Stanya Pārshva, Trik, Ūrū 1, Ūrū 2, Vankshana, Vrukka, Vrushana, Yoni Jihvā, Yoni Oshtha

Table 43: Mental Disturbances

Condition	General Marmāni
Stress	Adhah Skandha, *Ājñā*, Amsa, Ashrū, Brahmarandhra, Bhrūh 3, Grīvā, Hanu, Hridayam, Hrid, Kapāla, Karnapāla, Karnapālī, Kūrcha, Krikātikā, Mūrdhni, Nāsā Mūla, Pāda Madhya, Shankha, Shivarandhra, Ūrdhva Skandha, Vidhuram
Poor Memory	*Ājñā, Brahmarandhra*, Mūrdhni, Shankha, Shivarandhra
Poor Concentration	*Ājñā*, Mūrdhni, *Oshtha*, Tala Hrida
Attention Deficit Hyperactive Disorder (ADHD)	*Ājñā*, Brahmarandhra, Karnapāla, Karnapālī, *Mūrdhni, Oshtha*, Pāda Madhya, Shivarandhra, Tala Hrida
Insomnia	*Ājñā*, Ashrū, Brahmarandhra, Bhrūh, Kapāla, Mūrdhni, Nāsā Mūla, Pāda Kshipra, *Pāda Madhya*, Shivarandhra, Ūrdhva Skandha

Yoga Therapy and Marmāni

The term yoga stems from the root *yuj,* which means to yoke or unite. Yoga is that which unites the lower self with the higher Self through the practical discipline of tuning and purifying the physical body, stilling the mind, and knowing the Self. It is the union of body, mind and spirit. The practices of Yoga—postures (*āsana*), breath control (prānāyāma), moral discipline (*yama* and *niyama*) and so forth—constitute a path that allows the limited, bounded individual to merge with the unbounded infinite. Ultimately, Yoga is the divine union or merging of Prakruti (creative manifestation) with Purusha (universal pure awareness).

The object of both Yoga and Āyurveda is to achieve the four goals of life, known as the *purushārthas.* These are: *dharma* (righteous duty), *artha* (wealth and material comfort), *kāma* (fulfillment of positive desires) and *moksha* (liberation). Without complete health, these four pillars of human life cannot be attained. Thus, Yoga and Āyurveda, each with a vision of the integration of body, mind and spirit, are sister disciplines that complement each other. Just as the Ayurvedic clinician integrates yoga therapy for healing, the yogi can also learn the principles of Āyurveda to augment his or her yoga practice.

Pātañjali, traditionally considered the founder of the science of Yoga, set forth in his *Yoga Sūtra,* a system of personal development that includes eight limbs or branches, known as *ashtānga yoga.* These eight facets of Yoga form an elegant and comprehensive path of growth. They are:

* **Yama** ~ Abstinences, Austerities

* **Niyama** ~ Observances

* **Āsana** ~ Postures

* **Prānāyāma** ~ Breath Awareness and Control

* **Pratyāhāra** ~ Withdrawal of the Senses

* **Dhārana** ~ Concentration

* **Dhyāna** ~ Meditation

* **Samādhi** ~ Spiritual Absorption

Yama and niyama encompass the basic rules of conduct and behavior. The five yama are abstinences that help every human being—whether practicing Yoga or not—to live a better life: abstaining from violence, possessiveness, sexual misconduct, lying and stealing. The five niyamas are observances to sincerely practice purity, austerity, self-inquiry, contentment and surrender to God or ultimate reality. Generally, these first two limbs are considered prerequisites for practice of the other six limbs of Yoga.

The next limb is āsana, the physical postures that comprise the most well-known aspect of Yoga. The word āsana is derived from the root *asa,* existence or stability. Practice of āsana develops physical and mental stillness. The stability of the physical body is closely connected to the stability of the mind, reflecting the intimate relationship of mind and body. It is unfortunate that the popularization of Yoga in the West, a very positive trend in itself, has tended to emphasize the practice of āsana at the expense of the other seven limbs, for the integration of āsana with the other limbs is the surest path towards spiritual fulfillment.

There are thousands of postures within the system of Yoga—ancient texts suggest 840,000, an astonishing number—but it is far from necessary to learn all of them. Indeed, tradition holds that only Shiva, Lord of Yoga, can do them all. It is quite sufficient to learn and practice daily only eight to twelve postures that are most beneficial for one's health and spiritual development.

The diversity of āsanas reflects the richness of this discipline. Ancient rishis (enlightened seers) carefully observed the elements in nature and created āsanas that reflect the way the sun or moon rises, a tree stands or a lotus flower floats in water. They also observed the physical behaviors of various animals in their environment and named another class of āsanas correspondingly. Hence, āsanas mimic the way a cobra raises its hood, a lion opens its mouth, a camel stands or a cat or dog stretches. When we perform a particular pose, we may feel the subtle healing energetics of those animals or aspects of nature.

Many treat Yoga as little more than a system of physical exercise that tones the muscles, promotes flexibility and benefits the cardiovascular system—all of which is true, but it is more than that. The yogāsanas influence the seven dhātus, especially the nerve and connective tissues. More significantly, Yoga is highly beneficial for the mind. Every āsana offers the opportunity to sharpen one's concentration and awareness, and to gently still a turbulent mind.

The fourth limb of Yoga, prānāyāma, is the science and control of the breath. Prānāyāma is such a vast and profound field of knowledge that many instructors do not teach this until students are well-advanced and have mastered some of the basics of āsana.

Only human beings can breathe consciously, although most of the time our respiration is unconscious. Conscious breathing is conscious living and unconscious breathing is unconscious living. Unconscious living often gives rise to negative thoughts, feelings and emotions. If these negative mental states—anger, jealousy, resentment, fear, anxiety, depression, and all their cousins—do not get resolved and cleared from the system, they accumulate and stagnate in the deep connective tissues and nādīs.

Thoughts, feelings and emotions are the subtle manifestation of prāna in the body. Where prāna is accumulated and stagnated, pathological lesions, called khavaigunya, are created. Prānāyāma helps, by force of breath, to open the channels, remove the stagnation and eradicate the pathological process. Thus, the vital breath, prāna, is the bridge between body, mind and consciousness. By performing different types of prānāyāma (there are many) we can purify the nādīs (the pathways), detoxify the organs, and awaken certain marma energies in order to bring total health.

As we have explained, the accumulation of toxins (āma) in the subtle and gross levels of the body, whether originating in negative thoughts and emotions, eating unhealthy or excess food, poor digestion, etc. is considered by Āyurveda to be the primary cause of disease. Most of the modalities of Āyurvedic medicine are devoted to preventing this toxic buildup from occurring using right diet, healthy lifestyle and daily routine, yogāsanas, meditation, and so on; and by eliminating impurities, if and when they accumulate, via panchakarma, yogāsanas, marma chikitsā, etc. One of the best preventative measures—a daily-life meditative awareness that is a function of alert, conscious living—is to observe negative feelings when they arise, and to con-

tinue to observe them, innocently allowing them to increase and then subside.[1]

> **An Intriguing Hypothesis:** It has been theorized that prānāyāma, which brings an influx of oxygen and subtle energy to every cell, may stimulate the creation of new stem cells, which, in turn, regenerate the organs. It is known that four days after fertilization, one single stem cell develops into the brain, the heart and so on. If performing prānāyāma helps to generate stem cells, could this simple process of conscious breathing reverse or slow the aging process? Is this why legends abound of yogis in the Himalayas who live hundreds of years? This would be a fascinating subject for medical research.

Pratyāhāra, the fifth limb of Yoga, involves the withdrawal of the senses from sensory objects. Sānkhya philosophy has described (see chapter 1, page 9) how the five tanmātrās (subtle elements of sound, touch, vision, taste, and smell) are created and form a basis for human perception and interaction with the world. By learning to withdraw the senses, one begins to detach from the physical world and ceases to be inundated constantly with sensory input. This is a crucial step toward deep, settled meditative awareness.

Withdrawal of the senses is achieved by double-arrowed attention. When you look at a tree, one arrow of attention goes out to touch the tree; simultaneously, a second arrow goes inside to the heart of the observer. While watching the tree, you are watching the watcher; watching the watcher while watching the tree, or listening to the listener while listening to a sound, is double-arrowed awareness or pratyāhāra.

Ahar means food. Vision is food for the eyes, sound is food for the ears, touch is the food for skin. *Prati* means opposite, or reverse. So, the practice of pratyāhāra means that, in the course of our daily experiences and perceptions, when the senses are going toward their food, the objects of perception, one should also be aware of the perceiver. Instead of being turned totally outward perceiving only objects, one should perceive the perceiver in the act of perception. This automatically draws the mind inward.

Dhārana is concentration, focus on a single object such as a mantra or visual image. Typical objects of attention have also included the tip of the nose, the navel and the "third eye" point between the eyebrows. It could simply be looking at a tree, or a distant star in the sky. Whatever the object of focus, a yogi's concentration has strength, intensity and one-pointedness. The attention is unbroken, non-stop, continuous.

Dhyāna or meditation is the flow of the concentrated mind in moment-to-moment awareness. As dhārana involves intense attention on an unchanging object or

---

1. These guidelines for healthy living and purification are explained in detail in Dr. Lad's book, *The Complete Book of Ayurvedic Home Remedies.*

fixed point, in dhyāna the mind remains focused, but in fluid, moment-to-moment awareness, like the flow of pouring oil. It is like listening to beautiful, absorbing music, where there is a continuous flow in which the mind remains focused and absorbed.

Ultimately, the observer—the meditator, the watcher—merges into the observed. This is the final limb of Yoga, samādhi or spiritual absorption. In samādhi, there is a complete ending of the meditator as a separate observer or actor. Subject and object unite in a state of no-mind and no-time. It is a merging of individuality into universality, in which what remains is pure awareness, pure presence of totality.

We get flashes of samādhi in meditation, moments of timelessness. However, in samādhi, there is complete merging of the individual meditator into the totality. Samādhi is endless, boundless, timeless existence. Meditation is the means and samādhi is the end, a fully awake transcendental state of awareness where individual consciousness merges into universal consciousness.

Samādhi is the culmination and essence of all the previous limbs of Yoga. Only accomplished yogis experience the divine state of samādhi after long dedication to knowing the Self. They become absorbed in the inner light of awareness that leads to full enlightenment.

The table at right shows the wide ranging effect of Yoga on healing and strengthening mind and body.

The eight limbs of Yoga reflect a progression from the external world of action and behavior to the inner world of the mind and Self. The yamas and niyamas form a general code of conduct designed to regulate and uplift our actions and interactions in the external world. Āsanas are physical postures that engage the body, yet require mental discipline; thus āsanas become a bridge between the physical and mental levels. Prānāyāma is also a physical action, more subtle than āsanas, that becomes increasingly internal. It is based on the mind's ability to control the breath. Pratyāhāra, dhārana and dhyāna are all conscious, active experiences that lead the practitioner's awareness ever deeper inward. They reflect diminishing contact with the external world and physical activity. Lastly, samādhi, or spiritual absorption, is the deepest awareness of *Jyotis,* the flame of the Self. Jyotis is the inner light that burns brightly and is seen in meditation. The journey through the eight limbs of Yoga is identical to the journey towards the inner Self.

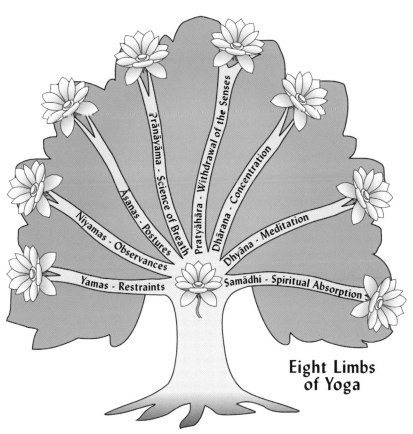

Eight Limbs of Yoga

Table 44: Yoga and Health

Branch of Yoga	Health Benefits
Yama and Niyama	Builds positive relationship with others and environment
Āsana	Strengthens and heals the physical body
Prānāyāma	Heals prāna body
Pratyāhāra	Sharpens sensory system
Dhārana	Promotes healthy mind
Dhyāna	Strengthens memory
Samādhi	Fosters health of the buddhi (intellect)

Āsana and Marmāni

Although Yoga is a vast and profound subject, the remainder of this chapter focuses on one limb, āsana, and its relationship to marmāni. Āsana practice and marma chikitsā are inextricably linked in that they both bridge the body and mind, bringing increased harmony and healing. Both enhance awareness and balance ojas, tejas and prāna.

Every āsana can be viewed in terms of its biomechanics and energetics. Biomechanics is the art of correct alignment and proper positioning, which are essential for gaining maximum therapeutic benefit. In general, initial emphasis is on form rather than on flexibility. With time and practice, flexibility and the ease of being in a particular posture increase.

Energetically, each āsana triggers the subtle flow of prāna and awareness into specific regions of the body, including the surface anatomy, organ systems and marmāni. Prāna is the intelligence that promotes optimal functioning of the body on every level from gross to subtle, including the cellular.

Because each āsana stimulates several marmāni, yoga can be considered a form of self-managed marma chikitsā. This occurs through three mechanisms:

1. Stretching of the connective tissue in which marmāni lie
2. Direct pressure on marmāni by the ground or other body parts
3. Flow of prāna to certain marmāni via the prāna nādīs (subtle channels)

This stimulation is comparable to the therapeutic application of physical pressure or massage to the marmāni. Hence, many benefits of marma chikitsā can be achieved through yoga postures. For example, āsanas that expand the chest stimulate local marmāni, many of which are related functionally to the lungs. Thus, a thorough knowledge of marmāni can deeply enhance any Yoga practice.

Yoga practice should also be combined with the Ayurvedic wisdom of selecting āsanas based on one's constitution. Certain poses either pacify or stimulate specific doshas, according to both the nature of the posture and how it is practiced. It is important that each person's yoga practice be unique to their doshic constitution and their present imbalances. Because of the influence of weather and seasons on the mind-body and the balance of the doshas, āsana practice would ideally vary with the seasons. For example, postures that increase heat would be avoided in summer and favored in winter. Understanding how an āsana is related to the doshas and to the marmāni is necessary for anyone who wishes to go deeply into yoga.

This chapter presents āsanas with postures that pacify vāta, pitta, kapha or all three equally. A select number of āsanas have been chosen to illustrate how certain marmāni are triggered in each āsana. Each āsana has a Sanskrit name, English translation, list of related marmāni and an illustration of the pose. The principal marmāni affected by a pose are emphasized. An āsana may activate all marmāni of a particular body region, but the list has been condensed to include only a few major points of that area.

Vāta Balancing Postures

Āsanas that are stabilizing and grounding calm vāta dosha. These postures focus on the pelvic cavity, lower abdominal region and low back. They also act on other regions governed by vāta dosha, including the colon, thighs, ears and extremities.

These āsanas increase clarity and stability, and pacify fluctuating emotions such as anxiety, nervousness and insecurity. Vāta individuals must avoid overexertion and strenuous exercises. In general, vāta moves upward, therefore inverted postures are beneficial because they help to pacify vāta dosha. Marmāni along the spine are stimulated in all these āsanas.

Vajrāsana
(Thunderbolt Pose)

Pāda Kshipra
Pāda Charana
Pārshni
Indrabasta
Jānu
Ūrū
Sakthi Ūrvī
Trik
Sphij

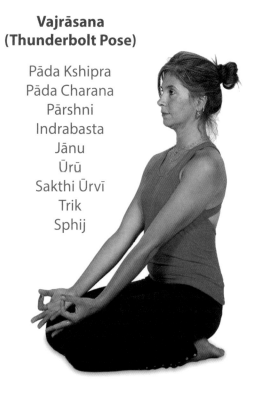

Bhujangāsana
(Cobra Pose)

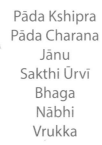

Pāda Kshipra
Pāda Charana
Jānu
Sakthi Ūrvī
Bhaga
Nābhi
Vrukka

Kukundara
Apastambha
Jatrū
Grīvā
Kūrpara
Marmāni
of the Hands

Shīrshāsana
(Head Stand)

Mūrdhni
Brahmarandhra
Shivarandhra
Kaksha
Kakshadhara
Nābhi
Kūrpara
Pāda Madhya
Marmāni of the Legs

Salabhāsana
(Locust Pose)

Hanu
Kantha
Grīvā
Ūrdhva Skandha
Yakrut
Plīhā

Nābhi
Bhaga
Jānu
Marmāni
of the Extremities

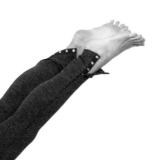

Pāvanmuktāsana
(Knee/Chest Pose)

Jatrū
Amsa
Yakrut
Plīhā
Vrukka
Kukundara
Kati
Trik
Jānu
Apastambha

Halāsana
(Plow Pose)

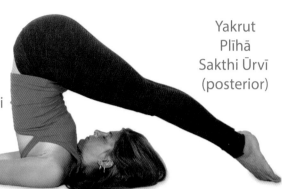

Shivarandhra
Jatrū
Grīvā
Amsa
Skandha marmāni
Kūrpara

Yakrut
Plīhā
Sakthi Ūrvī
(posterior)

Paschimottānāsana
(Forward Bend/Head To Knee Pose)

Pāda Madhya	Sphij
Gulpha	Vrukka
Indrabasta	Yakrut
Jānu	Plīhā
Sakthi Ūrvī	Kaksha
Trik	Mūrdhni

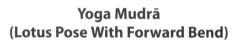

Yoga Mudrā
(Lotus Pose With Forward Bend)

Mūrdhni
Ājñā
Jatrū
Manyāmani
Nābhi
Bhaga
Vrukka
Trik
Sphij
Ūrū
Sakthi Ūrvī
Gulpha

Ūrdhva Padmāsana
(Elevated Lotus Pose)

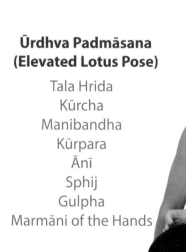

Tala Hrida
Kūrcha
Manibandha
Kūrpara
Ānī
Sphij
Gulpha
Marmāni of the Hands

Pitta Balancing Postures

Pitta pacifying āsanas focus on the solar plexus, navel and abdominal area, including the regions of the liver, spleen, stomach, small intestine and heart. All backward bends stretch these areas and are beneficial for pitta. Forward bends will increase pitta, as the blood rushes to the brain. Any inverted āsana should be done with moderation, because it stimulates pitta dosha. This is especially true of shīrshāsana (head stand). Caution should be taken to avoid āsanas that increase too much internal heat, as this will also aggravate pitta.

Jānu Shīrshāsana
(Head To Knee Pose)

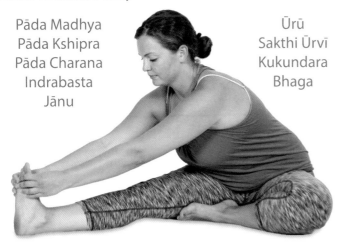

Pāda Madhya
Pāda Kshipra
Pāda Charana
Indrabasta
Jānu

Ūrū
Sakthi Ūrvī
Kukundara
Bhaga

Dhanurāsana
(Bow)

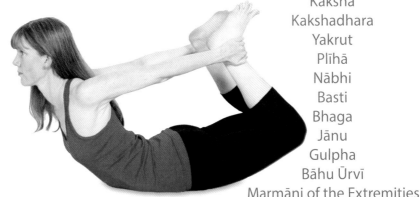

Manyāmani
Jatrū
Hrid
Kaksha
Kakshadhara
Yakrut
Plīhā
Nābhi
Basti
Bhaga
Jānu
Gulpha
Bāhu Ūrvī
Marmāni of the Extremities

Ardha Nāvāsana
(Half Boat)

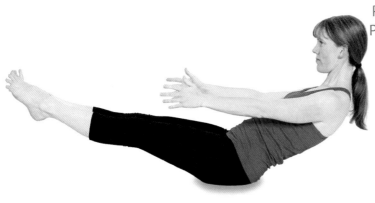

Pāda Madhya
Pāda Kshipra
Pāda Charana
Jānu
Ūrū
Trik
Bhaga
Vrukka
Nābhi
Yakrut
Plīhā

Ustrāsana
(Camel Pose)

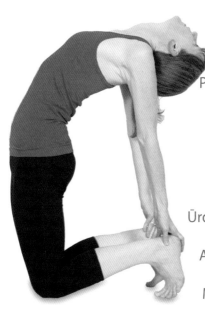

Pāda Kshipra
Gulpha
Jānu
Sphij
Trik
Vrukka
Amsa
Ūrdhva Skandha
Hrid
Apastambha
Jatrū
Manyāmani

Supta Padmāsana
(Hidden Lotus Pose)

Hanu   Bhaga
Kantha   Lohitāksha
Manyāmani   Trik
Ūrdhva Skandha Ūrū
Kakshadhara   Jānu
Nābhi   Pāda Madhya

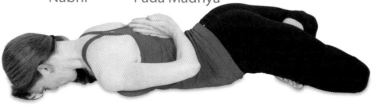

Sarvāngāsana
(Shoulder Stand)

Manyāmani
Kantha
Ūrdhva Skandha
Kūrpara
Vrukka
Sakthi Ūrvī
Pāda Madhya

Mūrdhni   Kaksha
Manyāmani   Kūrpara
Jatrū   Vrukka
Amsa Phalaka   Kati
Prushtha   Trik
Bruhatī   Pāda Madhya

Matsyāsana
(Fish Pose)

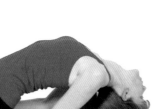

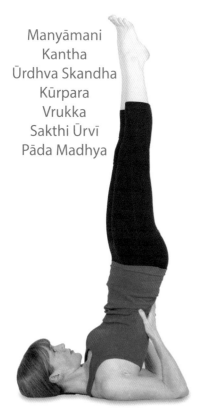

Setu Bandha Sarvāngāsana
(Bridge Pose)

Manyāmūla   Pārshni
Ūrdhva Skandha   Gulpha
Amsa   Pāda Kshipra
Kūrpara
Yakrut
Plīhā
Nābhi
Vrukka
Trik
Jānu

246

Kapha Balancing Postures

Āsanas should be stimulating, challenging and vigorous to pacify kapha dosha. These postures focus on the head, chest and stomach. They should be geared to increasing stamina, energy and heart rate. All standing poses and spinal twists are good for kapha dosha. Āsanas that open the chest especially by raising the arms over the head are beneficial. An overweight individual should use caution when putting weight or pressure on the joints.

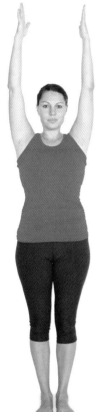

Tādāsana
(Palm Tree)

Pāda Madhya
Pāda Charana
Indrabasta
Jānu
Ūrū
Sakthi Ūrvī
Nābhi
Hrid
Jatrū
Ūrdhva Skandha
Kaksha
Manibandha
Tala Hrida
Mūrdhni

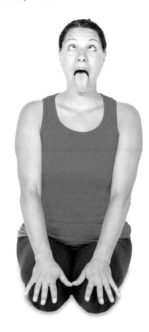

Simhāsana
(Lion)

Ājñā
Shankha
Ganda
Kapola Nāsā
Kapola Madhya
Oshtha
Chibuka
Hanu
Karnamūla
Kantha

Ardha Matsyendrāsana
(Half Spinal Twist)

Pāda Kshipra
Indrabasta
Jānu
Trik
Sphij
Yakrut
Plīhā
Nābhi
Vrukka
Prushtha
Bruhatī
Kakshadhara
Sīrāmantha

Vriksāsana
(Tree Pose)

Pāda Madhya
Pāda Kshipra
Pāda Charana
Bhaga
Nābhi
Hridayam
Kakshadhara
Kaksha
Ūrdhva Skandha
Bāhu Ūrvī
Tala Hrida

Paripūrna Nāvāsana
(Full Boat Pose)

Jatrū
Kakshadhara
Kaksha
Ānī
Tala Hrida
Nābhi
Yakrut
Plīhā
Bhaga
Ūrū
Sakthi Ūrvī
Jānu

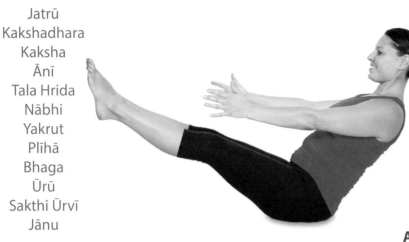

Adhomukha Svānāsana
(Downward Facing Dog Pose)

Pāda Kshipra
Pārshni
Indrabasta
Jānu
Ūrū
Nābhi
Hridayam
Ūrdhva Skandha
Kaksha
Mūrdhni
Marmāni of the hands

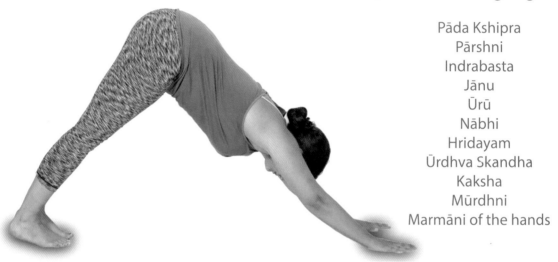

Gomukhāsana
(Cow Pose)

Kaksha
Kakshadhara
Ūrdhva Skandha
Kūrpara
Hridayam
Bruhatī
Sūrya
Bhaga
Jānu
Sakthi Ūrvī

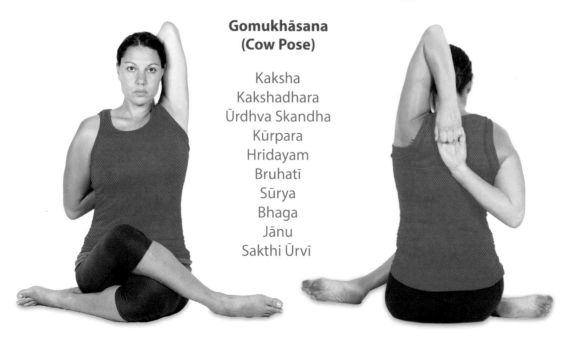

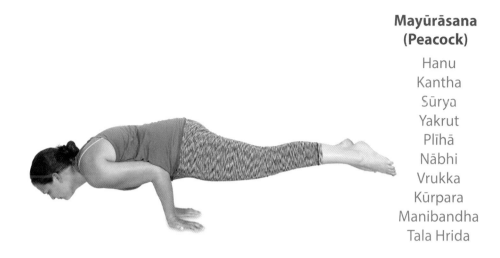

Mayūrāsana
(Peacock)

Hanu
Kantha
Sūrya
Yakrut
Plīhā
Nābhi
Vrukka
Kūrpara
Manibandha
Tala Hrida

Tridoshic Balancing Postures

All āsanas are tridoshic in nature, but some act upon one or two doshas more strongly than the others. The following three āsanas equally balance all three doshas and are appropriate for any constitution. Shavāsana is recommended at the end of a yoga practice to allow sufficient rest and rejuvenation. Padmāsana is considered the jewel of all āsanas and is the posture best suited for meditation.

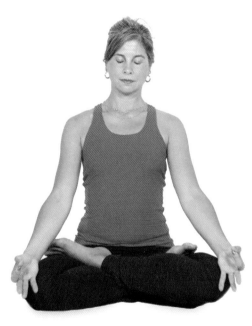

Padmāsana
(Lotus)

Sakthi Ūrvī
Trik
Sphij
Ūrū
Mūrdhni
Ājñā
Hridayam
Vrukka
Kukundara
Kati
Apastambha
Kantha

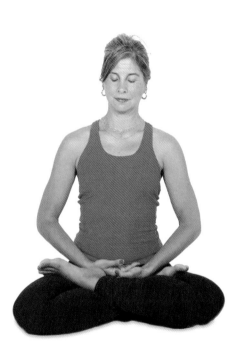

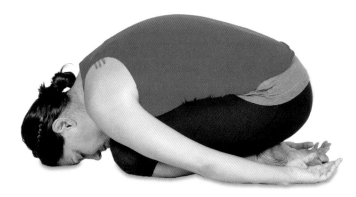

Balāsana
(Child's Pose)

Pārshni
Jānu
Ūrū
Yakrut
Plīhā
Kaksha
Ājñā
Tala Hrida
Pārshva Sandhi

Balāsana
(*Variation*)

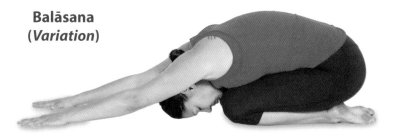

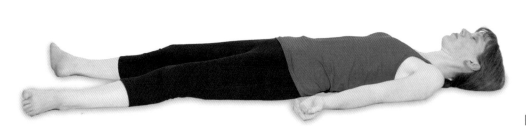

Shavāsana
(Corpse Pose)

Shivarandhra
Manyāmūla
Amsa
Bruhatī
Trik
Jānu
Indrabasta
Pāda Madhya

Appendix A
Specialized Āyurvedic Information

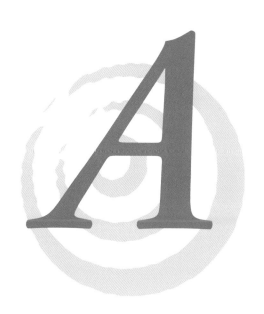

Table 45: The Five Elements and Manifestation in Āyurveda

	Space (Ether)	Air	Fire	Water	Earth
Season	Autumn	Autumn	Summer	Winter, rainy season	Spring
Direction	Above, down, everywhere	West	South	North	East
Type of Energy	Nuclear	Electrical	Radiant	Chemical	Physical/ mechanical
Sense	Sound	Touch	Vision	Taste	Smell
Sense Organs	Ears	Skin	Eyes	Tongue	Nose
Sound	Hām	Yam	Rām	Vam	Lam
Smell	No smell, ozone smell	Astringent	Burnt	Damp	Earthy smell
Emotions/ Functions Positive	Peace, freedom, expansion of consciousness	Creativity, flexibility, happiness, freshness, joy, excitation, clarity	Understanding, absorption, attention, comprehension, transformation, appreciation, recognition	Gentleness, love, contentment, compassion, forgiveness	Groundedness, support, stability, forgiveness, centeredness
Emotions/ Functions Negative	Loneliness, fear, separation, isolation, emptiness, insecurity, anxiety, ungroundedness	Isolation, grief, sadness, fear, anxiety, excess worrying, insecurity, restlessness, nervousness	Hate, envy, anger, criticism, ambition, discrimination	Attachment, greed, possessiveness, emotional hypersensitivity	Monotony, gloom, melancholy, depression, dullness, indecision, lack of clarity, pensiveness

Table 45: The Five Elements and Manifestation in Āyurveda (Continued)

	Space (Ether)	Air	Fire	Water	Earth
Gunas	Subtle, clear, light, cold, empty, soft, expansive, universal, formless, omnipresent, centrifugal, non-moving, all pervading, all enclosing, non-resistant	Mobile, dry, light, clear, subtle, rough, cold	Hot, sharp, light, dry, subtle, spreading, luminous, radiant, penetrating	Liquid, fluid, cold, aqueous, heavy, soft, spreading, dull, slow, oily, viscous, dense, smooth, cohesive, unctuousness	Heavy, gross, static, stable, hard, rough, firm, dense, resistant, centripetal
Doshas	Vāta	Vāta	Pitta	Pitta, kapha	Kapha
Dhātus	Asthi, majjā	Asthi, majjā	Rakta, māmsa	Rasa, rakta, meda, māmsa, shukra, ārtava	Asthi, māmsa, meda
Srotas	All spacious systems, ventricles of brain, bone porosities and cavities	Asthi, majjā	Rakta, māmsa, sveda, anna	Rasa, rakta, mūtra, sveda	Asthi, purīsha, māmsa
Color	Purple, indigo, twilight	Blue, purple	Red, orange, yellow	Colorless, white, pale blue	Brown, dark-reddish
Taste	Bitter	Bitter, astringent	Pungent, sour, salty	Salty, sweet	Sweet, sour, astringent
Three Gunas	Sattva	Rajas	Sattva, rajas	Sattva, tamas	Tamas
Chakras	Vishuddhi, throat	Anāhata, heart	Manipūra, solar plexus	Svādishthāna, splenic or navel plexus	Mūlādhāra, root
Expression of Consciousness	Expansion, all inclusiveness	Movement	Concentration	Liquefaction	Crystallization
Presence in Body	Empty spaces: colon, nose, respiratory tract, GI tract, nerve synapses, third ventricle, oral cavities, thoracic/abdominal cavities	Air fills space: in lungs, flatus in GI tract, CO_2 and O_2 in blood, impulse for sensory stimuli and motor responses	HCL, digestive enzymes, liver and pancreatic enzymes, neurotransmitters	Body is 70% water: blood, lymph, saliva, CSF, plasma, serum, urine, sweat, nasal secretions, cytoplasm, secretions in joints, mucus membrane	Minerals (Ca, Mg, etc.) for bones, hair, nails, teeth, cartilage, muscle tendons, skeleton, skin; movement of muscles, formation of bones and muscle structure
Cellular Level	Cellular vacuoles	Movement of cell	Nucleic acid and chemical compounds	Cytoplasm	Cell membrane

Table 45: The Five Elements and Manifestation in Āyurveda (Continued)

	Space (Ether)	Air	Fire	Water	Earth
Karmas, functions necessary for	Vibration, lightness, space creating and filling; produces cavitation, non-resistance, freedom, unconditional love, communication	Flow of thought, desire and will; all movement: movement of intestines, elimination, movement of muscles, heart pulsations, expansion and contraction of lungs, locomotion, sensory and neural impulses, breathing, ingestion and ejection, cleansing	Transformation of food into energy, metabolism: digestion, absorption & assimilation, intelligence & understanding, illumination, expression of color complexion, luster, eye color, upward movement, temperature regulation	Downward movement, nutrition, capillary action, water-electrolyte balance, percolation, lubrication, secretion, moisturizing, fluidity, flushing, cohesion, adhesion, binding, takes form of container	Strength, structure and stamina to body, gravitation, heaviness, compactness, growth, solidity, consolidation, fulfillment
Virtues	Bliss	Creativity	Knowledge	Compassion	Forgiveness
Related Finger	Thumb	Index finger	Middle finger	Ring finger	Little finger

Table 46: The Seven Dhātus (Bodily Tissues)

Dhātu	Tissue	Function	Size	Upa-dhātu	Dhātu Mala
Rasa	Plasma Lymph	Nutrition, affection (prīnana) Immunity	9 añjali	Top layer of skin Lactation (stanya) Menstruation (raja)	Poshaka kapha
Rakta	Red blood cells	Life function (jīvana) Oxygenation Enthusiasm	8 añjali	Blood vessels and granulation tissue (sirā) Small tendons and sinews (kandara)	Poshaka pitta
Māmsa	Muscle tissue	Plastering (lepana) Form, Movement, Support, Strength, Protection	varies	Six layers of skin (tvacha) Subcutaneous fat (vasā)	Ear wax, nasal crust, sebaceous secretions, teeth tartar, smegma (khāmala)
Meda	Adipose tissue	Lubrication (snehana) Personal love, Beauty, Bulk to body, Insulation	2 añjali	Tendons, ligaments, flat muscles (snāyu)	Sweat (sveda)
Asthi	Bone tissue	Support (dhārana) Structure Protection of vital organs	Approximately 365 bones	Teeth (danta) Cartilage (taruna asthi)	Hair (kesha) Nails (nakha)
Majjā	Bone marrow Nervous tissue Connective tissue	Fills bone spaces (purana), Sensation, Learning, Communication, Memory	2 añjali	Lacrimal secretions (ashru)	Oily secretions in eyes (akshi vitta sneha)
Shukra / Ārtava	Reproductive tissue	Reproduction (prajanama) Produce ojas Emotional release	½ añjali	Ojas	None

Table 47: Srotāmsi, the Systems and Channels of the Body

Srotāmsi	Functions	Mūla	Mārga	Mukha
Prāna Vaha Srotas	Respiration, Thinking, Emotion, Communication with higher self	Left chamber of heart, GI tract (maha srotas)	Respiratory tract, bronchial tree including alveoli	Nose (nāsā)
Ambu Vaha Srotas	Body temperature, Lubrication, Energy, Electrolyte balance, Selection of wastes	Pancreas (kloma), Soft palate (tālu), Choroid plexus	GI mucous membrane	Kidneys (vrukka), Tongue, Sweat glands (roma kūpa)
Anna Vaha Srotas	Digestion, Assimilation, Absorption	Esophagus, Stomach – greater curvature (fundus)	GI tract (maha srotas) – lips through ileocecal	Ileocecal valve
Rasa Vaha Srotas	Nutrition, affection (prīnana) Immunity	Right chamber of heart (where all venous blood comes), 10 great vessels	Venous system, Lymphatic system	Arteriole/venous junction
Rakta Vaha Srotas	Life function (jīvana) Oxygenation Enthusiasm	Liver (yakrut), Spleen (plīhā)	Arteriole circulatory system	Arteriole/venous junction
Māmsa Vaha Srotas	Plastering (lepana) Form, Movement, Support, Protection, Strength	Fascia and small tendons (snāyu), Mesoderm, 6 layers of skin (tvacha)	Entire muscle system incl. smooth, heart, involuntary muscles	Pores of skin
Meda Vaha Srotas	Lubrication (snehana), Personal love, Beauty, Bulk to body, Insulation	Omentum, Adrenal glands (vrukka)	Subcutaneous fat	Sweat glands (roma kūpa)
Asthi Vaha Srotas	Support (dhārana) Structure Protection of vital organs	Pelvic girdle, Sacrum	Skeletal system	Nails, Hair
Majjā Vaha Srotas	Fills bone spaces (pūrana) Sensation, Communication, Learning, Memory, Coordination	Brain, Spinal cord, Joints (sandhi)	Central, Sympathetic, & Parasympathetic Nervous Systems	Synaptic space, Neuromuscular cleft
Shukra Vaha Srotas	Reproduction (prajanama) Produce ojas Emotional release	Testicles, Nipples	Vas deferens, Epididymis, Prostate, Urethra, Urinogenital tract	Urethral opening
Ārtava Vaha Srotas	Reproduction (prajanama) Produce ojas Emotional release	Ovaries, Areola of nipples	Fallopian tubes, Uterus, Cervical canal, Vaginal passage (yoni)	Labia minor/major (yoni oshtha)
Purīsha Vaha Srotas	Absorption of minerals, Strength, Support, Formation and excretion of feces	Cecum, Rectum, Sigmoid colon	Large intestine	Anal orifice
Mūtra Vaha Srotas	Electrolyte balance, Maintain blood pressure, Excrete urine	Kidneys	Ureter (kidney to bladder), Bladder, Urethra	Urethral opening

Table 47: Srotāmsi, the Systems and Channels of the Body

Srotāmsi	Functions	Mūla	Mārga	Mukha
Sveda Vaha Srotas	Perspiration, Lubrication, Body temperature, Electrolyte balance, Elimination of liquid wastes	Sebaceous (sweat) glands	Sebaceous ducts	Sebaceous duct openings Pores of skin
Mano Vaha Srotas	Thinking, Feeling, Inquiring, Deciding, Discrimination, Desire, Communication, Memory, Contentment	Heart (cardiac plexus), 5 bilateral pairs (10) nādi (pathways) – 1 pair for each of the 5 senses	Entire body	Sense organs (ears, nose, skin, tongue, eyes), Marmāni (marma points)
Stanya Vaha Srotas	Lactation	Lactiferous glands	Lactiferous ducts	Duct openings in nipples

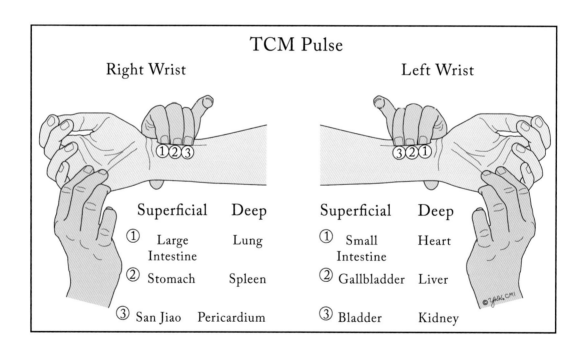

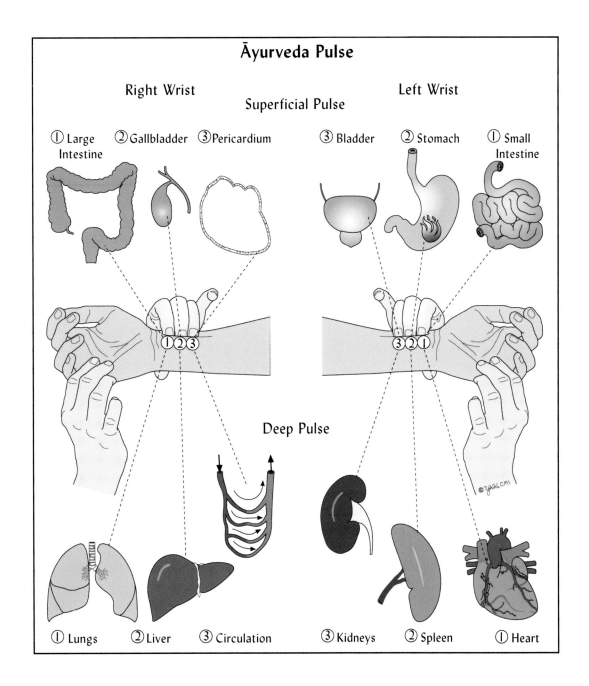

Āyurveda Pulse

Right Wrist   Left Wrist

Superficial Pulse

① Large   ② Gallbladder ③ Pericardium   ③ Bladder   ② Stomach   ① Small
Intestine   Intestine

① ② ③   ③ ② ①

Deep Pulse

① Lungs   ② Liver   ③ Circulation   ③ Kidneys   ② Spleen   ① Heart

Table 48: Properties of the Chakras

Chakra	Functions	Dysfunctions / Disorders	Nerve Plexus	Physiological / Endocrine System	Element
Mūlādhāra Root support Coccyx 4 petals	Survival, groundedness	Ungroundedness	Sacral Plexus	Reproductive / Gonads	Earth
Svādishthāna Self-place Hypogastric 6 petals	Self identity (lower self), self esteem, procreation	Repressed sexuality, fear, anxiety	Pelvic plexus	Genitourinary / Adrenals	Water
Manipūra Gem city Navel 10 petals	Ambition, achievement, power, domination	Anger, hate	Celiac plexus	Digestive / Pancreas (Islets of Langerhans)	Fire
Anāhata Unstruck sound Heart 12 petals	Love, immunity	Feels lack of love, immune problems	Cardiac plexus	Circulatory / Thymus	Air
Vishuddhi Purity Throat 16 petals	Communication, will	Lack of communication, suppressed emotions	Cervical plexus	Respiratory and metabolic / Thyroid and parathyroid	Ether (Space)
Ājñā Order Third eye 2 petals	Intuition (alpha meets omega)	Not wanting to see reality, hormonal imbalances	Optic chiasma	Autonomic nervous system / Pituitary	Consciousness
Sahasrāra Thousand petal lotus Crown 1000 petals	Spiritual quest, self realization, bliss	Psychosis, depression	Cerebral hemispheres	Central nervous system / Pineal (soma)	Bliss

Table 49: Subtle Healing and Balancing for the Chakras

Chakras	Herbs	Essential Oil	Sound/Seed Sound	Color, Note	Gem	Deity
Mūlādhāra	Triphala, Shatāvarī, Vidhari, Ashvagandha	Cedar	लं lam / gam	Red, Sa	Ruby	Ganesha, Kundalinī
Svādhishthāna	Punarnava, Licorice, Gokshura	Nutmeg	वं vam / klim	Orange, Re	Coral	Brahma (Creator), Dakini
Manipūra	Chitrak, Kutki, Neem	Hina	रं ram / shrim	Yellow, Ga	Topaz	Vishnu (Protector), Rakini or Parvati
Anāhata	Arjun, Licorice	Tulsi, Jasmine	यं yam / hrim	Green, Ma	Emerald, Rudraksha	Rudra (Transformer), Lakini or Lakshmi
Vishuddhi	Vacha, Shilajit, Gulvel Satva	Vacha, Eucalyptus	हं hām / aim	Blue, Pa	Diamond	Jīva (Life force), Sarasvati
Ājñā	Jatamāmsī, Jyotismati, Saffron	Sandalwood	सं क्षं sam ksham / sauhu	Indigo, Da	Alexandrite, Blue sapphire	Guru, Mahashakti
Sahasrāra	Brahmī, Gotu Kola, Gingko	Lotus	ॐ Aum (or So'ham)	Violet, Ni	Amethyst	Paramātman

Table 50: Chromotherapy

Color	Qualities	Doshic Influence	Acts On	Function	Organ	Psycho-spiritual Effect
Red	Hot, sharp, bright, penetrating, intense	V↑ P↓ K↑	Rakta, meda, majjā, shukra, ārtava	Erythrogenesis, decongestant, enhances circulation, colors complexion, heat promoter, blood builder, muscle relaxer	Skin, heart, lung, muscles, bone marrow, prostate, gonads, ovaries	Romantic heat, sex, anger, hate, irritability, violence
Orange	Warm, sharp, stimulant, antibacterial, energizing	V↑ P↓ K↑	Rasa, rakta, māmsa, majjā, ārtava	Decongestant, antibacterial, antidepressant, renunciation	Lymphatic system, heart, cervix, sex organs, ovaries, testicles, prostate, adrenals	Helps renunciation, antidepressant, mood elevator, enthusiasm, awakens kundalinī
Yellow	Warm, antibacterial, gastric stomach, enkindles agni, improves digestion	V↑ P↓ K↑	Gastro-intestinal (GI) tract, liver, spleen, pancreas	Treats anorexia and indigestion, stimulates metabolism, improves absorption, assimilation of food	Liver, GI tract, spleen, pancreas, stomach	Understanding, comprehension, cellular intelligence, aids concentration
Green	Heavy, refreshing, sedative, calming, relaxing, nutritive, grounding	V↓ P↓ K↑	Rasa, rakta, māmsa, majjā	Builds healthy kapha, muscle builder, anti-inflammatory, heals ulcer, diabetes, improves immune response	Gall bladder, lungs, heart, spleen, thymus, immune system	Happiness, joy, contentment, compassion, grounding
Blue	Cooling, calming, anti-inflammatory, relaxing, spacey	V↑ P↓ K↓	Rasa, rakta, māmsa, majjā, mind	Helps to heal jaundice, hemorrhoids, eczema, rash, stress	Calms nerves, thyroid, parathyroid	Peace, intuition, communication
Indigo	Expansive, etheric, cosmic, consciousness, meditation	V = P = K =	3rd Eye	Hormonal balance, insight, cellular communication	Pituitary, hormones	Meditation, tranquility
Violet	spiritual wisdom, higher consciousness	V = P = K =	Brain	Pineal gland, neuro-transmitter, cellular bliss, bliss molecule	Pineal, brain, cerebral cortex	Bliss, enlightenment

Table 51: Guidelines For Determining Your Constitution

Observations	V	P	K	Vāta	Pitta	Kapha
Body size	☐	☐	☐	Slim	Medium	Large
Chin	☐	☐	☐	Thin, angular	Tapering	Rounded, double
Cheeks	☐	☐	☐	Wrinkled, sunken	Smooth, flat	Rounded, plump
Eyes	☐	☐	☐	Small, sunken, dry, active, black, brown, nervous	Sharp, bright, gray, green, yellow/red, sensitive to light	Big, beautiful, blue, calm, loving
Nose	☐	☐	☐	Uneven shape, deviated septum	Long pointed, red nose tip	Short rounded, button nose
Lips	☐	☐	☐	Dry, cracked, black/brown tinge	Red, inflamed, yellowish	Smooth, oily, pale, whitish
Teeth	☐	☐	☐	Stick out, big, roomy, thin gums	Medium, soft, tender gums	Healthy, white, strong gums
Skin	☐	☐	☐	Thin, dry, cold, rough, dark	Smooth, oily, warm, rosy	Thick, oily, cool, white, pale
Hair	☐	☐	☐	Dry, brown, black, knotted, brittle, scarce	Straight, oily, blond, gray, red, bald	Thick, curly, oily, wavy, luxuriant
Nails	☐	☐	☐	Dry, rough, brittle, break easily	Sharp, flexible, pink, lustrous	Thick, oily, smooth, polished
Neck	☐	☐	☐	Thin, tall	Medium	Big, folded
Chest	☐	☐	☐	Flat, sunken	Moderate	Expanded, round
Belly	☐	☐	☐	Thin, flat, sunken	Moderate	Big, pot-bellied
Belly-button	☐	☐	☐	Small, irregular, herniated	Oval, superficial	Big, deep, round, stretched
Hips	☐	☐	☐	Slender, thin	Moderate	Heavy, big
Joints	☐	☐	☐	Cold, cracking	Moderate	Large, lubricated
Body weight	☐	☐	☐	Low	Medium	Overweight
Appetite	☐	☐	☐	Irregular, scanty	Strong, unbearable	Slow but steady
Digestion	☐	☐	☐	Irregular, forms gas	Quick, causes burning	Prolonged, forms mucous
Taste	☐	☐	☐	Sweet, sour, salty	Sweet, bitter, astringent	Bitter, pungent, astringent
Thirst	☐	☐	☐	Changeable	Surplus	Sparse
Elimination	☐	☐	☐	Constipation	Loose	Thick, oily, sluggish
Physical Activity	☐	☐	☐	Hyperactive	Moderate	Slow
Mental Activity	☐	☐	☐	Hyperactive	Moderate	Dull, slow
Emotions	☐	☐	☐	Anxiety, fear, uncertainty	Anger, hate, jealousy	Calm, greedy, attachment
Faith	☐	☐	☐	Variable	Extremist	Consistent
Intellect	☐	☐	☐	Quick but faulty response	Accurate response	Slow, exact
Recollection	☐	☐	☐	Recent good, remote poor	Distinct	Slow and sustained
Dreams	☐	☐	☐	Quick, active, many, fearful	Fiery, war, violence	Lakes, snow, romantic
Sleep	☐	☐	☐	Scanty, broken up, sleeplessness	Little but sound	Deep, prolonged
Speech	☐	☐	☐	Rapid, unclear	Sharp, penetrating	Slow, monotonous
Financial	☐	☐	☐	Poor, spends on trifles	Spends money on luxuries	Rich, good money preserver
Total						

To Fill Out the Constitution Chart

Instructions: To determine your constitution it is best to fill out the chart twice. First, base your choices on <u>what is most consistent over your lifetime</u> (your prakruti); then fill it out a second time responding to <u>how you have been feeling more recently – the past 30–90 days</u> (your vikruti). Sometimes it helps to have a friend ask you the questions and fill in the chart with you, as they may have insight (and impartiality) to offer. Each time, add up the number of marks under vāta, pitta and kapha. This will help you discover your own ratio of doshas in your prakruti and vikruti. Most people have one dosha predominant; a few have two approximately equal; even fewer have all three in equal proportion.

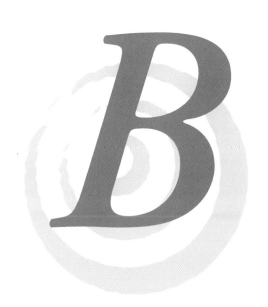

Appendix B
Specialized TCM
Information

Table 52: The Five Elements and Manifestation in Traditional Chinese Medicine

	Wood	Fire	Earth	Metal	Water
Season	Spring	Summer	Late Summer	Autumn	Winter
Direction	East	South	Middle	West	North
Sense	Vision	Speech	Taste	Smell	Hearing
Sense Organ	Eye	Tongue	Mouth	Nose	Ear
Emotion	Anger	Joy	Pensive	Grief	Fear
Color	Green	Red	Yellow	White	Black
Taste	Sour	Bitter	Sweet	Pungent	Salty
Sound	Shouting	Laughing	Singing	Crying	Lamenting
Odor	Rancid	Burnt	Fragrant	Rotten	Putrid
Development	Birth	Growth	Transformation	Manifestation	Death
Direction of Movement	Upwards	Peripherally	Balance	Downwards	Center
Climate	Wind	Heat	Damp	Dry	Cold
Substance	Blood	Spirit	Fluids	Qi	Essence
Tissues	Tendons	Vessels	Muscle	Skin/hair	Bones
Virtue	Kindness	Humility	Faithfulness	Fairness	Wisdom
Manifestation	Nails	Complexion	Lips	Body hair	Head hair
Secretion	Tears	Sweat	Saliva	Mucus	Urine
Yin Organ	Liver	Heart	Spleen	Lung	Kidney
Yang Organ	Gall bladder	Small intestine	Stomach	Large intestine	Bladder

Huatuojiaji Extra Points

• •

Huatuojiaji are the extra points located 0.5 to 1 cun lateral to the depression below the spinous process at the level of the cervical, thoracic, and lumbar vertebrae. Some authors classically refer to only the thoracic and lumbar points, excluding those in the cervical region. For this discussion, all forty-eight points will be considered. These points are attributed to Hua Tuo, a famous physician from the Han dynasty, who routinely used them in his clinical practice.

Each of these extra points treats pain and stiffness locally as well as herpes zoster at the level of the affected segmental nerve. Needling these points affects the spinal nerves and sympathetic ganglion at that vertebral level. These points also have a profound influence on calming the sympathetic and parasympathetic nervous systems. There are specific indications for the Huatuojiaji points depending on the vertebral level at which they are located. For example, many at the level of the thoracic and lumbar vertebrae influence the twelve principal organs that are the focus of the Chinese medical system. These indications are summarized below:

Vertebral Level	Region Affected
C1 to C4	Head
C4 to C7	Upper limbs
C1 to C7	Neck
C3 to T9	Chest wall, thoracic cavity
T1 to T4	Lungs and upper limbs
T4 to T7	Heart
T7 to T10	Liver and gallbladder
T10 to T12	Spleen and stomach
T5 to L5	Organs in the abdominal cavity
T11 to L5	Lumbar and sacral regions
L1 to L2	Kidneys
L2 to L5	Lower limbs
L3 to L5	Bladder, large and small intestines, uterus, lower limbs
L1 to S4	Pelvic cavity

Table 53: Marmāni that Correspond to Huatuojiaji Points

Vertebra	Marma Point	Region affected
C1	Vidhuram	Spinal cord, spinal nerves
C2	Krikātikā	Spinal cord, spinal nerves
C3	Grīva	Thoracic duct, vocal cord, cerebrospinal meninges
C4	Grīva	Thyrold and parathyroid
C5	Grīva	Thyroid and parathyroid
C6	Grīva	Trachea, intestines, colon

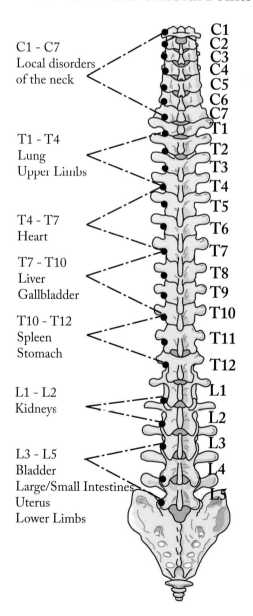

Huatuojiaji Points (M-BW-35)
Hua Tuo's Paravertebral Points

C1 - C7
Local disorders
of the neck

T1 - T4
Lung
Upper Limbs

T4 - T7
Heart

T7 - T10
Liver
Gallbladder

T10 - T12
Spleen
Stomach

L1 - L2
Kidneys

L3 - L5
Bladder
Large/Small Intestines
Uterus
Lower Limbs

The 14 Principal Meridians

Traditional Chinese Medicine has 12 principal meridians that correspond to the 12 organs. Each of these is listed in the table below. In addition, two of the extraordinary vessels—the Du and the Ren meridians—are included to comprise the 14 principal meridians.

Table 54: TCM Abbreviations for the 14 Principal Meridians

Organ	Abbreviation	Yin/yang	Element	Chinese Name
Lung	LU	Yin	Metal	Hand Taiyin
Large Intestine	LI	Yang	Metal	Hand Yangming
Stomach	ST	Yang	Earth	Foot Yangming
Spleen	SP	Yin	Earth	Foot Taiyin
Heart	HT	Yin	Fire	Hand Shaoyin
Small Intestine	SI	Yang	Fire	Hand Taiyang
Bladder	BL	Yang	Water	Foot Taiyang
Kidney	KD	Yin	Water	Foot Shaoyin
Pericardium	PC	Yin	Fire	Hand Jueyin
San Jiao	SJ	Yang	Water	Hand Shaoyang
Gallbladder	GB	Yang	Wood	Foot Shaoyang
Liver	LR	Yin	Wood	Foot Jueyin
Conception Vessel	CV (also known as REN, stands for Ren meridian)			
Governing Vessel	GV (also known as DU, stands for Du meridian)			

Yin Organs	Paired Yang Organs
Heart	Small Intestine
Pericardium	San Jiao
Spleen	Stomach
Lung	Large Intestine
Kidney	Bladder
Liver	Gallbladder

TCM Pulse Diagram.

TCM Pulse

Right Wrist

Left Wrist

	Superficial	Deep
①	Large Intestine	Lung
②	Stomach	Spleen
③	San Jiao	Pericardium

	Superficial	Deep
①	Small Intestine	Heart
②	Gallbladder	Liver
③	Bladder	Kidney

Acupuncture Points, Anterior View

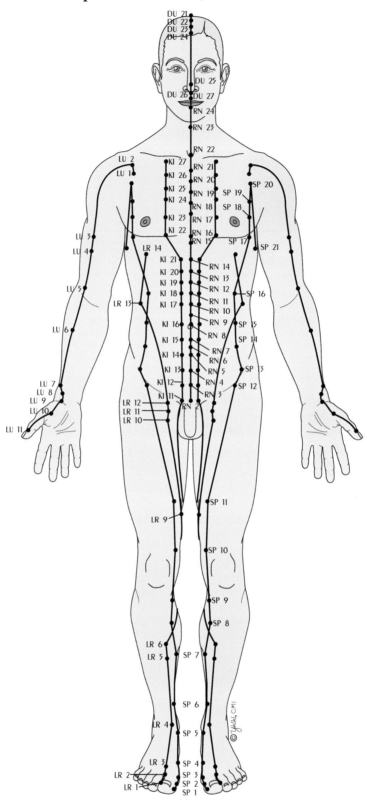

Acupuncture Points, Posterior View

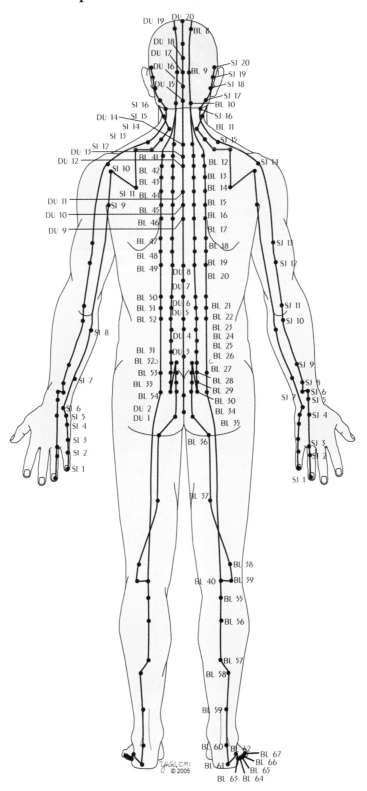

Acupuncture Points, Lateral View

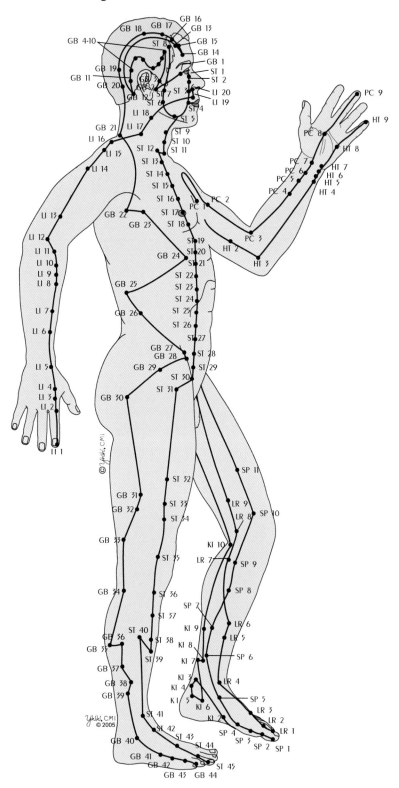

Appendix C
Marma Illustrations

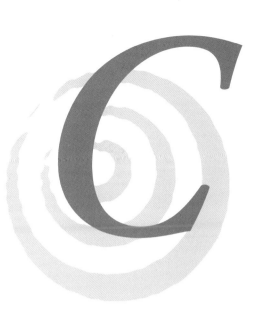

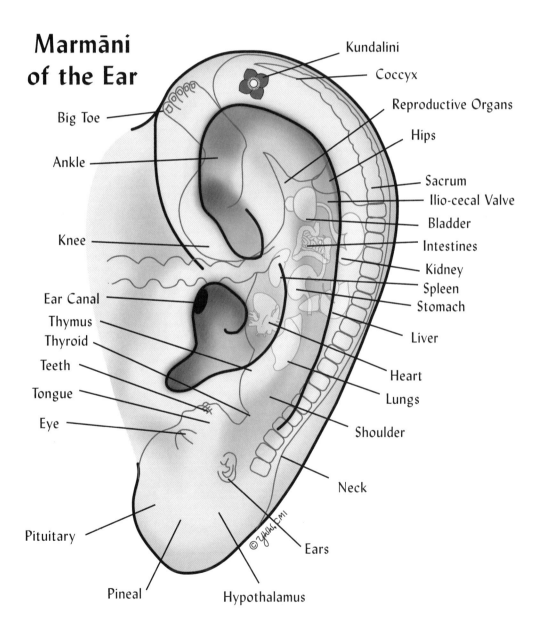

Marmāni of the Ear

Kundalini
Coccyx
Reproductive Organs
Hips
Sacrum
Ilio-cecal Valve
Bladder
Intestines
Kidney
Spleen
Stomach
Liver
Heart
Lungs
Shoulder
Neck
Ears
Hypothalamus
Pineal
Pituitary
Eye
Tongue
Teeth
Thyroid
Thymus
Ear Canal
Knee
Ankle
Big Toe

Marmāni, Anterior View

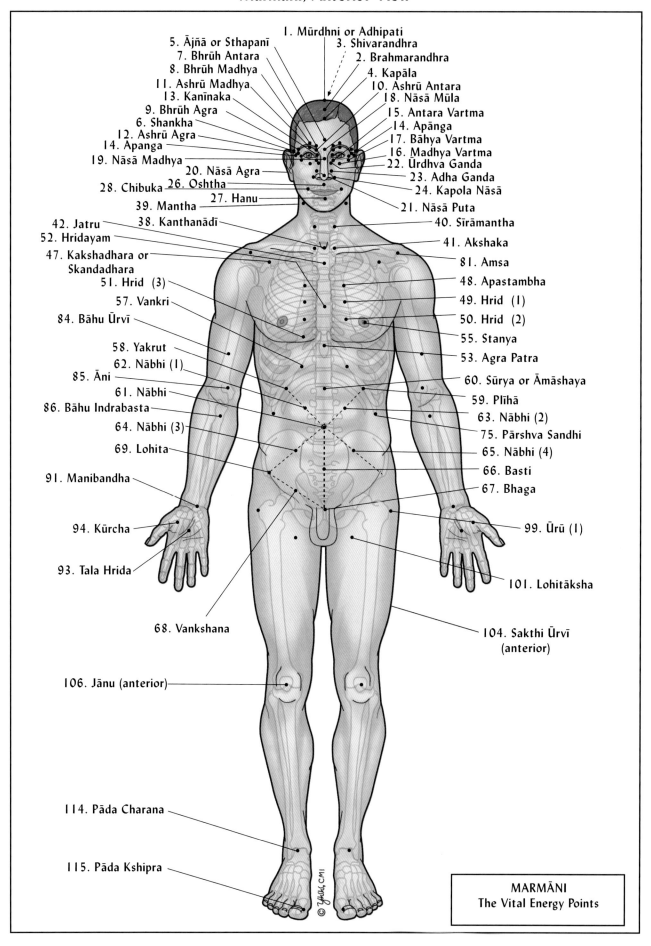

1. Mūrdhni or Adhipati
5. Ājñā or Sthapanī
3. Shivarandhra
7. Bhrūh Antara
2. Brahmarandhra
8. Bhrūh Madhya
4. Kapāla
11. Ashrū Madhya
10. Ashrū Antara
13. Kanīnaka
18. Nāsā Mūla
9. Bhrūh Agra
15. Antara Vartma
6. Shankha
14. Apānga
12. Ashrū Agra
17. Bāhya Vartma
14. Apanga
16. Madhya Vartma
19. Nāsā Madhya
22. Ūrdhva Ganda
20. Nāsā Agra
23. Adha Ganda
28. Chibuka   26. Oshtha
24. Kapola Nāsā
27. Hanu
39. Mantha
21. Nāsā Puta
42. Jatru   38. Kanthanādī
40. Sīrāmantha
52. Hridayam
41. Akshaka
47. Kakshadhara or
    Skandadhara
81. Amsa
51. Hrid (3)
48. Apastambha
57. Vankri
49. Hrid (1)
84. Bāhu Ūrvī
50. Hrid (2)
58. Yakrut
55. Stanya
62. Nābhi (1)
53. Agra Patra
85. Āni
60. Sūrya or Āmāshaya
61. Nābhi
59. Plīhā
86. Bāhu Indrabasta
63. Nābhi (2)
64. Nābhi (3)
75. Pārshva Sandhi
69. Lohita
65. Nābhi (4)
66. Basti
91. Manibandha
67. Bhaga
94. Kūrcha
99. Ūrū (1)
93. Tala Hrida
101. Lohitāksha
68. Vankshana
104. Sakthi Ūrvī
    (anterior)
106. Jānu (anterior)
114. Pāda Charana
115. Pāda Kshipra

MARMĀNI
The Vital Energy Points

270

Marmāni, Posterior View

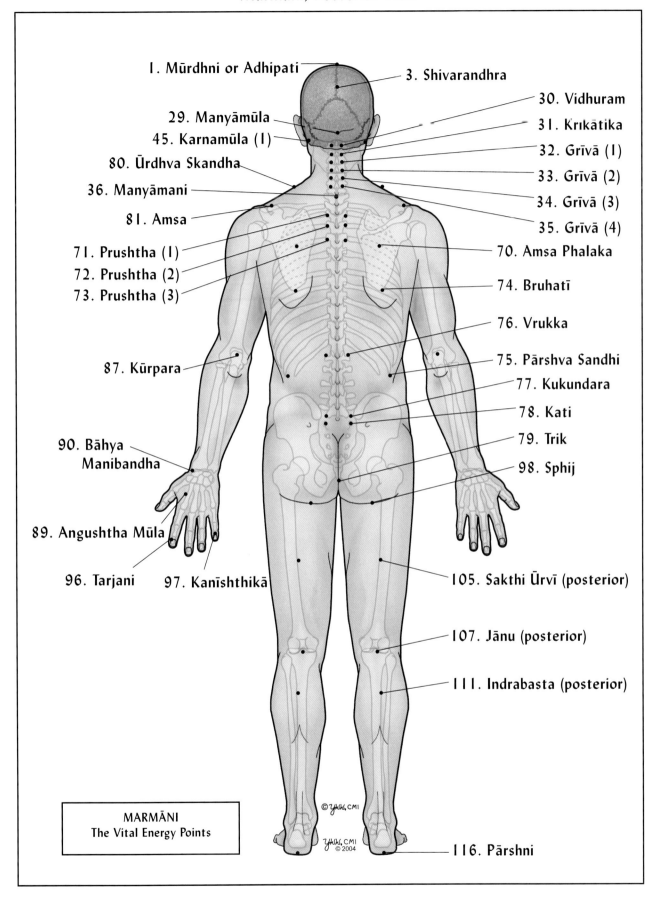

1. Mūrdhni or Adhipati
3. Shivarandhra
29. Manyāmūla
45. Karnamūla (1)
80. Ūrdhva Skandha
36. Manyāmani
81. Amsa
71. Prushtha (1)
72. Prushtha (2)
73. Prushtha (3)
87. Kūrpara
90. Bāhya Manibandha
89. Angushtha Mūla
96. Tarjani
97. Kanīshthikā

30. Vidhuram
31. Krikātika
32. Grīvā (1)
33. Grīvā (2)
34. Grīvā (3)
35. Grīvā (4)
70. Amsa Phalaka
74. Bruhatī
76. Vrukka
75. Pārshva Sandhi
77. Kukundara
78. Kati
79. Trik
98. Sphij
105. Sakthi Ūrvī (posterior)
107. Jānu (posterior)
111. Indrabasta (posterior)
116. Pārshni

© Yhshi CMI
© 2004

MARMĀNI
The Vital Energy Points

271

Marmāni, Lateral View

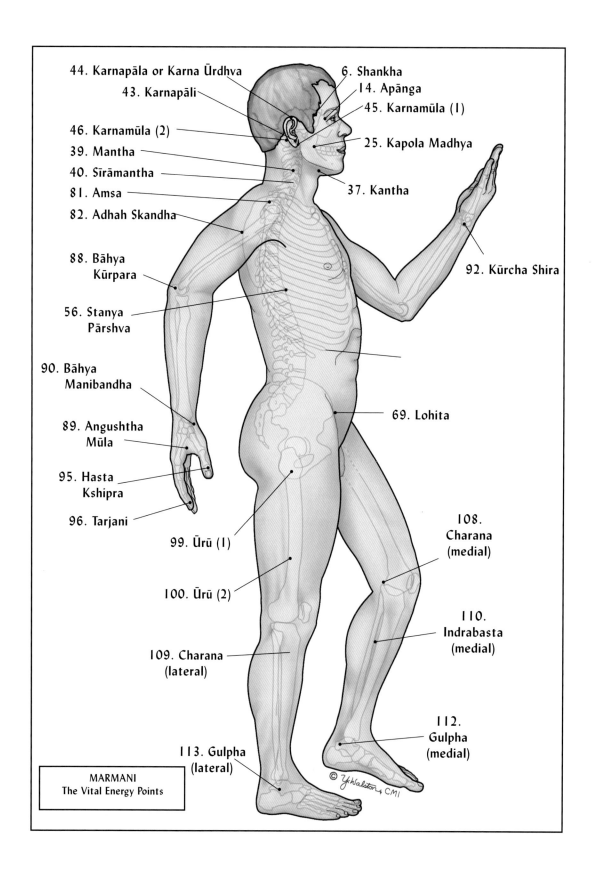

44. Karnapāla or Karna Ūrdhva
43. Karnapāli
46. Karnamūla (2)
39. Mantha
40. Sīrāmantha
81. Amsa
82. Adhah Skandha
88. Bāhya Kūrpara
56. Stanya Pārshva
90. Bāhya Manibandha
89. Angushtha Mūla
95. Hasta Kshipra
96. Tarjani
99. Ūrū (1)
100. Ūrū (2)
109. Charana (lateral)
113. Gulpha (lateral)

6. Shankha
14. Apānga
45. Karnamūla (1)
25. Kapola Madhya
37. Kantha
92. Kūrcha Shira
69. Lohita
108. Charana (medial)
110. Indrabasta (medial)
112. Gulpha (medial)

© Y. Halston, CMI

MARMANI
The Vital Energy Points

272

Marma Points, Lateral View Head and Neck

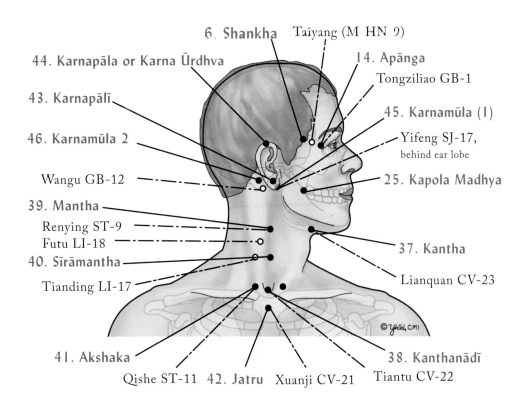

6. Shankha

Taiyang (M HN 9)

44. Karnapāla or Karna Ūrdhva

14. Apānga

Tongziliao GB-1

43. Karnapālī

45. Karnamūla (1)

Yifeng SJ-17, behind ear lobe

46. Karnamūla 2

Wangu GB-12

25. Kapola Madhya

39. Mantha

Renying ST-9

Futu LI-18

37. Kantha

40. Sīrāmantha

Tianding LI-17

Lianquan CV-23

41. Akshaka

38. Kanthanādī

Qishe ST-11   42. Jatru   Xuanji CV-21   Tiantu CV-22

Marma Points, Eye Area

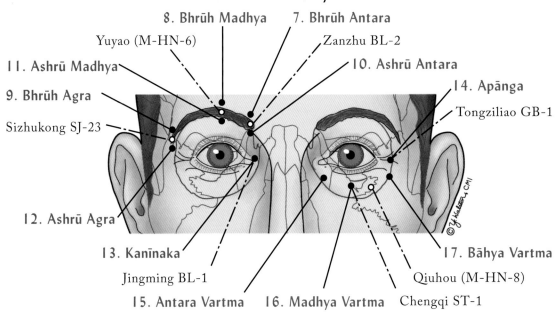

8. Bhrūh Madhya
7. Bhrūh Antara
Yuyao (M-HN-6)
Zanzhu BL-2
11. Ashrū Madhya
10. Ashrū Antara
9. Bhrūh Agra
14. Apānga
Sizhukong SJ-23
Tongziliao GB-1
12. Ashrū Agra
13. Kanīnaka
17. Bāhya Vartma
Jingming BL-1
Qiuhou (M-HN-8)
15. Antara Vartma
16. Madhya Vartma
Chengqi ST-1

Marma Points, Face

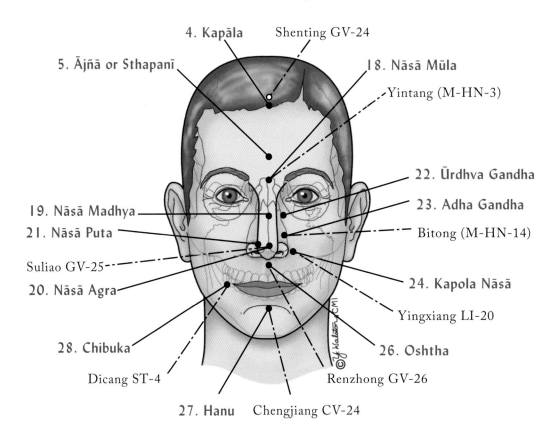

4. Kapāla
Shenting GV-24
5. Ājñā or Sthapanī
18. Nāsā Mūla
Yintang (M-HN-3)
22. Ūrdhva Gandha
19. Nāsā Madhya
23. Adha Gandha
21. Nāsā Puta
Bitong (M-HN-14)
Suliao GV-25
24. Kapola Nāsā
20. Nāsā Agra
Yingxiang LI-20
28. Chibuka
26. Oshtha
Dicang ST-4
Renzhong GV-26
27. Hanu
Chengjiang CV-24

Marma Points, Superior Aspect of Head

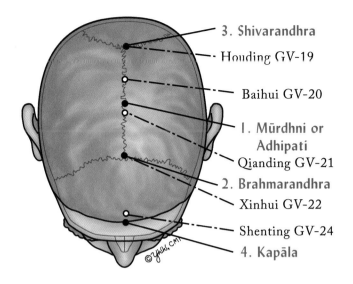

- 3. Shivarandhra
- Houding GV-19
- Baihui GV-20
- 1. Mūrdhni or Adhipati
- Qianding GV-21
- 2. Brahmarandhra
- Xinhui GV-22
- Shenting GV-24
- 4. Kapāla

Marma Points, Posterior View Head and Neck

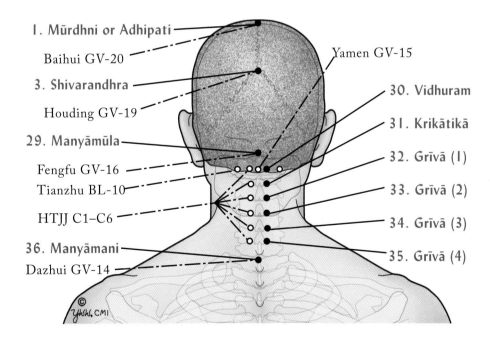

- 1. Mūrdhni or Adhipati
- Baihui GV-20
- 3. Shivarandhra
- Houding GV-19
- 29. Manyāmūla
- Fengfu GV-16
- Tianzhu BL-10
- HTJJ C1–C6
- 36. Manyāmani
- Dazhui GV-14
- Yamen GV-15
- 30. Vidhuram
- 31. Krikātikā
- 32. Grīvā (1)
- 33. Grīvā (2)
- 34. Grīvā (3)
- 35. Grīvā (4)

Marma Points, Chest

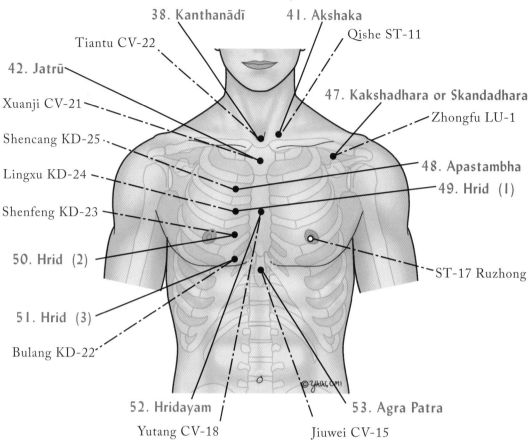

38. Kanthanādī
41. Akshaka
Tiantu CV-22
Qishe ST-11
42. Jatrū
Xuanji CV-21
47. Kakshadhara or Skandadhara
Shencang KD-25
Zhongfu LU-1
Lingxu KD-24
48. Apastambha
Shenfeng KD-23
49. Hrid (1)
50. Hrid (2)
ST-17 Ruzhong
51. Hrid (3)
Bulang KD-22
52. Hridayam
53. Agra Patra
Yutang CV-18
Jiuwei CV-15

Marma Points, Upper and Lower Abdomen

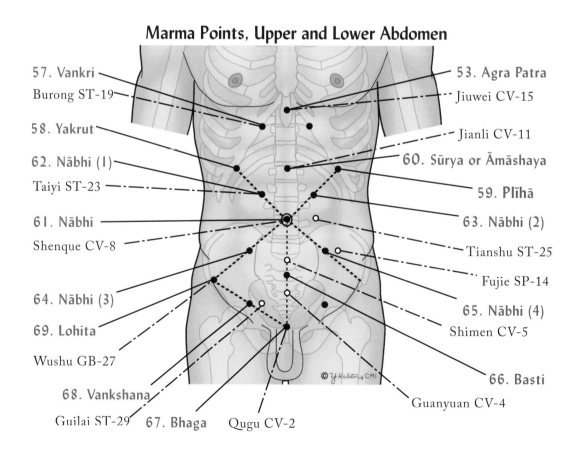

57. Vankri
53. Agra Patra
Burong ST-19
Jiuwei CV-15
58. Yakrut
Jianli CV-11
62. Nābhi (1)
60. Sūrya or Āmāshaya
Taiyi ST-23
59. Plīhā
61. Nābhi
63. Nābhi (2)
Shenque CV-8
Tianshu ST-25
Fujie SP-14
64. Nābhi (3)
65. Nābhi (4)
69. Lohita
Shimen CV-5
Wushu GB-27
66. Basti
68. Vankshana
Guanyuan CV-4
Guilai ST-29
67. Bhaga
Qugu CV-2

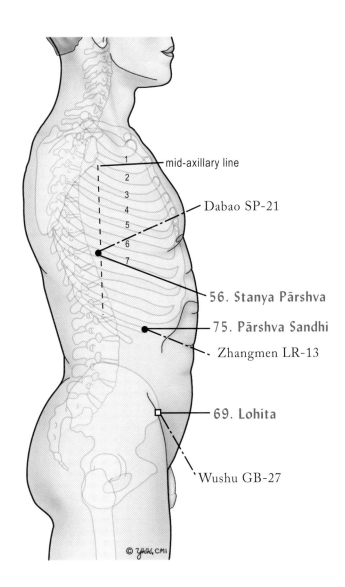

mid-axillary line

Dabao SP-21

56. Stanya Pārshva

75. Pārshva Sandhi

Zhangmen LR-13

69. Lohita

Wushu GB-27

© Yhthi, CMI

Marma Points, Back

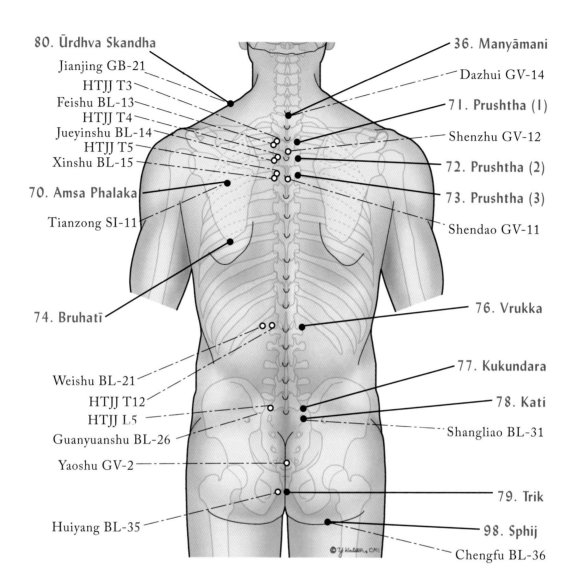

80. Ūrdhva Skandha

Jianjing GB-21
HTJJ T3
Feishu BL-13
HTJJ T4
Jueyinshu BL-14
HTJJ T5
Xinshu BL-15

70. Amsa Phalaka

Tianzong SI-11

74. Bruhatī

Weishu BL-21
HTJJ T12
HTJJ L5
Guanyuanshu BL-26
Yaoshu GV-2
Huiyang BL-35

36. Manyāmani

Dazhui GV-14

71. Prushtha (1)

Shenzhu GV-12

72. Prushtha (2)

73. Prushtha (3)

Shendao GV-11

76. Vrukka

77. Kukundara

78. Kati

Shangliao BL-31

79. Trik

98. Sphij

Chengfu BL-36

Marma Points, Upper Extremities

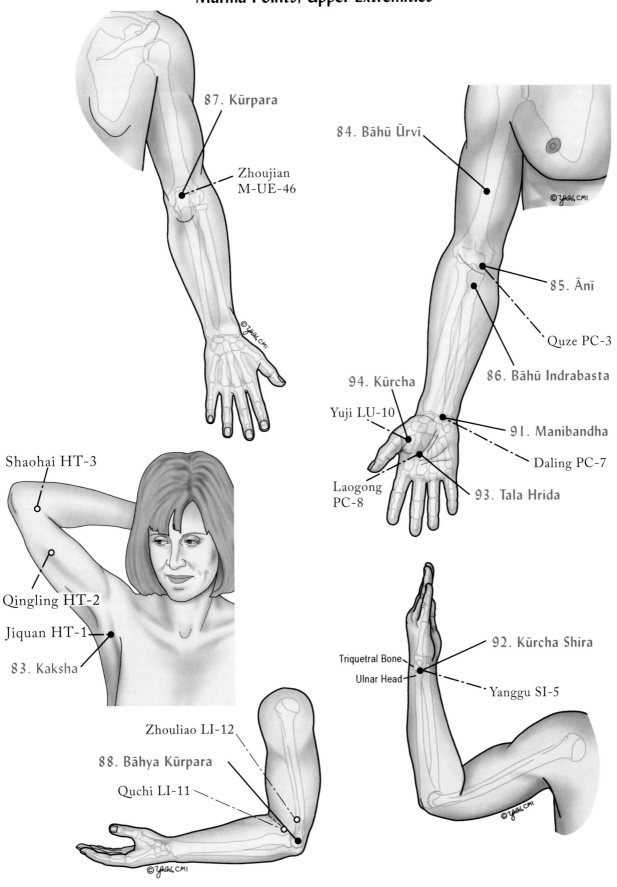

87. Kūrpara

Zhoujian M-UE-46

84. Bāhū Ūrvī

85. Ānī

Quze PC-3

86. Bāhū Indrabasta

94. Kūrcha

Yuji LU-10

91. Manibandha

Daling PC-7

Laogong PC-8

93. Tala Hrida

Shaohai HT-3

Qingling HT-2

Jiquan HT-1

83. Kaksha

Zhouliao LI-12

88. Bāhya Kūrpara

Quchi LI-11

92. Kūrcha Shira

Triquetral Bone

Ulnar Head

Yanggu SI-5

Marma Points, Upper Shoulder and Lateral Arm and Dorsal Hand

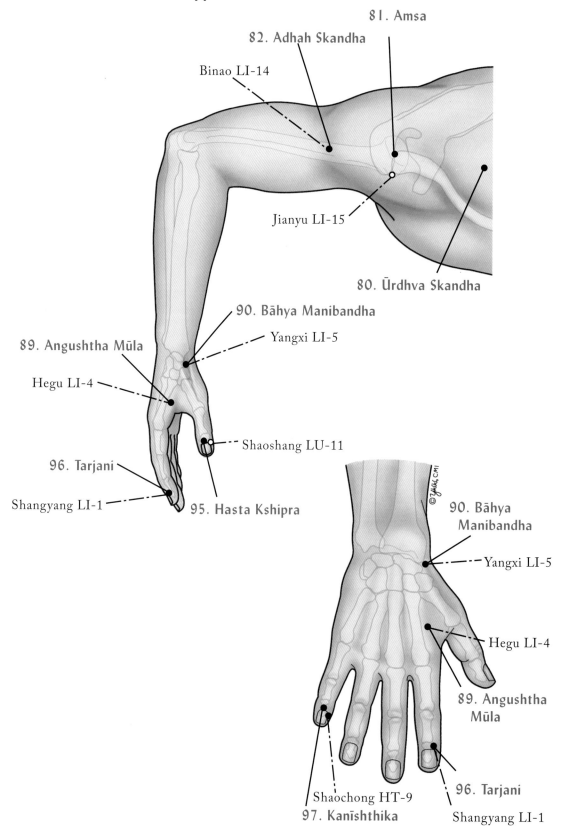

81. Amsa

82. Adhah Skandha

Binao LI-14

Jianyu LI-15

80. Ūrdhva Skandha

90. Bāhya Manibandha

Yangxi LI-5

89. Angushtha Mūla

Hegu LI-4

Shaoshang LU-11

96. Tarjani

Shangyang LI-1

95. Hasta Kshipra

90. Bāhya Manibandha

Yangxi LI-5

Hegu LI-4

89. Angushtha Mūla

96. Tarjani

Shaochong HT-9

97. Kanīshthika

Shangyang LI-1

Marma Points, Lower Extremities

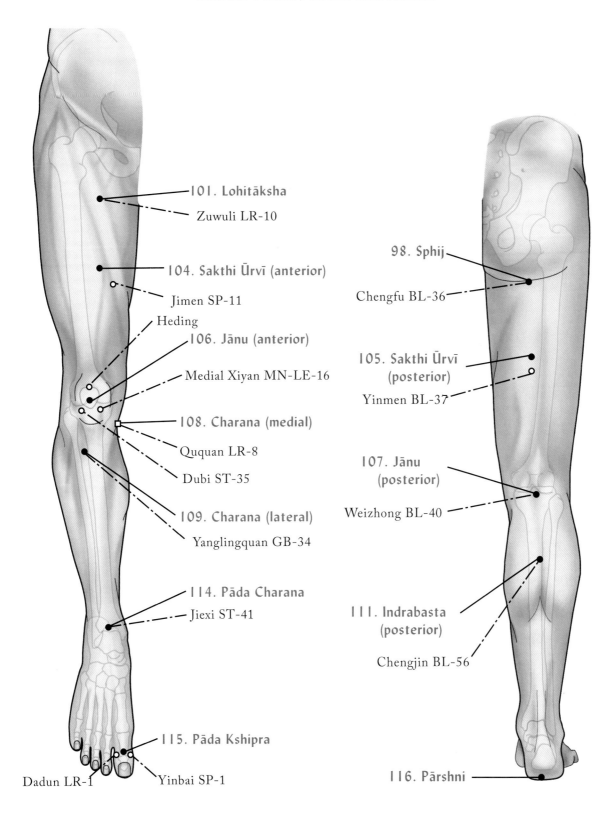

101. Lohitāksha
Zuwuli LR-10

104. Sakthi Ūrvī (anterior)
Jimen SP-11

Heding

106. Jānu (anterior)

Medial Xiyan MN-LE-16

108. Charana (medial)

Ququan LR-8

Dubi ST-35

109. Charana (lateral)
Yanglingquan GB-34

114. Pāda Charana
Jiexi ST-41

115. Pāda Kshipra

Dadun LR-1   Yinbai SP-1

98. Sphij
Chengfu BL-36

105. Sakthi Ūrvī
(posterior)
Yinmen BL-37

107. Jānu
(posterior)
Weizhong BL-40

111. Indrabasta
(posterior)
Chengjin BL-56

116. Pārshni

281

Lower Extremities (Cont'd.)

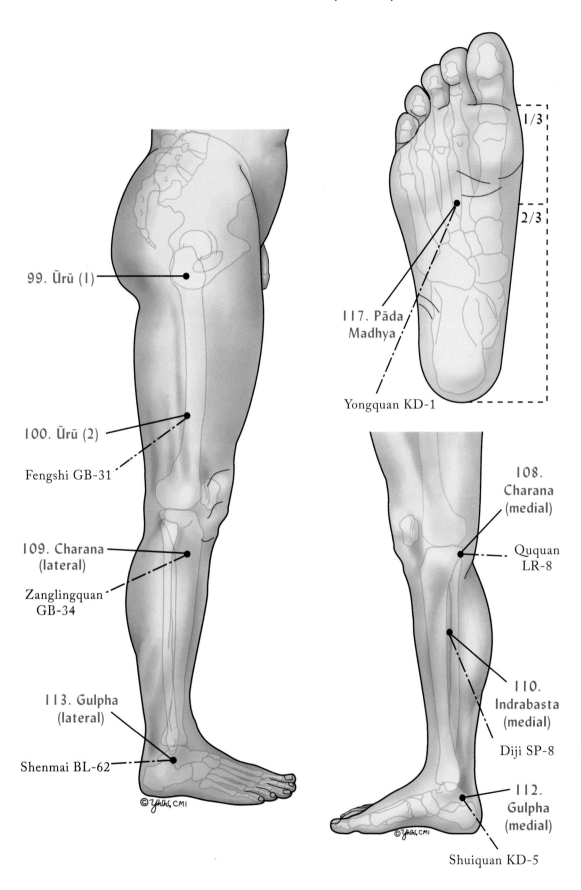

99. Ūrū (1)

100. Ūrū (2)

Fengshi GB-31

109. Charana (lateral)

Zanglingquan GB-34

113. Gulpha (lateral)

Shenmai BL-62

117. Pāda Madhya

Yongquan KD-1

1/3

2/3

108. Charana (medial)

Ququan LR-8

110. Indrabasta (medial)

Diji SP-8

112. Gulpha (medial)

Shuiquan KD-5

© Yhthf, CMI

Marma Points, Breasts

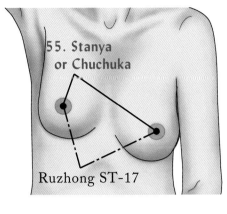

55. Stanya or Chuchuka

Ruzhong ST-17

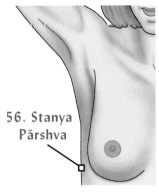

56. Stanya Pārshva

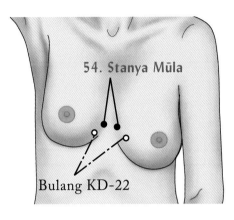

54. Stanya Mūla

Bulang KD-22

Marma Points, Genitals

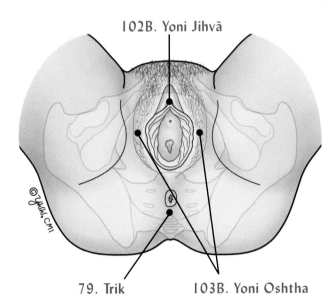

102B. Yoni Jihvā

79. Trik

103B. Yoni Oshtha

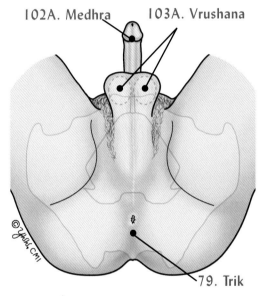

102A. Medhra

103A. Vrushana

79. Trik

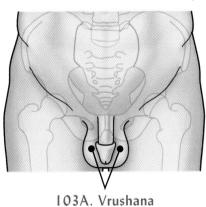

103A. Vrushana

Marma Massage Series

If you are not very experienced with Ayurvedic marma therapy, before attempting the following procedure please review chapter 8, especially "Guidelines for Touch and Pressure" on page 75 that offers specific information about massaging marmāni.

The instructions here refer to the drawings on these pages. The numbers are for use with these massage drawings only; they are different from the numbering system for the marma points used throughout the book. To look up details on a particular marma point, refer to the beginning pages of each chapter and the tables that reference all the marma points and their page numbers.

Apply a few drops of essential oil to the tips of the fingers. Start with gentle pressure on the marma points, and gradually increase according to the capacity of the individual. If you use too much pressure, the person will show facial expressions, such as wrinkling of the face. Pressure on all marmāni should be held for approximately one to two minutes. If you feel that stronger pressure is needed, you can apply it when the patient exhales.

Marma Head and Facial Massage

A. Ask the patient to lie in supine position and be at the head end of the patient. Begin with gentle pressure on Mūrdhni marma **(1)** with both thumbs. Then move up towards Brahmarandhra **(2)**, back to Mūrdhni and then to Shivarandhra **(3)**, applying pressure on each point for one minute.

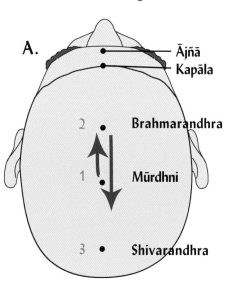

B. Next, massage Kapāla marma **(4)** on the forehead with both thumbs. Massage the entire midline of the scalp from Kapāla all the way to Shivarandhra **(3)**. Give emphasis to Kapāla **(4)** briefly again and then move down the forehead to Ājñā marma **(5)** and apply pressure.

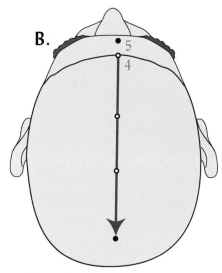

C. Repeat this motion three times, then move from Ājñā **(5)** to Bhrūh Antara **(6)** above the eyebrows, then Bhrūh Madhya **(7)**, all the way across to Bhrūh Agra **(8)**. Repeat this gentle, relaxing motion three times. Sweep the fingers from Ājñā **(5)** across the eyebrows until the thumbs land in a natural depression at Shankha marma **(9)**. Pressure should be held longer here, with a gentle counterclockwise rotation done to pacify pitta individuals.

Note: Here and in other instances, some people may not feel comfortable using the thumb; in that case, they may use the index or middle finger.

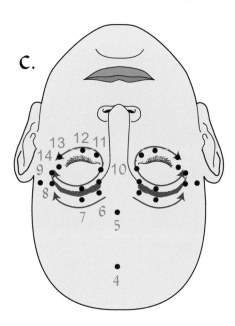

Next, apply light pressure on Kanīnaka **(10)** directed towards the inner side of the eyeball, then gradually move the fingers along the eye orbit. Then pinch the eyebrows at the medial end and release, repeating this technique towards the lateral end of the eyebrows to stimulate all Bhrūhu **(6, 7, 8)** and Ashrū marmāni **(inner 6, 7, 8)** simultaneously. This technique can be repeated several times. Use caution not to pull the eyelid or place pressure on the eyeball.

Gently move downwards from Kanīnaka **(10)** to the Vartma marmāni **(11, 12, 13)**, applying very light pressure to avoid discomfort. Start at the medial point and move laterally from the Vartma marmāni to Apānga **(14)** and then to Shankha **(9)**. With both middle fingers stimulating Shankha **(9)**, place the thumbs on Ājñā marma **(5)**, followed by Kapāla **(4)**. Pressure should be held for a slightly longer duration if the patient has a vāta constitution.

D. From Ājñā **(5)** move downwards to Nāsā Mūla **(15)**, Nāsā Madhya, Nāsā Agra **(16)** and Nāsā Puta, applying extremely light pressure. Then move to Kapola Nāsā **(17)**, followed by pressure on Ganda marmāni. Next, move the thumbs from Ganda marmāni downwards, until they fall in the natural groove at Kapola Madhya, followed by Chibuka **(18)**. Stimulate Oshtha with the thumb and then circle the fingers around the mouth, giving emphasis to Chibuka again.

Move to Hanu marma **(19)** at the chin and apply firm deep pressure with both thumbs. Grasp the chin between the thumbs and the index fingers and move from Hanu along the length of the mandible. Repeat this motion three times. After the last repetition, gently move upwards towards Shankha and hold. From Shankha return to Ājñā and hold the pressure for one minute. From Ājñā, let both thumbs slide upwards and hold Mūrdhni. Then move the fingers from the midline to the side of the head to complete the facial massage.

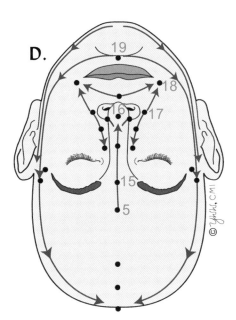

Marma Massage for Back of the Head and Neck

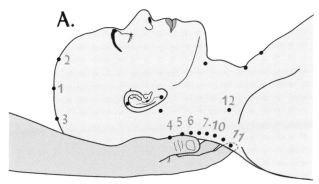

A. Let the patient lie in the supine position with the practitioner at the head. Begin by applying gentle pressure on Mūrdhni marma **(1)** at the crown with both thumbs. Then move up to Brahmarandhra **(2)**, back to Mūrdhni, and then Shivarandhra **(3)**, applying pressure on each marma for one minute. From here, apply pressure down the midline until Manyāmūla **(4)** at the base of the occiput. Move the fingers to Vidhuram **(5)** on each side of C1, then to Krikātikā **(6)** at C2, followed by Grīvā marmāni **(7–10)** from C3 to C6. Steady pressure should be held at each pair for roughly one minute, or longer if there is tenderness. Return to Manyāmūla and repeat this sequence a second time, until reaching Manyāmani **(11)** at C7, applying clockwise or counterclockwise pressure according to need. Generally, clockwise pressure increases pitta and relieves kapha and vāta, while counterclockwise pressure increases vāta and kapha and relieves or pacifies pitta. If the pain is pitta type, massage with a counterclockwise motion, and if it is vāta and kapha type, the motion should be clockwise. After massaging the back of the neck, stimulate Ūrdhva Skandha.

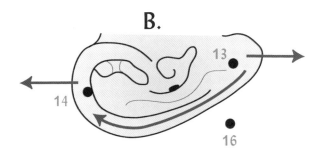

B and C. To massage the ears, begin at Karnapālī **(13)**. Squeeze the ear lobes between the thumbs and index fingers and gently pull them downwards. Then slowly massage along the ear lobes towards Karnapāla **(14)** at the apex and pull upwards. This sequence can be repeated several times. From the apex, move to Karnamūla marmāni, which are posterior to the ear. From Karnamūla 1 **(15)** move the fingers along the posterior border of the sternocleidomastoid muscle, activating

Mantha **(16)**, then Sīrāmantha **(17)** and then Akshaka **(18)**. Repeat this sequence three times.

When the patient is in the supine position, the marmāni on the front of the neck can be gently stimulated. This is an extremely sensitive area and should be handled delicately. Lightly touch Kantha **(20)**, followed by Kanthanādī **(21)** and then Jatrū marma **(22)**.

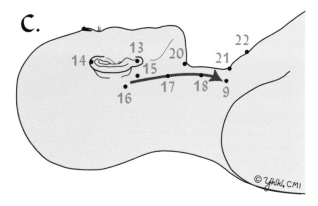

Marma Massage for the Trunk

A and B. Ask the patient to lie in supine position (face up) and stand at the head. Begin by stimulating Ūrdhva Skandha marma **(1)**. Then apply gentle pressure on Kakshadhara marma **(2)** with the thumbs. Both of these marmāni are often tender and require deeper stimulation if the patient can tolerate it.

Start with:
Ūrdhva Skandha

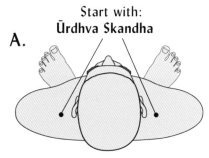

Move to the patient's side and apply pressure to Apastambha **(3)**, followed by each of the Hrid marmāni **(4–6)** for one minute. Slide from Hrid to Hridayam marma **(7)**, followed by Agra Patra **(8)**, Stanya Mūla **(9)** and then Vankri **(10)**. Move along the outer margin of the breast to Stanya Pārshva **(11)** at the lateral aspect of the breast. Repeat this sequence on the other side of the patient.

C. Next, from Agra Patra **(8)** slide along the costal margin over Vankri **(10)** towards Yakrut **(12)** and Plīhā **(13)** and apply pressure to both simultaneously. Then slide towards the midline and Sūrya marma **(14)**. From Sūrya, move outwards to Nābhi 1 and 2 **(15, 16)**, followed by Nābhi 3 and 4 **(17, 18)**. In general, points over the descending colon should be massaged first, followed by those over the ascending colon.

Finally, stimulate Basti **(19)**, Lohita **(20)** and Vankshana **(21)** to complete the abdominal massage.

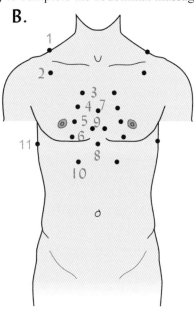

Repeat this sequence on the
left side of the patient.
(Can do both sides at the same time)

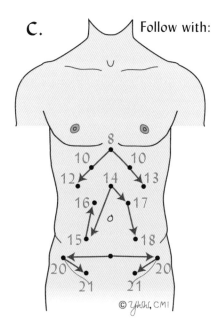

Marma Massage for the Back

A. Ask the patient to lie in a prone position (face down) and stand at the head end. This massage naturally follows massaging the back of the neck. Because the muscles of the back are strong and relatively stiff, it requires deeper pressure with the thumbs.

Begin by stimulating Ūrdhva Skandha **(1)** and then slide to Amsa Phalaka **(2)**. Repeat this three times. Move medially towards Manyāmani **(3)** at C7, and then slide the thumbs down along both sides of the spine all the way to the lumbar area. Repeat this motion three times.

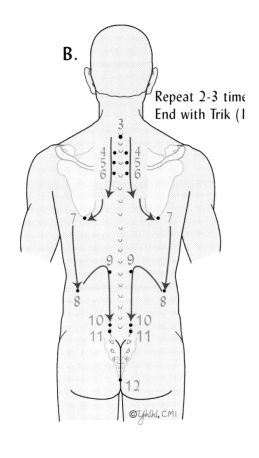

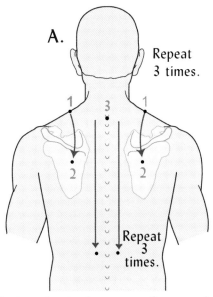

B. Next, apply steady pressure for one minute each from Manyāmani **(3)** to Prushtha marmāni **(4, 5, 6)** located at T3, T4 and T5. Slide the fingers along the medial border of the scapula until they reach Bruhatī marma **(7)**. Continue from Bruhatī to Pārshva Sandhi **(8)**, and from there move towards the spine and stimulate Vrukka **(9)**, then Kukundara **(10)** and Kati **(11)**. Repeat this motion two or three times. End the massage by giving added emphasis to Trik marma **(12)**.

Marma Massage for the Arms and Hands

Have the patient lie in supine position (face up) with the practitioner at the head. Begin by stimulating Ūrdhva Skandha marma (1). Then apply gentle pressure on Kakshadhara marma (2) with the thumbs. Both of these marmāni are often tender and require deep stimulation if the patient can tolerate it. Then move to the patient's left side and pull the left arm slightly away from the body. Stimulate Kaksha marma (3) at the armpit with the thumb and hold for one minute. Then move to Amsa marma (4). Massage the deltoid muscle with a "squeezing" motion, giving special emphasis to Adhah Skandha (5), and then apply either a clockwise or a counterclockwise rotation. Clockwise pressure increases pitta and relieves kapha and vata, while counterclockwise pressure increases vata and kapha and relieves or pacifies pitta. So if the pain or discomfort is pitta type, massage with a counterclockwise motion, and if it is vata and kapha type, the motion should be clockwise.

With the elbow in a flexed position, slide downwards to Bāhu Ūrvī (6), followed by Ānī (7) and then Bāhū Indrabasta (8). Slide the thumb gently along the midline of the forearm from Ānī (7) to Manibandha (9) at the wrist crease. Use gentle circular rotation to relax the patient. Massage Kūrcha Shira (10), followed by Bāhya Manibandha (11). Continue towards Angushtha Mūla (12) and hold for one minute. Turn the hand over and apply pressure to Kūrcha (13). Next, firmly hold Tala Hrida (14) at the center of the palm. Massage each finger from the base to the tip, starting with the little finger. Give special emphasis to Kanīshthika (15), Tarjani (16) and Hasta Kshipra (17).

Repeat on the opposite side.

While standing again at the head, end the massage with both thumbs applying deep pressure on Kakshadhara marma (2).

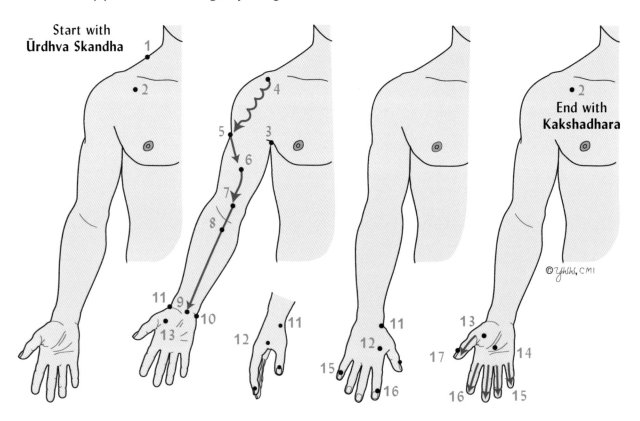

Marma Massage for the Legs And Feet

It's possible to perform the Prone Position series on both legs simultaneously but you can do one leg at a time as well. The Supine Position series should be done on one leg at a time.

Prone Position. Ask the patient to lie in prone position to massage the posterior aspect of the legs. These large muscles require greater pressure to be exerted with the thumbs. Begin at Sphij marma **(1)** and hold for one minute. Slide down the midline from Sphij to Posterior Sakthi Ūrvī **(2)**, and then Posterior Jānu **(3)**. Repeat this sequence three times. Slide down the midline again from Posterior Jānu **(3)** to Posterior Indrabasta **(4)** and hold. Repeat this sequence two or three times as well.

From Posterior Jānu **(3)**, move to Medial Charana **(5)** and slide down the medial aspect of the calf with a "squeezing" motion. Next, move from Posterior Jānu (3) to Lateral Charana **(6)** and repeat the "squeezing" technique down the lateral aspect of the calf. Massage Lateral and Medial Gulpha **(7, 8)** together at the ankle. Apply pressure on Pārshni **(9)**, followed by Pāda Madhya **(10)**.

Supine Position. Next, ask the patient to lie in supine position so the anterior aspect of the legs can be massaged. Begin by stimulating Ūrū 1 **(11)** and sliding the thumb towards Lohitāksha **(12)**. Next apply pressure on Ūrū 2 **(13)**, followed by Anterior Sakthi Ūrvī **(14)**. Slide down the midline from Lohitāksha **(12)**, to Anterior Sakthi Ūrvī **(14)**, and then Anterior Jānu **(15)**. Repeat this procedure three times.

From Lateral Charana **(16)**, apply the squeezing technique down the lateral aspect of the calf. Repeat the squeezing technique down the medial aspect of the calf. Give emphasis to Medial Indrabasta followed by Medial Charana **(5)**. Continue towards the ankles and massage both Gulpha marmāni **(7, 8)** simultaneously, followed by Pāda Charana **(18)** and Pāda Kshipra **(19)**.

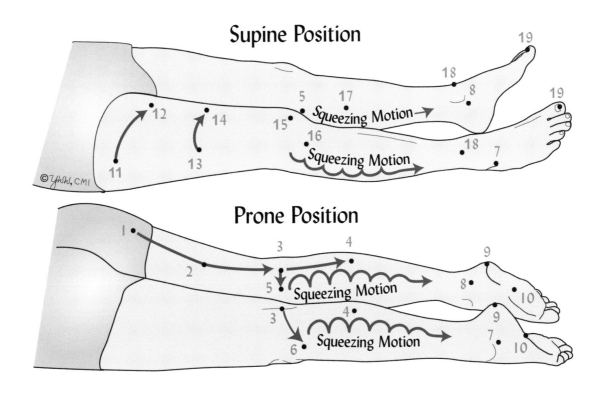

289

Appendix D
Marmāni and Acupoints: Correspondences, Locations and Lists

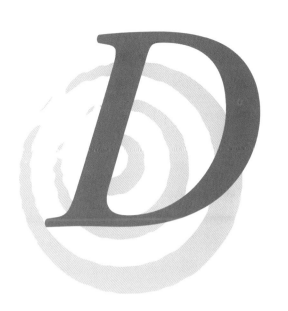

Table 55: Marma Point List, Alphabetical

Marma Point Names	Sanskrit (Devanagari)	Full Transliteration	Page
Āni	आणि	āṇi	175
Adha Gaṇḍa[a]	अधो गण्ड	adho gaṇḍa	104
Adhah Skandha	अधः स्कन्ध	adhaḥ skandha	172
Agra Patra	अग्र पत्र	agra patra	141
Ājñā or Sthapanī	आज्ञा or स्थपनी	ājñā or sthapanī	89
Akshaka	अक्षक	akṣaka	127
Amsa	अंस	aṃsa	171
Amsa Phalaka	अंस फलक	aṃsa phalaka	160
Angushtha Mūla	अंगुष्ठ मूल	aṅguṣṭa mūla	180
Antara Vartma	अन्तर वर्त्म	antara vartma	97
Apānga	अपांग	apāṅga	96
Apastambha	अपस्तम्भ	apastambha	137
Ashrū	अश्रू	aśrū (3)	94
Bāhya Kūrpara	बाह्य कूर्पर	bāhya kūrpara	179
Bāhya Manibandha	बाह्य मणिबन्ध	bāhya maṇibandha	181
Bāhya Vartma	बाह्य वर्त्म	bāhya vartma	97
Bāhu Indrabasta[b]	बाहु इन्द्रवस्त	bāhu indravasta	176
Bāhu Ūrvī	बाहु ऊर्वी	bāhu ūrvī	174
Basti	बस्ति	basti	152
Bhaga	भग	bhaga	153
Bruhatī	बृहती	bruhatī	162
Brahmarandhra	ब्रह्मरन्ध्र	brahmarandhra	84

Table 55: Marma Point List, Alphabetical

Marma Point Names	Sanskrit (Devanagari)	Full Transliteration	Page
Bhrūh Agra	भ्रूः अग्र	bhrūḥ agra	92
Bhrūh Antara	भ्रूः अन्तर	bhrūḥ antara	92
Bhrūh Madhya	भ्रूः मध्य	bhrūḥ madhya	92
Charana (lateral)	चरण	caraṇa	200
Charana (medial)	चरण	caraṇa	200
Chibuka	चिबुक	cibuka	110
Grīvā	ग्रीवा	grīva	121
Gulpha (lateral)	गुल्फ	gulpha	203
Gulpha (medial)	गुल्फ	gulpha	203
Hanu	हनु	hanu	108
Hasta Kshipra	हस्त क्षिप्र	hasta kṣipra	186
Hridayam	हृदयम्	hṛdayam	140
Hrid	हृद्	hṛd	140
Indrabasta (medial)	इन्द्रबस्त	indravasta	202
Indrabasta (posterior)	इन्द्रबस्त	indravasta	202
Jānu (anterior)	जानु	jānu	199
Jānu (posterior)	जानु	jānu	199
Jatru	जत्रू	jatrū	128
Kaksha	कक्ष	kakṣa	173
Kakshadhara or Skandhadhara	कक्षधर or स्कन्दधर	kakṣadhara or skandhadara	136
Kanīnaka	कनध्नक	kanīnaka	95
Kanishthaka	कनिष्टक	kaniṣṭhaka	188
Kantha	कण्ठ	kaṇṭha	123
Kanthanādī	कण्ठनाडी	kaṇṭhanāḍī	124
Kapāla	कपाल	kapāla	88
Kapola Madhya	कपोलमध्य	kapolamadhya	106
Kapola Nāsā	कपोल नासा	kapola nāsā	105
Karnamūla	कर्णमूल	karṇamūla	132
Karnapāla or Karna Ūrdhva	कर्णपाल or कर्णू ऊर्ध्व	karṇapāla or karṇa ūrdhva	131
Karnapāli	कर्णपालि	karṇapāli	130
Kati	कटि	kaṭi	165
Kurcha	कूर्च	kūrca	185

Table 55: Marma Point List, Alphabetical

Marma Point Names	Sanskrit (Devanagari)	Full Transliteration	Page
Kurcha Shira	कूर्चशिर	kūrchashira	183
Krikāṭikā	कृकाटिक	krikāṭika	120
Kukundara	कुकुन्दर	kukundara	164
Kūrpara	कूर्पर	kūrpara	178
Lohita	लोहित	lohita	155
Lohitākṣa	लोहिताक्ष	lohitākṣa	195
Madhya Vartma	मध्य वर्त्म	madhya vartma	97
Manibandha	मणिबन्ध	maṇibandha	182
Mantha	मन्थ	mantha	125
Manyāmani	मन्यामणि	manyāmani	122
Manyāmūla	मन्यामूल	manyāmūla	116
Medhra	मेढ्र	meḍhra	196
Mūrdhni or Adhipati	मूर्ध्नि or अधिपति	mūrdhni or adhipati	82
Nābhi	नाभि	nābhi (5)	150
Nāsā Agra	नासा अग्र	nāsā agra	101
Nāsā Madhya	नासा मध्य	nāsā madhya	100
Nāsā Mūla	नासा मूल	nāsā mūla	99
Nāsā Puṭa	नासा पुट	nāsā puṭa	102
Oshtha	ओष्ठ	oṣṭha	107
Pāda Madhya	पाद मध्य	pāda madhya	207
Pāda Charana	पाद चरण	pāda caraṇa	204
Pāda Kshipra	पाद क्षिप्र	pāda kṣipra	205
Pārshni	पार्ष्णि	pārshni	206
Pārshva Sandhi	पार्श्व सन्धि	pārśva sandhi	145
Plīhā[c]	प्लीहा	plīhan	148
Prushtha	पृष्ठ	pṛṣṭha (3)	161
Sakthi Ūrvī (anterior)	सक्थि ऊर्वी	sakthi ūrvī (anterior)	198
Sakthi Ūrvī (posterior)	सक्थि ऊर्वी	sakthi ūrvī (posterior)	198
Shankha	शङ्ख	shaṅkha	91
Shivarandhra	शिवरन्ध्र	śivarandhra	86
Sīramantha	सीरामन्थ	sīramantha	126
Sphij	स्फिज्	sphij	193

Table 55: Marma Point List, Alphabetical

Marma Point Names	Sanskrit (Devanagari)	Full Transliteration	Page
Stanya	स्तन्य	stanya	143
Stanya Mūla	स्तन्य मूल	stanya mūla	142
Stanya Pārshva	स्तन्य पार्श्व	stanya pārśva	144
Sūrya or Āmāshaya	सूर्य or आमाशय	sūrya or āmāśaya	149
Tala Hrida	तल हृद	tala hṛda	184
Tarjani	तर्जनि	tarjani	187
Trik	त्रिक्	trik	166
Ūrdhva Ganda	ऊर्ध्व गण्ड	ūrdhva gaṇḍha	103
Ūrdhva Skandha	ऊर्ध्व स्कन्ध	ūrdhva skandha	170
Ūrū	ऊरू	ūrū (2)	194
Vankri	वङ्क्रि	vankri	146
Vankshana	वङ्क्षण	vankṣaṇa	154
Vidhuram	विधुरम्	vidhuram	118
Vrukka	वृक्क	vṛkka	163
Vrushana	वृषण	vṛṣaṇa	197
Yakrut	यकृत्	yakṛt	147
Yoni Jihvā	योनि जिह्व	yoni jihva	196
Yoni Oshtha	योनि ओष्ठ	yoni oṣṭha	197

a. This is the common form of this word. It's more formal spelling is Adho Ganda, अधः गण्ड.
b. In northern India, Indrabasta is spelled with a "v" instead of the "b," e.g., इन्द्रवस्त.
c. Like marma vs. marman, plīhā is commonly used versus its correct spelling, e.g., plīhān.

Table 56: Translations of Marma Point Names

Marma Point	Translation	Marma Point	Translation
Āmāshaya	Stomach	Kūrpara	Corner
Amsa	Top part of shoulder, fragment or part of shoulder blade, lung	Lohita	Blood
Amsa Phalaka	Switchboard of lung	Lohitākṣa	Eyes are peeping into blood
Angushtha Mūla	Root of thumb	Madhya Vartma	Middle eyelid
Antar Amsa	In between lungs	Manibandha	Point where woman ties jewelry to wrist
Antara Vartma	Inner eyelid	Mantha	Churning
Apānga	Outer corner, angle of the eye	Manyāmani	Jewel of the neck
Apastambha	Pillar that supports or stabilizes	Manyāmūla	Root or beginning of neck
Ashrū	Tears	Medhra	Penis
Bāhya Kūrpara	Outer corner	Mūrdhni	Movement from moment to moment, momentary time
Bāhya Manibandha	External point where woman ties her jewelry	Nābhi	Umbilicus, central part of body axis, place of no fear
Bāhya Vartma	Outer eyelid	Nāsā Agra	Tip of nose
Basti	Bladder	Nāsā Madhya	Middle of nose
Bhaga	Sexual experience	Nāsā Mūla	Root of nose
Bruhatī	Expansion to promote easy breathing	Nāsā Puta	Nose petal, doorway to nose
Brahmarandhra	Opening to creator and cosmic creative energy	Oshtha	Upper lips, self-expression, energy rising to brain
Bhrūh Agra	External tip of eyebrow	Pāda Charana	Movement of the foot
Bhrūh Antara	Inner eyebrow	Pāda Madhya	Center arch of foot
Bhrūh Madhya	Middle of eyebrow	Pārshni	Heel
Charana	Movement	Pārshva Sandhi	Joint on side, joint of rib
Chibuka	Prāna of oral cavity	Plīhā	Spleen, that which filtrates
Ganda	Maxillary bone	Prushtha	Back
Grīvā	Neck, responsibility	Sakthi Ūrvī	Energy of thighs
Gulpha	Dimple or ditch	Shankha	Conch
Hanu	Mandible, chin, pride	Shivarandhra	Opening to cosmic transformer and destructive energy
Hridayam	Heart	Sīrāmantha	Rope that does churning
Hrid	Heart	Skandhadhara	That which holds the shoulder, shoulder joint
Indrabasta	Inner door of colon, stable crown of Indra	Skandha	Shoulder, support, responsibility
Jānu	Knee	Sphij	Gluteal fold

Table 56: Translations of Marma Point Names

Marma Point	Translation	Marma Point	Translation
Jatrū	To preserve or maintain	**Stanya**	Breast
Kaksha	Armpit	**Stanya Mūla**	Root of the breast
Kanīnaka	Inside of the eye, controller of water	**Stanya Pārshva**	Side of the breast
Kanīshthika	Small finger	**Sthapani**	Establishment, steadiness, stability
Kanthanādī	Channel of throat	**Sūrya**	Sun
Kapāla	Throat	**Tala Hrida**	Heart of palm
Kapola	Ruler of time, forehead	**Tarjani**	To show, indicate, or point out
Kapola Madhya	Middle of cheek	**Trik**	Triangle
Kapola Nāsā	Between nose and cheek	**Uru**	Origin of thigh
Karna Ūrdhva	Pinnacle or top of the ear	**Ūrvī**	Raise energy, vitality
Karnamūla	Root of ear	**Vankri**	Curved bone or bony curvature
Karnapālī	Ear lobule	**Vankshana**	Groin, the joint of the thigh
Kati	Hip or waist	**Vidhuram**	That which holds the base of the skull, that which holds consciousness
Kūrcha	Ligaments or fascia	**Vrukka**	Kidney, filters water
Kūrcha Shira	Head of ligaments	**Vrushana**	Testicle
Krikātikā	Axis that facilitates rotation of skull, quadriplegic, responsibility	**Yakrut**	Liver
Kshipra	Instantaneous, immediately acting	**Yoni Jihvā**	Clitoris
Kukundara	That which supports vertebral column and back	**Yoni Oshtha**	Female opening

Marma Points and Corresponding Acupoints

Mukha (Face) and Shiro (Head) Marmāni (28)

#	Marma Points	Page	Acupoint
1	Mūrdhni or Adhipati	82	≈GV 20 ≈GV 21
2	Brahmarandhra	84	GV 22
3	Shivarandhra	86	GV 19
4	Kapāla	88	≈GV 24[a]
5	Ājñā or Sthapanī	89	≈Yintang
6	Shankha	91	≈Taiyang
7	Bhrūh Antara	92	≈BL 2
8	Bhrūh Madhya	92	≈Yuyao
9	Bhrūh Agra	92	≈SJ 23
10	Ashrū Antara	94	≈BL 2
11	Ashrū Madhya	94	≈Yuyao
12	Ashrū Agra	94	≈SJ 23
13	Kanīnaka	95	BL 1
14	Apānga	96	GB 1
15	Antara Vartma	97	≈ST 1, BL 1
16	Madhya Vartma	97	ST 1
17	Bāhya Vartma	97	Qiuhou, ≈GB 1
16	Nāsā Mūla	99	Yintang
19	Nāsā Madhya	100	_____[b]
20	Nāsā Agra	101	GV 25
21	Nāsā Puta	102	-----------
22	Ūrdhva Ganda	103	≈Bitong
23	Adhah Ganda	104	Bitong
24	Kapola Nasa	105	LI 20
25	Kapola Madhya	106	----------
26	Oshtha	107	GV 26
27	Hanu	108	CV 24
28	Chibuka	110	ST 4

a. ≈ means marma is in close proximity to this acupoint.
b. The dashed line means there are no acupoints that correspond to this marma point.

Shiro (Back of Head) and Grīva (Neck) Marmāni (5)

#	Marma Points	Page	Acupoint
29	Manyāmūla	116	GV 16
30	Vidhuram	118	HTJJ C1
31	Krikātikā	120	HTJJ C2
32	Grīvā (1)	121	HTJJ C3
33	Grīvā (2)	121	HTJJ C4
34	Grīvā (3)	121	HTJJ C5
35	Grīvā (4)	121	HTJJ C6
36	Manyāmani	122	GV 14

Jatrū Ūrdhva (Front of Neck) Marmāni (6)

#	Marma Points	Page	Acupoint
37	Kantha	123	CV 23
38	Kanthanādī	124	CV 22
39	Mantha	125	ST 9
40	Sīrāmantha	126	≈LI 17, LI 18
41	Akshaka	127	ST 11
42	Jatru	128	CV 21

Karna (Ear) Marmāni (4)

#	Marma Points	Page	Acupoint
43	Karnapālī	130	Eye point on ear
44	Karnapāla or Karna Ūrdhva	131	Ear apex point
45	Karnamūla 1	132	SJ 17
46	Karnamūla 2	132	≈GB 12

Urah (Chest) Marmāni (11)

#	Marma Points	Page	Acupoint
47	Kakshadhara or Skandadhara	136	LU 1
48	Apastambha	137	KD 25
49	Hrid 1	138	KD 24
50	Hrid 2	138	KD 23
51	Hrid 3	138	KD 22
52	Hridayam	140	CV 18
53	Agra Patra	141	CV 15
54	Stanya Mūla	142	≈KD22
55	Stanya/Chuchuka	143	ST 17
56	Stanya Pārshva	144	SP 21
75	Pārshva Sandhi	145	LR 13

Udara (Abdominal) Marmāni (12)

#	Marma Points	Page	Acupoint
57	Vankri	146	ST 19
58	Yakrut	147	----------
59	Plīhā	148	----------
60	Sūrya/ Āmāshaya	149	CV 11
61	Nābhi	150	CV 8
62	Nābhi 1	150	ST 23
63	Nābhi 2	150	ST 23
64	Nābhi 3	150	≈SP 14
65	Nābhi 4	150	≈SP 14
66	Basti	152	≈CV 4, CV 5
67	Bhaga	153	CV 2
68	Vankshana	154	≈ST 29
69	Lohita	155	GB 27

Prushtha (Back) Marmāni (10)

#	Marma Points	Page	Acupoint
70	Amsa Phalaka	160	SI 11
71	Prushtha 1	161	HTJJ T3
72	Prushtha 2	161	HTJJ T4
73	Prushtha 3	161	HTJJ T5
74	Bruhatī	162	----------
76	Vrukka	163	HTJJ T12
77	Kukundara	164	HTJJ L5
78	Kati	165	BL 31
79	Trik	166	BL 35

Bahu (Arm) Marmāni (9)

#	Marma Points	Page	Acupoint
80	Ūrdhva Skandha	170	GB 21
81	Amsa	171	≈LI 15
82	Adhah Skandha	172	LI 14
83	Kaksha	173	HT 1
84	Bāhu Ūrvī	174	≈HT 2
85	Ānī	175	PC 3
86	Bāhū Indrabasta	176	≈HT 3, PC 3
87	Kūrpara	178	Zhoujian
88	Bāhya Kūrpara	179	≈LI 11

Hasta (Hand) Marmāni (9)

#	Marma Points	Page	Acupoint
89	Angushtha Mūla	180	LI 4
90	Bāhya Manibandha	181	LI 5
91	Manibandha	182	PC 7
92	Kūrcha Shira	183	SI 5
93	Tala Hrida	184	PC 8
94	Kūrcha	185	LU 10
95	Hasta Kshipra	186	LU 11
96	Tarjani	187	LI 1
97	Kanīshthika	188	≈HT 9

Sakthi (Thighs) Marmāni (14)

#	Marma Points	Page	Acupoints
98	Sphij	193	BL 36
99	Ūrū 1	194	----------
100	Ūrū 2	194	GB 31
101	Lohitāksha	195	LR 10
102	Medhra/Yoni Jihvā	196	----------
103	Vrushana/ Yoni Oshtha	197	----------
104	Sakthi Ūrvī (anterior)	198	≈SP 11
105	Sakthi Ūrvī (posterior)	198	≈BL 37
106	Jānu (anterior)	199	≈Heding, ≈medial Xiyan, ≈ST 35
107	Jānu (posterior)	199	BL 40
108	Charana (medial)	200	LR 8
109	Charana (lateral)	200	GB 34
110	Indrabasta (medial)	202	SP 8
111	Indrabasta (posterior)	202	BL 56

Pada (Foot) Marmāni (6)

#	Marma Points	Page	Acupoint
112	Gulpha (medial)	203	KD 5
113	Gulpha (lateral)	203	BL 62
114	Pāda Charana	204	ST 41
115	Pāda Kshipra	205	≈SP 1, LR 1
116	Pārshni	206	---------
117	Pāda Madhya	207	KD 1

Glossaries: Āyurvedic, Chinese and Medical

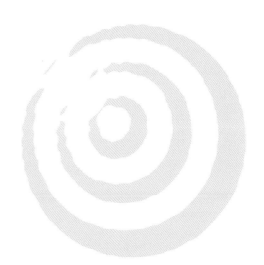

Āyurvedic Glossary

A

āhāra rasa. Nutritive juice that is the end product of digested food, formed about 12 hours after eating; the nutritional precursor of all bodily tissues; asthāyi (unstable, unprocessed) form of rasa dhātu.

ājñā. The center point between the eyebrows related to the pituitary gland; the point where right hemisphere meets with left, alpha meets with omega, intuition meets with logic; the highest end point of human polarity; the center of cognition which is activated by light.

ākāsha. Ether or space element, the first of the five basic elements; the first expression of Consciousness; the subtle, light, expansive element which serves as the common factor or "home" for all objects in the universe and manifests as nuclear energy.

ālochaka pitta. One of the subtypes of pitta dosha, situated in the sense organ of seeing; it is responsible for vision and color perception.

āma. Raw, uncooked; toxins; a toxic substance that impairs bodily or mental functions and can be physical, as in undigested food, or mental, as in any incomplete thought, experience or emotion; āma always arises from physical or mental indigestion. It is considered the root cause of many diseases.

āmāshaya. The stomach; literally, the receptacle for undigested food.

ānanda. Bliss.

ānandamaya kosha. The sheath made of bliss.

āpas. Water; the Water element.

ārtava. Female reproductive tissue, including ovaries, uterus, cervix, vagina and the ova; closely associated with rasa dhātu due to its functional integrity with menstruation and lactation.

ārtava vaha srotas. The channels carrying nutrients for ārtava dhātu, or female reproductive tissue. The roots or governors of this channel are the ovaries and areola of the nipples. The pathway includes the fallopian tubes, uterus, cervical canal, and vaginal canal, and the opening is the labia of the vagina.

āsana. Yoga posture; one of the eight limbs of Yoga Philosophy; that which brings stability, strength and ease to the body and mind.

ātman. The soul or Self.

āvila. Cloudy; characterized by cloudiness; confusion, loss of sensory perception; it increases kapha, decreases pitta and vāta.

āyuh. Life; longevity.

abhyantara mārga. Abhyantara: inner; mārga: pathway; the innermost pathway of the body, it includes the GI tract and is the site of the first two stages of disease according to the Āyurvedic model of pathology.

abhrak bhasma. Mica ash.

abhyanga. Full-body oil massage commonly given before pañchakarma to move doshas and toxins into the gastrointestinal tract where they can be removed by cleansing procedures; abhyanga is also done as part of a daily routine.

adho jatru granthi. The thymus gland.

agni. Fire element, the second of the five basic elements in the body; it regulates temperature, performs digestion, absorption and assimilation of ingested food, and transforms food into energy or consciousness.

Agnideva. The ancient Vedic deity of fire, both creative and destructive in nature; the energy of physical fire.

agni karma. Application of local heat, comparable to moxibustion in TCM, especially effective in kapha related conditions or poor circulation.

ahamkāra. A continuous feeling of "I am;" a center in the daily operating consciousness from where each individual thinks, feels and acts as an independent being from his or her individual accumulated experience.

ahimsā. Non-violence; one of the prerequisite attitudes of a yogi according to Yoga philosophy; one of the primary tenets of Buddhism, it prevented the widespread use of acupuncture in India.

ambu. Water; the Water element.

Glossaries: Āyurvedic, Chinese and Medical

ambu vaha srotas. The bodily channels carrying water. The roots or governors of this channel are the pancreas, soft palate, and choroid plexus in the brain. Its pathway is the mucus membrane of the gastrointestinal tract, and the openings are the kidneys, tongue, and sweat glands.

anāhata. The heart chakra; related to the thymus gland; the center of unconditional love; related to immunity; also denotes the cardiac plexus which governs heart activity.

angula. Form of measurement for locating marma points. One angula is the width of the patient's middle finger measured across the proximal interphalangeal joint.

añjali. A measurement formed when two hands meet together to make an empty bowl.

anna vaha srotas. The bodily channels that take in and carry food. This channel begins at the lips of the mouth, is governed by the esophagus and greater curvature of the stomach, continues through the entire gastrointestinal tract, and opens at the ileocecal valve.

annamaya kosha. Literally, the sheath made of food; the physical body.

anu. Atom; also individual (as opposed to universal).

anu vaha srotas. The atomic channel or pathway; the pathway of atoms, which is the cell.

apāna vāyu. The energy that governs outward movement; one of the subtypes of vāta dosha functioning mainly in the colon, it governs the elimination of feces, flatus, urine, menstrual blood and other gross wastes as well as subtle or cellular wastes.

apāna vāyu dushti. Disorder or disturbance of apāna vāyu; known by such symptoms as abdominal distention, diarrhea or constipation, gas, bloating, pain and accumulation of wastes.

apakti. Indigestion; impaired digestion.

apara ojas. Unstable, less processed form of ojas that circulates throughout the body.

apunarbhava chikitsā. Preventative approach to medicine that emphasizes living with awareness and following a daily routine and diet appropriate to one's prakruti and vikruti as well as the current season.

artha. The second of the four goals of human life (see "purushārtha"), artha is the universal human goal of attaining proper means of support or wealth. Artha also means having proper goals and objectives.

ashru. Lacrimation, tears; the superior by-product of majjā dhātu.

ashtānga yoga. The path of yoga as explained by Pātañjali in the second century BC, which divides the practice of yoga into eight (ashta) limbs (anga). The first two (yama and niyama) deal with establishing the right attitudes and behaviors in the practitioner, the third (āsana) relates to the postures of hatha yoga, the fourth (prānāyāma) deals with breath observance, and the last three (dhārana, dhyāna and samādhi) relate to cultivating one-pointed awareness, meditation and union with cosmic consciousness.

asthi dhātu. One of the seven bodily tissues, asthi relates to bone tissue. Its major functions are supporting the body frame, giving protection, shape and longevity, and making movement possible.

asthi vaha srotas. The channel carrying nutrients for asthi dhātu or bone tissue; its roots or governors are the pelvic girdle and sacrum. Its passageway is the entire skeletal system, and the openings or mouths of the channel are the nails and hair.

Atharvaveda. The fourth of the four Vedas, ancient scripture of India.

avalambaka kapha. The functions of kapha that are specifically related to the lungs and heart, it protects and moisturizes the entire pleural space.

avyākta. Unmanifested; the pre-"big bang" state.

B

bāhya mārga. Outer (bāhya), pathway (mārga); the superficial pathway of the body, it includes the channels that carry rasa and rakta and is associated with the prasara (spreading) stage of pathogenesis, during which the doshas spread throughout the body and affect superficial areas such as the skin.

basti. Enema, one of the five important cleansing measures of pañchakarma, it eliminates excess vāta dosha via the colon, using medicated substances such as herbal tea or oil.

bhakti. Unconditional, selfless and causeless love; devotion; reverence.

bhakti yoga. One of the main paths to liberation, the path of devotion leading to realization of the Divine in oneself.

bheda. Destruction; differentiation; the last stage out of six in the Āyurvedic system of pathogenesis (see "samprāpti"), bheda stage is the stage in which complicated symptoms can be observed, and damage or destruction of bodily tissues takes place.

bhrājaka pitta. One of the five types of pitta, located in the skin of the entire body. Its function is to give tactile sensation, color complexion and luster to the skin as well as digestion of any medications that are applied to the skin, such as oils, salves, or plasters.

bhrājaka agni. The fire component of bhrājaka pitta, which governs and organizes its functions.

bhūta. Element; the five basic elements of Ether, Air, Fire, Water and Earth; that which manifests as matter.

bhūta agni. The fire component of the five elements based in the liver, which manifests as the liver enzymes. It converts the five elements present in ingested food into biologically available forms of the elements that can be utilized by the body. There are five bhūta agnis, one for each of the five elements.

bīja mantra. Seed sound; a potent sound that sprouts like a seed and conveys a meaning that is beyond the scope of the intellectual or verbal mind, manifesting a reality that is aligned with its particular vibration and application.

Brahmā. Creative potential; the first in the Hindu trinity of gods: the creator of the universe.

brāhma. The expansive, all-pervasive, universal consciousness; eternal timeless existence.

brahmī. An herb similar to gotu kola.

buddhi. The individual intellect.

C

chakra. The energy centers in the body, related to nerve plexus centers that govern the bodily functions. Each chakra is a separate reservoir of consciousness connecting the physical body to the astral body.

chala. Mobile; an attribute characterized by mobility and changeability; increases vāta and pitta, and decreases kapha.

chikitsā. Treatment.

chitta. The mind; psychic energy; the psyche as a whole.

D

dashamūla. A classical Āyurvedic herb formula specifically used for vāta dosha, dasha is ten and mūla is root. Dashamula is comprised of the roots of ten herbs.

dhārana. The sixth limb in the Yoga system of Patañjali; the act of focusing attention on one object and mentally holding the object; one-pointed awareness.

dhātu. The elemental structural tissues that constitute the human body. There are seven basic tissues defined in Āyurveda: plasma, blood, muscle, fat, bone, nerve and bone marrow, and reproductive tissue.

dhātu agni. The agni component of each dhātu, located in the membrane that separates one dhātu from another. It nourishes the tissue, maintains tissue metabolism, and transforms immature tissue into mature tissue.

dhamanī. Artery.

dhanurveda. The science of archery; one of the four *upavedas*.

dharma. The first of the four goals of human beings (see "purushārtha"), dharma is the universal human goal of finding one's true path in life and doing what is uniquely proper for oneself. It is often translated as righteousness

dhī. Cognition; one of the faculties of buddhi, or intellect.

dhruti. Retention; one of the faculties of buddhi, or intellect.

dhyāna. The seventh limb in the Yoga system of Patañjali; meditation; a continuous flow of attention without words or thoughts; a state of moment-to-moment, choiceless, passive awareness, or witnessing, without judgment, liking, or disliking.

dīpana. The action of kindling agni.

dosha. Referring to vāta, pitta and kapha; the three psychophysiological functional principles of the body, the ratio of which determines an individual's constitution at the time of conception. When functioning normally and present in normal quantities, the doshas maintain all healthy bodily processes. When out of balance, they create disease.

dosha gati. The vector or direction in which a dosha moves.

dravya. Matter; substance; defined as that which has attribute and action, or guna and karma, dwelling inseparably.

duhkha. Literally, 'bad space'; a state of misery, pain, disease, unhappiness, or suffering of any kind.

G

gandha. Odor; the tanmātrā relating to earth element; the subtle quality of the earth element that exists in objects, allowing them to be sensed by smell.

Ganesha. The big-bellied elephant-headed deity who is the son of Shiva and Pārvatī, he is said to be the remover of obstacles and governs the mūlādhāra chakra and the initial rising of the kundalinī energy coiled there. He is always the first deity to be approached at the beginning of a ceremony or any enterprise.

gharshana. A dry massage treatment especially good for kapha, in which the skin is brushed with powder or a skin brush, creating friction and stimulating circulation and exfoliation.

ghrita. A preparation of ghee (clarified butter) in which herbs are infused or boiled into the ghee.

granthi. 1. Gland 2. A swelling or hardening of the vessels or an abnormal growth in the body.

guna. Attribute or quality; one of the twenty qualities or attributes used to describe substances and determine their effects; also, one of the three universal qualities that are present in creation and that cause all phenomena. These are: sattva, the quality bringing essence, light, balance and understanding; rajas, the energy of movement and activity; and tamas, the quality bringing darkness, inertia, heaviness and materialism.

guru. Teacher; one who removes the darkness of ignorance; the channel through which understanding of the Divine comes to one; also: heavy, an attribute characterized by heaviness and bulk, it increases kapha and decreases pitta and vāta.

H

Hanuman. The monkey god who served Rāma with extraordinary strength and prowess during his exile in the forest, Hanuman represents the essence of true friendship, the path of loving and serving God as a friend.

hrid. The heart; cardiac muscle.

I

īdā. One of the three primary subtle energy channels in an individual, īdā flows along the left side of the central channel (sushumna nādī). Īdā controls the parasympathetic nervous system, is associated with feminine, lunar energy, and is primarily yin. Stimulating this channel by breathing through the left nostril increases relaxation and cools the body.

Indra. An ancient Vedic deity; cosmic prāna.

Glossaries: Āyurvedic, Chinese and Medical

indriya. Inner doors of perception, including sensory and motor organs and their pathways in the brain.

indriya agni. The fire component present in each of the five sense faculties, it converts sensory input into understanding, experience, and knowledge.

J

jāthara agni. The central fire of the digestive system, responsible for digestion and assimilation of ingested food; it nourishes all bodily agni.

jatru agni. The fire component present in the thyroid gland; it is the bridge between bhūta agni and dhātu agni.

jihva. Tongue; one of the openings of ambu vaha srotas.

jīvātman. The individual soul.

jīva. Individual life; individual consciousness; the pure sense of "me".

jīvana. Life-giving (a special function of rakta dhātu).

jñāna. Wisdom or knowledge.

jñāna yoga. One of the main paths to liberation; the path of knowledge or wisdom to realize the Divine in oneself.

jñānendriya. The five sensory faculties; the inner doors of perception, including sensory organs and their pathways in the brain.

Jyotis. Light, luster; the inner light of the self.

K

kāma. Joy, happiness; the third of the four goals of human beings (see "purushārtha"), kāma is the universal human goal of fulfilling positive desires and attaining a lasting state of joyfulness.

Kāpila. The name of the sage who founded the Sānkhya school of philosophy.

kāya chikitsā. Internal medicine, one of the eight branches of Āyurvedic medicine along with pediatrics, psychiatry, E.N.T., surgery, dentistry, geriatric medicine and virilization/rejuvenation.

kandara. One of the superior by-products of rakta dhātu; small tendons and sinews, such as hamstring muscles.

kapha. One of the three doshas, combining the water and earth elements; the psycho-physiological energy that forms the body's structure and holds the cells together.

karma. Action; the law stating that for every action there is an equal and opposite reaction; specific action of a substance or herb; along with guna (attribute), karma makes up the inherent nature of a substance, according to Vaisheshika.

karma yoga. One of the main paths to liberation; the path of taking positive action and surrendering the fruits of all actions to the Divine.

karmendriya. The five motor faculties; the faculties of action, including motor organs and their pathways in the brain.

kathina. Hard quality; hardness; increases vāta and kapha and decreases pitta; associated with strength, rigidity, self-ishness, callousness, and insensitivity. Also associated with things like pneumonia, callouses, and hardening of the arteries.

kati. Pelvic girdle, waist, lumbosacral area, lumbar spine.

kesha. Hair; the inferior by-product of asthi dhātu.

khā. Space.

khavaigunya. Any weak or defective space in the body that exists because of past trauma, chronic disease, or hereditary influence and becomes a place where aggravated doshas can easily lodge and create disorder.

khamala. The inferior by-products of māmsa dhātu, including nasal crust, earwax, sebaceous secretions, tartar, and smegma.

khāra. Rough quality; roughness, which is connected with dryness, absorption, constipation, and which aggravates vata and decreases pitta and kapha.

kitta. Waste product or inferior by-product; feces; the non-essential component of ingested food that is excreted from the body.

kleda. Liquefaction, hydration, water; sebaceous secretions, mucus, and other liquid secretions associated with kapha dosha.

kledaka kapha. One of the kapha subtypes; its function is to liquefy ingested food in the stomach; it also protects the stomach wall from the digestive enzymes and acids; the gastric mucous membrane.

kloma. Pancreas; the root of the water carrying channels; kloma also refers to the choroid plexus in the brain.

kloma agni. The digestive energy of the pancreas. It works in conjunction with bhūta agni from the liver and assists in the digestion of proteins, carbohydrates, and fats.

kosha. Sheath. There are five sheaths: the sheath of bliss, the sheath of knowledge, the sheath of mind, the sheath of prāna, and the sheath of food.

kshaya. Decrease of anything, used to describe depletion of bodily tissues or doshas.

kundalinī. The coiled, serpentine, spiritual energy, which, for most people, lies dormant at the base of the spine.

kundalinī shakti. The power of pure energy; the term used in describing the awakening of spiritual energy.

L

laghu. Light; an attribute characterized by radiance and/or lightness, it aids in digestion, cleansing, and promotes freshness and alertness. In excess it may cause insomnia and ungroundedness; an attribute of both vāta and pitta doshas.

lepana. Plastering; holding; one of the main important functions of māmsa dhātu.

M

māmsa dhātu. One of the seven bodily tissues, māmsa consists of all types of muscle. Its functions include movement, coordination, "plastering," protection, maintenance of body temperature and body shape, ambition, confidence, and strength.

māmsa vaha srotas. The channel carrying nutrients for māmsa dhātu, or muscle tissue. The roots or governors of this channel are the fascia and small tendons. The passageway of the channel is the entire musculature system, and the opening of the channel is the pores of the skin.

mārga. Passageway; a synonym for the word srotas.

madhyama mārga. Madhyama: middle; mārga: pathway; The central pathway of the body, it includes the deep connective tissue, seven dhātus and visceral organs. It is often the site of the last stages of disease according to the Āyurvedic model of pathology, at which point the doshas affect the deep tissues and vital organs.

mahā marmāni. A category of the most vital marma points.

mahā srotas. The largest channel in the body, the digestive tract

Mahad. The great principle; cosmic intelligence; the cosmic aspect of the intellect, it contains buddhi, the individual intellect, ego, and mind.

majjā dhātu. One of the seven bodily tissues, majjā consists of bone marrow, connective tissue and nerve tissue, and associated with the endocrine system and erythrogenesis. Its main functions are communication and filling space in the body, especially the spaces within the bones.

majjā vaha srotas. The channel carrying nutrients for majjā dhātu, or bone marrow and nervous tissue. The roots or governors for this channel are the brain, spinal cord, and joints. The pathway is the central, sympathetic, and parasympathetic nervous system. The opening is the synaptic space.

mala. Any impurity; the waste products that get produced in the body through the processes of digestion and tissue nutrition, malas must constantly be moving out of the body as they are produced. Deficiencies or excesses in the production of any mala reflect some disturbance in the particular metabolic process to which the mala is related.

mala vaha srotas. Another name for the channel carrying feces, or the purīsha vaha srotas.

manas. Mind; one of the causative substances according to the Vaisheshika philosophy; the faculty arising from sattva guna according to the Sānkhya school of thought; the sensory-feeling part of the mind that manifests thoughts and emotions, as contrasted with buddhi, the intellectual faculty of mind. Manas can be anu (individual) and vibhu (universal).

manas prakruti. Mental constitution, which is manifested at the time of fertilization and described in terms of the three gunas—sattva, rajas, and tamas. In the cosmic mind, equilibrium of the gunas is maintained; in an individual mind, these three are in unequal proportion, according to the karmas expressing in that individual's consciousness.

manda. Slow quality; an attribute that increases kapha and decreases vāta and pitta, creates sluggishness, slow action, relaxation and dullness as well as calm, quiet and silence.

manda agni. Slow digestion; one of the three categories of disturbed agni; digestion affected by the heavy, slow, and cool qualities of kapha dosha, causing slow metabolism.

mano vaha srotas. The channel that carries the mind. The roots or governors of this channel are the heart and the sensory pathways. Its pathway is the entire body, and the opening or mouth of this channel is the sense organs and the marmāni.

manomaya kosha. The sheath made of mind; related to manas, the sensory and emotional mind.

mantra. A form of vocal or silent suggestion, usually repetitive; a syllable, word, or group of words that illuminate consciousness, bringing clarity, understanding, stillness, peace, prolonged concentration, and eventually samādhi; words uttered from the heart of a wise being. Mantra must be spoken, heard, or felt; a written mantra has no power.

mardana. A very deep, strong massage especially good for kapha type individuals, mardana breaks up stagnation and stimulates circulation.

marmāni. The plural form of marma; vital energy points, similar to acupuncture points, where consciousness is most expressive.

marma. A vital point on the body that is used therapeutically and diagnostically.

maya. "Made of" as in prāna maya kosha, the sheath made of prāna.

meda dhātu or medas. One of the seven bodily tissues, meda is a loose connective tissue that includes fat, steroids such as cholesterol, and other types of lipids. Its functions include storing energy, giving shape, beauty and insulation to the body, sweet tone to the voice, and lubrication and protection of all bodily systems.

medo vaha srotas. The bodily channel carrying nutrients for the fat tissue. The roots or governors of this channel are the omentum and the adrenals. The passageway is the subcutaneous fat tissue, and the opening is the sweat glands.

mithuna. Male and female energy merging together; sex.

moksha. Freedom, liberation; the final aim of all knowledge, work, and activity; the ultimate aim of life; the ending of involuntary and unconscious participation in the relative world

mrudu. Soft quality; softness, delicacy; promotes mucus, adipose tissue, relaxation, tenderness, love, care, promotes kapha and pitta and decreases vāta.

mudrā. A gesture or positioning of the fingers practiced in devotional worship or yogic practice that allows for communication between the individual and the deity or the mind and body.

mukha. Face; mouth; opening; in the bodily srotāmsi, the mukha is identified as the place where the srotas system opens.

mukta. The free or liberated mind that is completely aware, clear, attentive, and blissful; one of the five states of mind.

mukta triveni. One of the significant points at which the īdā, pingalā and sushumnā nādīs meet, associated with the third eye region and ājñā marma.

mūla. Root; governor; in the bodily srotāmsi, the mūla is identified as the place from which the srotas originates physically, or the place where its functions are primarily governed.

mūlādhāra chakra. The first chakra, associated with the perianal area or the base of the spine and related to survival, stability, security and instincts, it is also associated with Ganesha, the deity with whose grace one may awaken the kundalinī energy that lies dormant in mūlādhāra chakra.

mūrdhni. The head, the primary site of prāna vāyu.

mūtra. Urine; one of the three primary wastes of the body along with feces and sweat.

mūtra vaha srotas. The channel that carries urine; the root or governor of this channel is the kidneys. The pathway of this channel is the ureters, urethra, and bladder. The opening or mouth of this channel is the opening of the urethra.

N

nādī. Literally, a river; a channel or passageway; the pulse; there are innumerable nādis in the human body, from the very subtle to the very gross, all carrying substances into, out of, or throughout the body.

nasya. The nasal administration of herbal powders, oil, medicated oil, or other therapeutic substances, nasya is done to eliminate residual doshas in the head, especially as part of the pañchakarma process.

netra basti. A treatment in which the eyes are bathed in ghee.

nirvāna. State of pure existence; no-mind state.

niyama. The five habits or codes of ethical/moral conduct expounded as the second limb in the eight-limbed Yoga system of Pātañjali; the means of putting oneself into harmony with nature and establishing harmony in all relationships, niyama consists of: physical and mental purity, contentment, self-discipline/austerity, self-study, and surrender to God.

O

ojas. The subtle, positive energy of kapha dosha, it maintains immunity, strength, integrity, and vitality and has a functionally integrated relationship with tejas and prāna.

oshtha yoni. The labia, or lips of the vagina

P

pāchaka. One of the five subtypes of pitta, located in the stomach and small intestine. It includes hydrochloric acid, digestive enzymes, pepsin, and intestinal juices secreted from the villi of the small intestine.

pāka . Digestion.

Pārvatī. "Daughter of the Mountain," she is the goddess whose father is the Himālayas. Parvati is the mother of Ganesha and wife of Shiva, and represents the spine, which is the anchor by which the human being manifests in the body and interacts with the environment, and which becomes the channel for the movement of kundalinī.

Pātañjali. Name of the celebrated sage who created *The Yoga Sūtras*.

pakti. Digestion, absorption, and assimilation of food and sensory experience; one of the functions of agni.

pañchakarma. The five methods for eliminating excess dosha and/or āma from the body for internal purification: vomiting (vamana), purgation (virechana), decoction or oil enema (basti), bloodletting (rakta moksha), and nasal administration (nasya). In the pañchakarma process, excessive dosha and/or āma is brought back to its main site in the body and then eliminated through one or more of the five measures.

pañcha mahābhūta. The five great elements from which all substances arise: ether/space, air, fire, water and earth.

Para Brāhman. The highest self, beyond the body and the mind.

paramātman. The higher self; cosmic soul.

para ojas. The superfine or fully processed form of ojas, eight drops of which are stored in the heart to maintain life.

parināma. Transformation; change; growth; dimension or expansion, one of the qualities or functions of tejas is in expansion due to heat.

patha. Path; a synonym for the word srotas.

pīdana. The application of localized deep pressure adjusted according to the patient's pain tolerance. A bluntly tapered object, called a shalākā, is sometimes used for this.

pīlu agni. The digestive fire present in the membrane of every cell, it maintains semi-permeability of the cell membrane and governs the selection of cellular nutrients.

pīlu pāka. The process of cellular digestion and nutrition which takes place in the cell membrane and in the cytoplasm outside the cell nucleus.

pingalā. One of the three primary subtle energy channels in an individual, pingalā flows along the right side of the central channel (sushumna nādī). Pingalā controls the sympathetic nervous system, is associated with masculine, solar energy, and is primarily yang. Stimulating this channel by breathing through the right nostril stimulates energy, vigor and stamina.

pithara agni. The fire component in the nucleus of the cell; the purest manifestation of tejas in the body; it governs the transformation of cellular food into consciousness.

pitta. One of the three doshas, made up of the fire and water elements; governs digestion, absorption, assimilation, nutrition, metabolism, and body temperature.

poshaka. The essential component of ingested food, separated from the non-essential component to nourish bodily tissues. Literally, one who nourishes and supports; a name for asthāyi (unstable) dhātu, which nourishes the sthāyi (stable) dhātu; also a name for the precursors of each dosha.

poshaka kapha. The physical precursor or nourisher of kapha dosha, produced by rasa dhātu.

poshaka pitta. The physical precursor or nourisher of pitta dosha, produced by rakta dhātu; bile.

prājñāparādha. "Crime against wisdom," going against the body's innate intelligence; for example, indulging a mental craving for a food or substance that undermines the body's health. *Prājñāparādha* powerfully contributes to doshic disturbance.

prānāyāma. The control of life-energy by various techniques that regulate and restrain breath, helping one to control the mind and improve the quality of awareness and perception; this assists meditation.

prāna. The vital life force without which life cannot exist and which is primarily taken in through the breath; the flow of cellular intelligence that governs cellular communication, sensory perception, motor responses, and all subtle electrical impulses of the body; the subtle essence of vāta dosha. Prāna has a functionally integrated relationship with ojas and tejas.

prāna vāyu. One of the five subtypes of *vāta dosha*, *prāna* moves inward and downward and is associated with the nervous system, where it governs all sensory functions and maintains attention, and with the lungs, where it governs the inhalation aspect of respiration.

prāna vaha srotas. The bodily channels that take in and carry prāna, or life force. The roots or governors of this channel are the left chamber of the heart and the entire gastrointestinal tract. The channel continues along the respiratory tract and bronchial tree, including the alveoli, and opens at the nose.

prānamaya kosha. The sheath made of electromagnetic energy or vital essence. The etheric body.

prajanana. Producing, creating; function of shukra and ārtava dhātus.

prakopa. Literally, "enraged;" "provocation," the second stage of six in the Āyurvedic model of pathogenesis (see "*samprāpti*"), *prakopa* is the stage in which the doshas have already increased in their own sites and are easily provoked to manifest increasingly intense symptoms.

prakruti. Primordial matter, the Cosmic Mother or cosmic womb, the root cause of the creation of the universe; on an individual level, prakruti is the psychosomatic, biological constitution of an individual, the unique combination of the three doshas that forms the person's constitution at the time of conception and creates the inborn tendencies that influence how one experiences life.

prasāda. Clarity, purity; an offering of holy food to a deity; the essence of food.

prasara. Spreading or creeping; the third stage of six in the Āyurvedic model of pathogenesis (see "*samprāpti*"), prasara is the stage in which the provoked doshas enter into the circulatory system and move around the body.

pratyāhāra. Withdrawal of the senses; the fifth limb in Pātañjali's eight-limbed system of Yoga; the act of bringing consciousness deeper inside the body, drawing the psychic energy from peripheral sense organs to the inner movements of the mind.

prīnanam. Nutrition, the main function of rasa dhātu.

pruthivī. Earth element.

purīsha agni. The fire component of the membranous structure surrounding the organs of the excretory system, it governs the elimination of feces. It also helps to absorb liquids and minerals, forms the stools, and maintains the temperature and color of the feces.

purīsha vaha srotas. The bodily channel that carries feces; the root or governor of this channel is the cecum, rectum, and sigmoid colon. The pathway of the channel is the large intestine, and the opening or mouth of this channel is the anal orifice.

purushārthas. Purusha (human being), artha (goals), the four universal aims of human life: dharma (duty, proper path), artha (procurement of resources), kāma (joy) and moksha (liberation).

Purusha. Pure, undifferentiated, infinite consciousness; choiceless, passive awareness; consciousness that dwells in the "city of senses," which is the human being.

pūrana. Filling up, completing; a major function of majjā dhātu and vāta dosha, especially prāna vāyu.

pūrana. The act of filling space, a function of vāta dosha.

R

rāga. Affection; enthusiasm; coloration; one of the functions of healthy agni.

rajah. Menstruation; one of the superior by-products of rasa dhātu.

rajas. One of the three universal gunas or qualities of consciousness; the principle of kinetic energy; active, mobile, and responsible for all movements.

rakta agni. The fire component present in the blood, it is responsible for the digestion and assimilation of nutrients that nourish blood tissue.

rakta dhātu. Blood; one of the seven bodily tissues, rakta consists of red blood cells, and in Āyurveda is a separate tissue from the plasma (rasa dhātu). Its main functions include maintenance of life, oxygenation, and transportation of nutrients. Rakta is said by Sushruta to be the fourth dosha because ultimately all untreated disorders will affect the blood, and because unhealthy blood causes systemic problems in the same way that an aggravated dosha does.

rakta moksha. Bloodletting or blood cleansing, one of the five cleansing actions of pañchakarma; a specific treatment for removing excess pitta and purification of the blood.

rakta vaha srotas. The bodily channel that maintains the functions of rakta dhātu, or red blood cells. The root or governor of this channel is the liver and spleen. It extends throughout the arteriole circulatory system, and opens at the arteriovenous junction.

rañjaka pitta. One of the subtypes of pitta dosha located in the liver and spleen, it gives color to the blood and is responsible for the formation of blood.

rasāyana chikitsā. Rejuvenation therapy which brings about renewal, regeneration, and restoration of all bodily cells, tissues and organs; enhances immunity and stamina and gives longevity.

rasa. Taste; the tanmātrā relating to water element; the subtle quality of the water element that exists in objects, allowing them to be sensed by taste; the first experience of food in the mouth; there are six tastes in our diet: sweet, sour, salty, pungent, bitter and astringent.

rasa dhātu. Plasma, the first of the seven dhātus, it includes lymph fluid, white blood cells, and the plasma component of blood. Rasa is the first tissue to be nourished from ingested food and provides nutrition to every cell and tissue of the body.

rasa vaha srotas. The bodily channel that maintains the functions of rasa dhātu, the lymph and plasma tissue. The roots or governors of this channel are the right chamber of the heart and the ten great vessels of the heart, the passage is the venous and lymphatic systems, and it opens at the juncture between the arteries and veins.

Rigveda. The oldest of the four Vedas, the ancient scriptures of India, the rig veda is said to have been produced from fire.

rishi. A seer or sage; the beings who perceived and/or recorded the Vedic hymns; the enlightened sages who shared their knowledge, medicine, philosophy and spiritual teachings.

roma kūpa. Sweat glands; one of the openings of ambu vaha srotas.

rūksha. Dry quality; creates dehydration and causes choking, constriction, spasm, pain, and dryness of the skin as well as isolation, separation, fear, nervousness and loneliness.

rūpa. Form; the tanmātrā relating to fire element; the subtle quality of the fire element that exists in objects, making objects visible; color.

S

sādhaka pitta. One of the five subtypes of pitta; responsible for intelligence, memory, mental digestion, enthusiasm and other functions of the higher mental faculties.

sākshin. Witness, observer, a name for the supreme being (purusha) according to Sānkhya philosophy.

Sāmaveda. The third of the four Vedas.

sānkhya. Number; a particular quality or function of tejas by which cellular division takes place and the proper number of chromosomes, tissues, doshas and malas are maintained.

Sānkhya. A major school of Indian philosophy founded by the sage Kāpila. It gives Āyurveda a systematic account of cosmic evolution according to 25 categories: purusha, cosmic spirit; prakruti, creative energy; mahad, cosmic intelligence; ahamkāra, the individuating principle or "I-maker"; manas, the individual mind; indriyāni, the 10 sense and motor facilities; tanmātrās, the five subtle elements; and pañcha mahā bhūtas, the five gross elements.

sadyah prānahara. Most vital marmas—see also maha marmāni.

sahasrāra. The seventh or crown chakra, located at the topmost part of the skull and related to the pineal gland; the "thousand petaled lotus"; "Sa" means soma, lunar, female energy; "Ha" means solar, male energy. This chakra is where male and female energies merge into one and all definitions dissolve into the undefined.

sakthi. The thigh or thigh bone; one of the sites of vāta dosha.

samādhi. Cosmic consciousness; an expansive state of choiceless, passive awareness that is all-inclusive equilibrium; a balanced state of body, mind and consciousness.

samāna vāyu. One of the five subtypes of vāta, its movement is linear and outward. It is mainly present in the small intestine and navel area, and stimulates appetite and the secretion of digestive juices, so is closely connected with agni (digestive fire). It is responsible for peristalsis and the opening and closing of the pyloric and ileocecal valves during the process of digestion.

sama agni. Balanced agni; the state of optimal, balanced metabolism that arises when all three doshas are in balance according to the individual's constitution.

samprāpti. The Āyurvedic model of pathogenesis, which involves six phases of dosha activity: sañchaya (accumulation of a dosha within its main site), prakopa (provocation of the dosha), prasara (spreading of the dosha throughout the body), sthāna samshraya (deposition of the dosha into a tissue), vyakti (manifestation of cardinal symptoms) and bheda (destruction or derangement of tissue).

sandhi. The joints of the body.

sandra. Dense; density; associated with substances like meat and cheese; increases kapha and decreases vāta and pitta; brings compactness to the body and makes a person more grounded; promotes solidity, density and strength.

sanga. Accumulation, stagnation; physiologically it can manifest as constipation, blood clots, lymphatic congestion, growths, or blockages.

sañchaya. Accumulation, the first of six stages in the āyurvedic model of pathogenesis (see "samprāpti"), sañchaya is the stage in which doshas accumulate in their own sites.

sattva. One of the three universal gunas or qualities of consciousness; the principle of equilibrium, intelligence, essence, consciousness and clarity of perception; potential energy; jñānshakti, the energy of wisdom, understanding and cognition; it gives rise to the mind and senses in Sānkhya Philosophy.

shākhā. Limbs; extremities.

shabda. Sound; the tanmātrā relating to ether element; the subtle quality of the ether element that exists in objects, allowing them to be sensed by hearing; speech; one of the four valid sources of knowledge according to Nyāya philosophy: testimony that is authentic and truthful. Sacred texts and realized masters have verbal authority; their words are shabda.

shabdendriya. The auditory pathways of hearing, including the ears as the related sense organs.

Shad Darshan. The six major schools of Indian thought, consisting of Sānkhya, Nyāya, Vaisheshika, Mīmāmsa, Vedānta and Yoga; these philosophies are incorporated and applied in Āyurveda.

shakti. Energy; the divine creative will; power, strength.

shalākā. Various kinds of rods or bluntly tapered instruments used to give stronger stimulation to a marma point, especially used in pīdana and agni karma therapies.

shamana. Therapeutic techniques that involve gently palliating the doshas in patients for whom intensive cleansing therapies are contraindicated.

shīta. Cold quality; associated with numbness, unconsciousness, contraction, fear and insensitivity in the body. Slows digestion and reduces immunity.

shīta vīrya. Cooling energy of a substance.

shilājit. A naturally occurring mineral resin used in Āyurvedic treatment.

shirodhāra. A therapy in which a warm stream of oil is poured continuously over the patient's third eye and forehead.

Shiva. The third in the Hindu trinity of gods: the destroyer; Infinite Consciousness; who transforms ego into bliss.

shiva granthi. The pineal gland.

shivarandhra. A small opening located at the posterior fontanel of the cranium bone and connected to sushumnā nādī; it is said that the consciousness of a yogi leaves the body at death through this opening.

shlakshna. Smooth quality; brings lubrication, flexibility and ease of movement to the body.

shleshma. Another name for kapha; the root of shleshma means "to hug." It is the nature of kapha molecules to hug together and create a compact mass.

shodhana. Cleansing therapies including the process of pañchakarma.

shukra. Male reproductive tissue, one of the seven bodily tissues; the word shukra also refers to the orgasmic fluid secreted by a woman.

shukra vaha srotas. The channel carrying nutrients for shukra dhātu, or male reproductive tissue. The roots or governors of this channel are the testicles and the nipples, the pathway includes the vas deferens, epididymis, prostate, urethra, and urinogenital tract, and the mouth is the urethral opening.

siddhi. The result or benefit of any yogāsana, meditation or endeavor; success; skill; supernatural power.

sirā. Blood vessels, veins; any tubular structure.

sirā granthi. Dilation, growth, swelling; one of the three general categories of sroto dushti.

smruti. Memory; one of the faculties of buddhi, or intellect.

snāyu. Tendons, sinews, ligaments, flat muscles.

snehana. The process of internal and external oil application that precedes and accompanies pañchakarma; snehana softens the tissues, helping them to let go of deep-seated toxins, doshas and emotional stresses.

snigdha. Oily quality; oiliness; unctuous; associated with nourishment, relaxation, smoothness, moisture, lubrication, love, compassion and vigor; increases pitta and kapha and decreases vāta.

soma. The subtlest essence of ojas; cosmic plasma; lunar energy; the most subtle form of matter; the food of cells and RNA/DNA molecules, which becomes consciousness.

sparsha. Touch; the tanmātrā relating to air element; the subtle quality of the air element that exists in objects, allowing them to be sensed by touch; one of the causes of suffering according to Buddhism; in this sense it means contact of objects with the senses.

sparshendriya. The faculty of tactile perception, including the skin as the related sense organ.

srotāmsi. The plural form of the word srotas, bodily channel.

srotas. Pathway; a subtle or gross channel made up of dhātus (tissues) that carries substances or energies from place to place in the body; one of the innumerable special systems in the body. Each channel has a root, which is a governing organ or area of the body, a pathway and an opening or outlet. Examples of srotāmsi (the plural form of srotas) are the gastrointestinal tract and the veins and arteries.

sroto agni. The fire component of a specific bodily srotas (channel). Located in the root of the srotas, it maintains the function of that channel.

sroto mārga. That portion of a specific srotas that is between the opening and the root, the entire tract of the srotas.

sroto mūla. The root, origin, or governor of a particular srotas.

sroto mukha. The opening, end, or "mouth" of a particular srotas.

stanya. Lactation; the superior by-product of rasa dhātu.

stanya vaha srotas. The channels carrying breast milk.

sthāna samsraya. Lodging or deposition; the fourth stage of the Āyurvedic model of pathogenesis (see "samprāpti"), the stage in which the aggravated dosha deposits into a weakened tissue or space in the body.

sthira. Static or stable quality; stability, promotes stability and support, associated with all supportive structures in the body, also with fixity, obstructiveness, constipation, stubbornness and lack of flexibility; increases kapha and decreases vata and pitta.

sthūla. Gross quality, grossness; associated with obstruction, obesity and substances like meat and cheese. The gross quality increases kapha and decreases vāta and pitta.

sukha. Literally: "good space," a word for health, often translated as happiness.

Sushruta. Literally "well-heard," or one who is versed in Vedas; Sushruta is the name of the author of the Sushruta Samhitā, one of the main three authoritative texts on Āyurveda.

sushumnā. The central channel for prāna currents in the body, sushumna carries kundalinī shakti from the base of the spine to the crown center, passing through all seven chakras; it is located in between the īdā and pingalā nādīs.

sūchi bharana. The insertion of needles at marma points, equivalent to the Chinese practice of acupuncture.

sūkshma. Subtle quality; associated with any subtle thing, including cells, thoughts, emotions, etc.

sūrya. The sun; solar energy that maintains life along with soma (lunar energy) and anila (cosmic prāna).

sūtra. A small, easily memorized phrase or aphorism that contains a great deal of knowledge and awakens the intuition. A sūtra is analogous to the seed of a tree, which contains within itself all the forms of the tree in its stages of growth.

svādhishthāna. The second chakra, located in the pelvic cavity; the seat of self-esteem, courage and self-confidence; where vital energy meets the vital organs; associated with prāna maya kosha, or the body of life-force.

sveda. Sweat.

sveda agni. The fire component of the organs and structures related to the excretion of sweat. It regulates body temperature, maintains the moisture, softness, oiliness and acid-alkaline (pH) balance of the skin, and helps govern the water-electrolyte balance in the body.

svedana. Sudation; the use of heat to loosen toxins, doshas and emotional stress from the deep tissues and encourage them to move into the gastrointestinal tract where they can be removed by cleansing procedures.

sveda vaha srotas. The bodily channels that carry sweat; this channel is governed by the sweat glands, it continues through the sweat ducts and opens at the pores of the skin.

T

tālu. The soft palate; one of the roots of ambu vaha srotas.

tada. A unit of measurement equivalent to 12 anguli used to locate marma points.

tamas. One of the three universal gunas or qualities of consciousness (along with sattva and rajas), tamas gives rise to the five elements and the tanmātrā (subtle qualities of the elements) in Sānkhya Philosophy. It is the principle of inertia and is responsible for sleep, heaviness, slowness, unconsciousness and decay. When it predominates in the mind, it brings ignorance, laziness, violence and inertness.

tanmātrā. Sound, touch, form, taste and smell; the objects of perception; the subtlest energy of the five elements, through which the gross elements are evolved.

tanmātrā chikitsā. Therapies that involve the five sensory faculties and act on a more subtle, mental or emotional level.

tantra. A spiritual path utilizing a set of demanding practices that require great discipline, strength and understanding.

tapasyā. Austerity, discipline, that which heats up and burns one's karmas.

tarpaka kapha. One of the five kapha subtypes. Associated with the white matter of the brain and the cerebrospinal fluid, it forms the protective and nourishing membranes and fluids of the nervous system. Tarpaka kapha is the film on which all experience, emotions, and knowledge are recorded in the form of memory.

taruna asthi. Cartilage.

tejas. The subtle essence of fire (agni) and pitta dosha, tejas governs digestion on both subtle and gross levels; the energy of intelligence, discrimination and of all bodily fire;

gives luminosity, brightness, brilliance, enthusiasm, passion; solar energy.

tīkshna. Sharp quality; associated with concentration, understanding, discrimination, appreciation and comprehension.

tikta. Bitter taste; made up of air and ether, it increases vāta dosha, and pacifies pitta and kapha.

tikta ghrita. Bitter ghee (clarified butter with bitter herbs).

trasana. A therapy that involves dry massage in which a brush or stone is rubbed against the skin, creating a gentle friction. Trasana enhances circulation and releases stagnant Qi or prāna. Equivalent to the Chinese practice of plum blossoming.

tridoshic. A word to describe something that affects or involves all three doshas, either in a beneficial or detrimental way.

tvacha. Skin; one of the superior by-products of māmsa dhātu.

U

udāna vāyu. One of the five subtypes of vāta dosha; the upward moving energy, it mainly moves through the diaphragm, lungs, bronchi, trachea and throat. It governs exhalation and is responsible for speech, expression and any action that requires effort. It also stimulates memory and helps a person rise from confusion, attachment, depression and other daunting experiences.

udvāhana. Upward movement; a function of udāna vāyu.

upadhātu. The superior by-product that results from the formation of a dhātu.

Upanishad. The later, higher teachings of the Vedas; implies sitting in the vicinity of an enlightened one and listening to him or her without any doubt, delusion, or comparison. The entire teaching of vedānta is upanishad.

Upa-vedas. Secondary or subordinate Vedas. Āyurveda is an upa-veda.

ushna. Hot quality; stimulates gastric fire, improving circulation, digestion, absorption and assimilation. Promotes cleansing, expansion, anger and irritability.

ushna vīrya. Heating energy of a substance.

V

vāta. One of the three doshas, vāta is associated with ether and air elements. It governs all movements and activities in the body.

vāyu. Air element, the second of the five basic elements; wind; another name for vāta.

vaigunya. Literally: lack of good qualities; defective; impairment.

vamana. Therapeutic vomiting, one of the five cleansing procedures of pañchakarma, it clears the stomach and especially deals with excessive kapha dosha.

vasā. Subcutaneous fat; one of the superior by-products of māmsa dhātu.

veda. Knowledge; teaching; also the name of the ancient scriptures of India.

veshtana. A therapy that involves applying firm steady pressure, often by binding the area with a cloth. The binding action is antagonistic to the mobile quality of vāta dosha that is responsible for creating cramps, spasms, tremors and pain.

vibhu. Universal.

vīrya. The energy or potency of a substance; the secondary action of an ingested substance, experienced after taste; two primary kinds: hot or cold.

vijñānamaya kosha. The sheath made of wisdom, knowledge, or cognition.

vikruti. Unnatural, imbalanced, or modified state; the current state of the individual, as opposed to prakruti, the original state of the constitution; a state of the body and mind in which the individual is more prone to disease.

vimārga gamanam. False passage; something passing through the wrong channel; one of the three general categories of sroto dushti.

vipāka. The final post-digestive effect of food that occurs in the colon and has an action on the excreta: urine, feces and sweat. Vipāka is described as sweet, sour, or pungent.

virechana. Purgation; one of the five important cleansing procedures used in pañchakarma, it eliminates excess pitta via the small intestine using purgative herbs.

vishāda. Confusion or deep grief.

vishada. Clear quality, associated with clarity, understanding, communication, cleansing.

Vishnu. The supreme all-pervading lord; the second in the Hindu trinity of gods: the preserver, whose qualities are knowledge, strength, power, virility and splendor; cosmic prāna, which is present in the atmosphere and protects global life.

vishuddhi. The fifth chakra, located at the throat; related to the thyroid and parathyroid glands; associated with communication, will and the vijñāna maya kosha.

vrukka. Kidney; one of the openings of ambu vaha srotas. (Vrukkau is the plural of vrukka.)

vrushana. Testicles.

vyāna. The subtype of vāta dosha that is primarily located in the heart and circulates all over the body. It is responsible for pulsation and circulation of venous blood and lymph fluid, and it maintains cardiac activity and oxygenation of cells, tissues, and organ systems, through the circulation of nutrients. Also responsible for all reflex actions and the movement of the joints and skeletal muscles through the reflex arc.

vyakti. Manifestation; the manifested universe; also, the 5th stage of pathogenesis during which the cardinal signs and symptoms of a disease manifest.

Y

Yajurveda. One of the four main Vedas, this is a collection of sacred ceremonies and rituals.

yakrut. The liver.

yama. The first limb of Pātañjali's eight limbed Yoga system; restraints or abstentions including non-violence, non-lying, non-misuse of sex energy, non-possessiveness; these restraints have the purpose of bringing the Yogi into a harmonious relationship with Nature and with all beings.

yantra. A mystical or astronomical diagram used for the worship of a deity; the āsana, or seat of the deity into which that deity can be invited and established for worship.

yogāsana. The third limb of Pātañjali's eight limbed Yoga system; the means of bringing awareness, stability and ease to the body through the use of physical postures and mūdrās for the purpose of supporting meditation.

Yoga. One of the six philosophies; the science expounded by celebrated sage Pātañjali including the practical means of uniting the higher and lower self and merging with cosmic consciousness through a gradual unfolding of inner strength and wisdom.

Yoga Sūtras (of Pātañjali). The garland of sūtras expounding the science of yoga.

yogi. One who practices yoga; a blissful or enlightened one.

yoni. Vagina.

Chinese Glossary

ashi points. Tender points that are painful to the touch and not a major acupoint located on the 14 principal meridians.

bi syndrome. Pain or blockage that is due to stagnant qi or blood in meridians, different types of "bi" related to heat, cold, wind, damp.

cun. Form of measurement for locating acupoints. One cun is considered to be the width of the patient's thumb.

De. Individual's unique nature or constitution that is expressed as a predominance of one of the five elements.

Eight Principles. Used to categorize disease and imbalance through 4 pairs of opposites: interior and exterior, deficiency and excess, hot and cold and yin and yang.

gu qi. Energy that is received from food.

jin ye. Body fluids that are subdivided into thin and thick fluids. One of the 5 vital substances.

jing. Essence that is inherited from the parents at birth. One of the 5 vital substances.

jing luo. Meridians and collaterals that are pathways through which energy flows.

moxibustion. Herbal heat therapy over an acupoint or meridian to reduce pain, unblock stagnation and eliminate cold and wind.

pericardium. The protective structure for the heart that is more susceptible to pathogenic influence.

Pernicious Influences. 6 pathogens that create disease are wind, dryness, summer-heat, fire, cold and damp.

qi. Energy, life force, flows within the body through channels called meridians. One of the 5 vital substances.

Qigong. Practice of cultivating energy either internally or externally for healing purpose.

qing qi. Energy of air.

rebellious qi. Energy that is flowing in the opposite direction of normal movement in the body, counterflow. Manifests as coughing, wheezing, hiccupping, acid reflux, etc.

san jiao. Also known as triple burner or triple heater that is divided into upper jiao, middle jiao and lower jiao. An energetic system of water regulation that includes the synergistic influence of many organs.

shen. Spirit that resides in the heart and is governed by that organ. One of the 5 vital substances.

shu points (5). Located on each of the 12 primary channels where the energy intensifies as it flows from point to point. Originate at the extremities and terminate at the elbows or knees. These points are named jing-well, ying-spring, shu-stream, jing-river and he-sea.

stagnation. Interrupted flow of qi or blood in the body that can occur at specific meridians.

tai ji. Means supreme ultimate. Image or symbol for yin and yang polarities contained into one.

Tao. Supreme Oneness that is undifferentiated potential. Also known as Wu-void.

TCM. Abbreviation for Traditional Chinese Medicine that includes the subsets of acupuncture, acupressure, moxibustion, Chinese herbs, tui na (massage) qigong (energy work), tai chi (therapeutic exercise) and diet and lifestyle.

wei qi. Immunity or protective energy.

Wu. Cosmic undifferentiated unity that is the void or emptiness from which all things arise. Also known as the Tao.

Wu Xing. 5 elements, also known as 5 movements or 5 principles of transformation, includes fire, earth, metal, water and wood.

xie qi. Pathogens that affect immunity and create imbalance in the body.

xue. Blood. One of the 5 vital substances.

yang. Exists in relation to it's polarity yin and symbolizes masculine aspects of nature.

yin. Exists in relation to it's polarity yang and symbolizes feminine aspects of nature.

ying qi. Nutritional energy.

yuan qi. Source energy, ancestral energy that is inherited from the parents at birth.

zang fu. 12 principal organs subdivided under yin or yang predominance. Yin organs include Heart, Pericardium, Lung, Liver, Spleen and Kidney. Yang organs are Large Intestine, Small Intestine, Stomach, Bladder, Gallbladder and Sanjiao.

zong qi. Energy of chest that circulates in the upper Jiao.

Medical Glossary

adenoids. Lymphoid tissue in the nasopharynx, also called pharyngeal tonsils.

adhesive capsulitis. An inflammatory thickening of the joint capsule limiting range of motion in the joint. When this affects the shoulder joint, it is commonly known as frozen shoulder.

adrenal insufficiency or hypocortisolism. Under-activity of the adrenal glands resulting in decreased production of corticosteroid hormones.

allergic rhinitis. A common type of allergic reaction to air-borne particles like pollens, molds and dusts that results in sneezing, an itchy, runny or congested nose and itchy eyes.

amenorrhea. Absence of menses.

anemia. A condition in which the number of red blood cells circulating or the amount of hemoglobin is less than normal. Hemoglobin is the protein in the blood that carries oxygen.

angina pectoris. Severe pain in the chest due to decreased blood supply to the heart muscle, resulting from coronary artery disease.

anhidrosis. Diminished or complete absence of sweating.

anorexia. Loss of appetite.

anosmia. Loss of the sense of smell.

arrhythmia. Abnormal heart rhythms such as bradycardia (slow heart rate) and tachycardia (fast heart rate).

Attention Deficit Hyperactive Disorder (ADHD). Child-hood disorder characterized by poor attention span and hyperactivity.

autoimmune disorders. Disorders involving immune reactions in which abnormal antibodies are produced that attack the body's own tissues.

Bell's palsy. Weakness of muscles on one side of the face due to facial nerve paralysis.

bipolar disorder. Psychiatric illness characterized by manic or manic and depressive episodes.

brachial plexopathy. Disorder involving the brachial plexus, which is a network of nerves that supply the shoulder, upper extremity, upper back and chest.

bradycardia. Abnormally slow heart rate (less than 60 heart beats per minute).

bronchodilatation. Dilatation of the bronchial passage. This is necessary to relieve the symptoms of asthma.

bronchospasm. An abnormal narrowing and partial obstruction of the bronchi due to spasms of the peribron-chial smooth muscle. Occurs in asthma and bronchitis.

bursitis. Inflammation of the bursa. A bursa is a sac or cavity found in connective tissue, usually in the vicinity of joints, lined with synovial membrane and containing fluid, synovia.

carpal tunnel syndrome. Compression of the median nerve at the wrist resulting in tingling, numbness and weakness of the hand.

cerebral ischemia. Decreased blood supply to the brain.

cerebral malaria. Complication of malaria involving the brain.

cerebrospinal fluid (CSF). Nourishing and protecting fluid that bathes the brain and spinal cord.

cerebrovascular accident (CVA). Cerebrovascular conditions that have either ischemic or hemorrhagic lesions, resulting in critical decrease of blood supply to the brain tissue. Commonly known as a stroke.

cervical spondylosis. Degenerative arthritis of the cervical spine.

cervicitis. Inflammation of the cervix.

chronic fatigue syndrome. An illness characterized by inca-pacitating fatigue. May be accompanied by low grade fever and swelling of the lymph nodes.

chronic obstructive pulmonary disease (COPD). A disorder that decreases the ability of the lungs to perform ventilation. Is associated with chronic bronchitis and emphysema resulting in chronic obstruction of the airways.

conjunctivitis. Inflammation of the conjunctiva, a mucus membrane covering the surface of the eyeball and the inner surface of the lid.

coronary artery disease. A condition in which fatty plaques are deposited in the walls of the coronary arteries. These arteries supply the heart muscle and critical obstruction of them results in myocardial infarction (heart attack).

costochondritis. Inflammation of the costal cartilage(s) characterized by pain and tenderness locally. This cartilage is present at the junction of the rib and sternum. (Tietze Syn-drome)

cystitis. Inflammation of the urinary bladder.

degenerative joint disease (DJD). Arthritis involving the joints.

diverticulosis. Presence of a number of diverticula, small herniations in the lining of the colon.

dysentery. Frequent watery stools that may be accompa-nied by blood or mucus and marked by inflammation of the mucous membrane.

dysmenorrhea. Difficult and painful menstruation.

dysphagia. Inability to swallow or difficulty in swallowing.

edema. An abnormal accumulation of fluid, most commonly seen in the legs. It is present in conditions such as congestive heart failure or renal failure.

enuresis. Involuntary discharge of urine.

epicondylitis. Inflammation and degeneration of the attachments of the muscle to the elbow. Commonly referred to as golfer's elbow (medial epicondylitis) and tennis elbow (lateral epicondylitis).

epididymitis. Inflammation of the epididymis. The epididy-mis is a part of the male genitalia that is a reservoir of sperm.

epilepsy. Disorder of cerebral function characterized by sud-den, brief attacks of altered consciousness, motor activity or sensory phenomena. Convulsive seizures are the most com-mon form of attack.

epistaxis. Nosebleed.

fissures (anal). A linear ulcer on the margin of the anus.

flatulence. Excessive amount of gas in the intestines.

gastritis. Inflammation of the stomach mucosal lining.

gastroesophageal reflux disease (GERD). A disorder thought to be due to a reflux of gastric or intestinal contents into the lower esophagus. This results in damage to the esophageal mucus lining.

glaucoma. Disorder characterized by increased intraocular pressure of the eye resulting in difficulty with vision and possibly blindness.

goiter. An enlargement of the thyroid gland.

hemorrhoids. Painful dilation of the hemorrhoidal veins, both external and internal, in the anal region.

hernia. Abnormal protrusion of an organ or part of an organ through the wall of the cavity that normally contains it.

hydrocele. An accumulation of fluid within the testis.

hyperthyroidism. An abnormal condition of the thyroid gland associated with elevated secretion of thyroxine.

hypothyroidism. An abnormal condition of the thyroid gland associated with deficient thyroid secretion.

hypoxia. An oxygen deficiency.

incontinence. Inability to restrain the discharge of excretions such as urine or feces.

inflammatory bowel disease. Chronic disorders characterized by inflammation of the intestinal wall. It can result in recurring abdominal cramps and diarrhea. The two main types are Crohn's disease and ulcerative colitis.

insomnia. Prolonged or abnormal inability to sleep.

iritis. Inflammation of the iris.

irritable bowel syndrome (IBS). A condition where the motility of the gastrointestinal tract is affected, resulting in abdominal pain, constipation or diarrhea.

keratitis. Inflammation of the cornea.

leukorrhea. Vaginal discharge that is characterized as white or yellowish in color.

lymphadenopathy. Any disease process affecting a lymph node(s). Cervical lymph nodes are those located in the neck region and axillary lymph nodes those in the armpits.

lymphedema. An abnormal increase of tissue fluid (potential lymph) in the interstitial spaces.

mastitis. Inflammation of the breast.

Ménière's disease. A condition involving recurrent attacks of vertigo, hearing loss and tinnitus.

meningitis. Inflammation of the membranes of the brain or spinal cord.

migraine. A severe headache occurring periodically and possibly accompanied by nausea, vomiting, vertigo or photophobia. Ophthalmic migraines are a type of migraine where the extraocular muscles of the eyes are affected.

myalgia. Tenderness or pain in the muscle.

myocardial infarction (MI). A medical emergency where blood supply to the heart is critically restricted. This results in death of the heart muscle. It is commonly referred to as a heart attack.

nasal polyp. Mass of tissue that develops within the nasal mucus membranes.

neuropathy. Any disease of the nerves. Can be due to injury (focal neuropathy) or a disease process (peripheral neuropathy), for example, diabetes. Symptoms can include tingling, numbness, pain and/or weakness.

night blindness. A disorder in which vision is affected at nighttime.

oophoritis. Inflammation of an ovary.

optic neuritis. Inflammation of the optic nerve.

orchitis. Inflammation of the testis.

otitis media. Inflammation of the middle ear.

palpitations. A condition in which the pulsations of the heart become faster than normal or irregular. The patient may perceive this as a "pounding" in the chest.

paresthesia. A sensation of numbness, prickling or tingling. Most commonly occurs due to nerve damage in conditions like neuropathy.

parotitis. An Inflammation of the parotid gland that commonly occurs in mumps.

pelvic inflammatory disease (PID). Infection of the uterus, fallopian tubes and contiguous pelvic structures that is not associated with surgery or pregnancy.

peptic ulcer disease. An ulcer created by the erosive action of digestive juices on the lining of the duodenum (duodenal ulcer) or stomach (gastric ulcer).

pericardial effusion. Fluid in the pericardial cavity.

Peripheral Neuropathy – See neuropathy..

peripheral vascular disease (PVD). A condition in which there is narrowing of the arteries and veins of the extremities leading to decreased blood flow.

photophobia. Sensitivity to light.

pleural effusion. An accumulation of fluid in the thoracic cavity surrounding the lungs.

postural hypotension. A reduction in blood pressure when a person goes from supine position to sitting or standing posture.

prolapse. A falling or dropping down of an organ or internal part, especially at a natural or artificial orifice. For example, a prolapsed uterus or bladder prolapse.

prostatitis. Inflammation of the prostate.

ptosis. A condition in which there is drooping of an organ or a part, such as an eyelid due to paralysis of the oculomotor nerve (third cranial nerve).

pyloric stenosis. Narrowing of the pyloric canal, which is the distal-most part of the stomach connecting to the duodenum.

quadriplegia. Paralysis of all four limbs.

radiculopathy. Disorder of the spinal nerve roots, commonly referred to as a pinched nerve. When this affects the nerve roots in the lumbosacral area, it is commonly referred to as sciatica.

renal colic. Excruciating pain originating in the kidneys and toward the thigh, often due to the presence of a stone (renal calculi).

retention of urine. Incomplete emptying of the bladder often due to a neurological condition such as spinal cord injury and diabetic polyneuropathy but with many other causes as well.

scleritis. Inflammation of the sclera.

sinusitis. Inflammation of the mucus membrane of a sinus, which are air cavities in the facial skeleton around the nose.

spasticity. An increase in muscle tone or contractions of muscles causing stiff or awkward movements. Commonly seen in neurological disorders such as strokes, traumatic brain injury and spinal cord injury.

spermatorrhea. An involuntary discharge of semen without orgasm.

stroke. see Cerebrovascular accident.

syncope. Transient loss of consciousness caused by diminished cerebral blood flow.

tachycardia. Rapid beating of the heart (over 100 beats per minute).

tendonitis. Inflammation of a tendon. Commonly affected tendons include rotator cuff and biceps tendons in the shoulder and patellar tendon in the knee.

tinnitus. Subjective ringing in the ears.

TMJ pain. Pain resulting from dysfunction in the temporo-mandibular joint(s). This joint is present on each side of the jaw.

trigeminal neuralgia. A disorder of the trigeminal nerve, which supplies sensation to the face. This results in severe pain.

ulcerative colitis. A chronic disease of the large intestine characterized by inflammation and ulceration. Symptoms may include abdominal cramps, bloody diarrhea and fever.

urethritis. Inflammation of the urethra.

vertigo. A sensation of one's self moving or spinning or of the surrounding objects moving or spinning. Commonly referred to as dizziness.

Bibliography and References

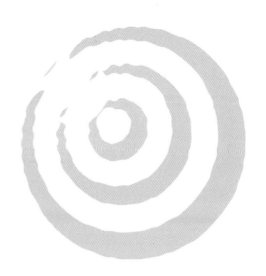

Āyurveda Texts

Bhishagratna, Kaviraj Kunjalal, editor-translator. *Sushruta Samhita.* 4th ed., 2 vols. Chowkhamba Sanskrit Series Office: Varanasi, India, 1991

Johari, Harish. *Chakras: Energy Centers of Transformation.* Inner Traditions India: 1987.

Lad, Vasant. *The Complete Book of Ayurvedic Home Remedies.* New York: Harmony Books 1998.

Lad, Vasant. *Secrets of the Pulse.* Albuquerque: The Ayurvedic Press 1996.

Lad, Vasant. *Textbook of Ayurveda: Fundamental Principles.* Albuquerque: The Ayurvedic Press 2002.

Shankaracharaya, H.H. Adi., author. Chinmayananda, H.H. Swami, commentary. *Atma Bodha.* Bombay: Central Cinmaya Mission Trust 1999.

Sharma, Priyavrat V. editor-translator. *Caraka Samhita.* 4 vols. Chowkhamba Sanskrit Series Office: Varanasi, India, 1981–1994.

Svoboda, Robert and Lade, Arnie. *Tao and Dharma: Chinese Medicine and Ayurveda.* Lotus Press: Twin Lakes, 1995.

Thatte, D.G. *Acupuncture, Marmas, and other Asian Therapeutic Techniques.* Chaukambha Oriental Publishers: Delhi, 1988.

Tigunait, Pandit Rajmani, Ph.D. *Seven Systems of Indian Philosophy,* Honesdale: Himalayan Institute Press, 1984.

Vagbhata. *Ashtanga Hridayam,* translated by K. R. Srikantha Murthy. 2 vols. Krishnadas Academy: Varanasi, India, 1991–1992.

Western Medical Texts

Descartes, Renee. *The Passions of the Soul.* Charles Scribner's Sons from Descartes Selections, edited by Ralph M. Eaton, 1927. Article 31–35.

Harrison's Principles of Internal Medicine. McGraw-Hill, Inc: 1991.

Berkow, Robert. Editor-in-chief. *Merck's Manual of Medical Information.* Pocket Books, 1997.

Ganong, William F. *Review of Medical Physiology.* Appleton and Lange: 1995.

Martini, Frederic H. and Timmons, Micheal J. *Human Anatomy.* Prentice Hall: Englewood Cliffs, 1995.

Moore, Keith L. *Clinically Oriented Anatomy.* Williams and Wilkins: 1992.

Oliver, Marcelo V. *Rapid Review: Anatomy Reference Guide.* Anatomical Chart Company: Skokie, 1996.

Stedman's Medical Dictionary. Lippincott Williams and Wilkins: 2000.

Traditional Chinese Medicine Texts

Deadman, Peter and Al-Khafaji, Mazin with Baker, Kevin. *A Manual of Acupuncture.* Journal of Chinese Medicine Publications: England, 1998.

Cheng, X.N. ed. *Chinese Acupuncture and Moxibustion.* Foreign Languages Press: Beijing, 1987.

Feng, G.F. and J. English. *Lao Tsu – Tao Te Ching.* Random House: New York, 1972.

Jarrett, Lonny S. *Nourishing Destiny: The Inner Tradition of Chinese Medicine.* Spirit Path Press: Stockbridge, 1988.

Maciocia, Giovanni. *The Foundations of Chinese Medicine: A Comprehensive Text for Acupuncturists and Herbalists.* Churchill Livingstone: London, 1989.

O'Connor, John and Bensky, Dan. *Acupuncture: A Comprehensive Text.* Eastland Press: Seattle, 1981.

Stux, G. and Pomeranz B. *Acupuncture: Textbook and Atlas.* Berlin: Springer-Verlag 1987.

Tyme. *Student Manual on the Fundamentals of Traditional Oriental Medicine.* Living Earth Enterprises: San Diego, 1997.

Tzu, Lao, translated by John C. H. Wu, *Tao Teh Ching.* Boston: Shambhala 1990.

Acknowledgments

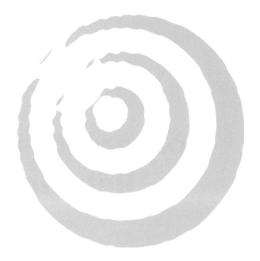

Vasant Lad

The author would like to acknowledge those whose dedication and insight brought the knowledge of Āyurveda to the world, especially his teachers who lovingly showed the way and shared their knowledge and experience.

He would also like to express his gratitude to the following people, without whose contributions this book would not exist: to his family for their love, patience and support during the writing of this book. To Wynn Werner, Laura Humphreys and the Ayurvedic Institute staff for their help with the original outline, the various drafts and for raising important points during this process. To Anisha Durve, for being my student, attending our school and being inspired by this and her acupuncture education to come to me with the idea of sharing the combined knowledge of these two great healing traditions. To Yvonne Walston for her creative talents in combining art and science. Her illustrations bring authenticity to this ancient wisdom.

Anisha Durve

My heartfelt thanks to everyone who has assisted at every level in the making of this work:

My parents, for giving me their blessings to always pursue higher knowledge and the inspiration to always follow my dreams. My sisters, Anuja and Namita, for their constant encouragement and patience. Special thanks to Anuja for her zealous commitment to review the manuscript at every stage of the work.

Dr. Vasant Lad, for his grace in accepting me as a student and his blessing to let our marma project bloom into a wonderful book. I have been deeply touched and inspired by Dr. Lad's mastery of Ayurveda and all related topics, his eloquence as a speaker, his amusing and refreshing sense of humor, and his humility as a healer.

Sonam Tarjee, for his time and expertise to edit sections on Traditional Chinese Medicine. Gillian Ehrlich, for her enthusiasm and commitment to review parts of the manuscript when I needed a fresh perspective. My acupuncture teachers, Dr. Qijian Ye and the late Lynsay Tunnell, for taking the time to offer advice on Traditional Chinese Medicine material.

Wynn Werner, Michele Schulz and the staff at the Ayurvedic Institute for their support. Chitra Giaque and the late Betheyla for their insights into the chapter on yoga. Yvonne Walston for her wonderful illustrations that bring the book to life.

Laura Humphreys, Project Manager

My thanks go to the technical readers who helped make this text more rounded and complete at several stages of the process, especially Jaisri Lambert, who has such a long-standing background in marma therapy, and Danielle Dorman, who gave us her gentle guidance. Barbara Cook provided us with excellent Sanskrit advice. Michele Schulz did excellent work on the yoga photos, interacted skillfully with so many people in the various phases of the project and kept me organized during the most challenging steps. Sonia Masocco gave us her expert advice on the aromatherapy chapter. Claudia Welch, DOM, helped me to place the points correctly on the illustrations. Yvonne Walston, illustrator, worked beautifully with Dr. Lad and Anisha Durve to bring forth their vision. And my gratitude goes to Jack Forem, who worked with Dr. Lad to give the manuscript the final polish that makes it shine so brightly today.

Credits

Yoga photos are © 2014 The Ayurvedic Institute, all rights reserved. Yoga photography by Chris Harris, thinkharris.com.

Photos listed here are © iStockphoto.com/ page 221, Terriana, page 221 alexluengo, page 221 leonello, page 221 Eraxion, page 221 AgnieszkaS; page 222 alexluengo, page 222 leonello, page 223 luchschen, page 223 (2) Eraxion; page 224 angelhell; page 226 alexluengo, page 226 leonello; page 227 janulla, page 227 alexluengo, page 227 Eraxion; page 228 (2) Eraxion.

Photos listed here are © 123rf.com/ page 223 and 225 by alila.

Illustrations on pages 58 and 60 are © 1994, 2014 The Ayurvedic Press, all rights reserved. Photo page 225 from *Atlas and Textbook of Human Anatomy Volume III*, Sobotta, Johannes.

All other illustrations are by Yvonne Wiley Walston, CMI, © 2008, 2014 Creative Imagery Inc.

Index

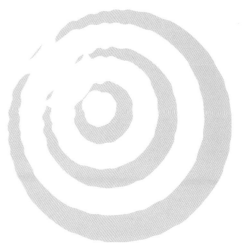

A

āhāra rasa, 221
Ājñā chakra, 29, 258, 259
Ājñā marma, 22, 89
ākāsha (space element), 10, 251
    marmāni regions associated with, 21
    compared to TCM elements, 38
Ākāshīya srotas, 51
ākruti parīkshā, 41
ālasya, 63
ālochaka pitta, 12, 21
āma (toxins), **62–64**, 150, 240
    detoxifying, 20
    pain associated with, 44
    symptoms of, 63
Āmāshaya marma, 149
ānandamaya kosha (bliss body), 27
āpas (water element), 11, 21, 251
ārtava dhātu, 14, 43, 254
    disturbances of, marmāni for, 237
    marmāni of, tissue disturbances of, 63
ārtava vaha srotas, 220
    disturbances of, treating, 226–227
    nādīs and organs associated with, 51
    systems associated with, 255
āsanas (yoga postures), 20, 31, **239–240**
    health benefits of, 241
    for kapha dosha, 247–250
    for pitta dosha, 245–246
    relationship to marmāni, 241–242
    for vāta dosha, 242–244
ātman, 40
Āyurveda, **1**, **7–9**
    channels in, 45, 50–52
    dhātus of. See dhātus
    diagnosis in, 19, 41–42
    doshas of. See doshas
    elements of, 9–11, 251
    etiology, 40, 57–58, 62

    health, definition of, 40
    limitations of, 2
    pain, types of, 43, 44
    pathogenesis. See samprāpti
    philosophy embraced by, 7
abdomen
    distention of, 147, 148, 150, 153, 154, 155, **235**
    pain in, 145, 147, 149, 150, 155, **232**, **233**
    pain in lower region of, 152, 153, 154
    pain in upper left quadrant of, 148
    pain in upper region of, 146
    pain in upper right quadrant of, 147
abhyanga (oil massage), 20
abhyantara mārga, 60, 61
abscesses, 84, 86
abscesses, breast, 142, 144, 173
abstinences (yama), **239**, 241
accumulation stage (sañchaya), 59
acidity, high, 91, 172
acupoints, TCM
    classification of, 52, 55
    compared to marmāni, 52–53
    illustrations of, 266
    marmāni corresponding to, 18, 297–298
    measurement units for locating, 53
    mechanism of action, 18
    See also specific acupoints
acupuncture, TCM, compared to marma chikitsā, 42, 71
Adhah Ganda marma, 104
Adhah Skandha marma, 172
adhesive capsulitis (frozen shoulder), 136, 170, 171, 172, 173
Adhipati marma, 82
Adhomukha Svānāsana (Downward Facing Dog Pose), 248
adipose tissue. See meda dhātu
adrenal disorders, **234**
    insufficiency, 150, 163
    pain, 163
    stress, 97
aggressiveness, 100

Index

agitation, 73
agni (digestive fire), **62**
    kindling with shamana, 66
    low, 150
    qualities of, 62
    stimulation of, 20
    See also fire element
agni karma (heat application), 19, 73
    equivalent to, in TCM, 71
    See also moxibustion
Agra Patra marma, 70, 141
ahamkāra, 7, 8, 25, 32, 219
ahimsā, 73
air element (vāyu), 10, 251
    compared to TCM elements, 38
    marmāni regions associated with, 21
    and sparsha, 9
air, energy of (qing qi), TCM, 33
Akshaka marma, 127
alambusha nādī, 51
allergies, 100, 105
    eye reactions to, 97
    itching caused by, 96
    rhinitis caused by, 97, 102
ambu vaha srotas, 220
    disturbances of, treating, 221
    systems associated with, 255
amenorrhea, 155
Amsa marma, 171
Amsa Phalaka marma, 160
Anāhata chakra, 29, 258, 259
ancestral energy (yuan qi), TCM, 33
anemia, 148, 150
anger, 100, 236
angina, 73, 126, 127, 138, 140, 161, 188
anguli, 53
Angushtha Mūla marma, 180
anhidrosis (lack of sweating), 173
Ānī marma, 175
anila mūdhata, 63
animal chakras, 29
ankle pain, 203, 204
anna vaha srotas, 220
    disturbances of, treating, 221
    systems associated with, 255
annamaya kosha (physical or food body), 27
anorexia, 141, 146, 149, 150, **235**
anosmia, 102, 105
antahkarana, 219
Antar Amsa marmāni, 161
Antara Vartma marma, 97
anterior cranial fossa conditions, 84
anu (cell, or individual mind), 26, 51
anu vaha srotas, 51
anxiety, 92, 97, 130, 188, 236
apāna vāyu, 12, 21, 27
Apānga marma, 70, 96

apakti, 63
apara ojas, 151
Apastambha marma, 70, 137
appetite, poor, 110, 149
apunarbhava chikitsā, 65, 66
Ardha Matsyendrāsana (Half Spinal Twist), 247
Ardha Nāvāsana (Half Boat Pose), 245
arms
    massage for, 189
    pain in, **232**, **233**
    See also elbow; forearm
aromatherapy (gandha chikitsā), 18, 69, 211
arrhythmia, 124, 125, 126, 127, 137, 138, 140, 141, 184, **235**
arterial circulation disorders, 234
arteries (dhamanī), 51
artha (wealth and material comfort), 239
arthritis, 73, 203, 204, 206
    hand, 180, 181, 182, 183, 184, 185, **236**
    hip, 194, 195, 198
    index finger, 187
    knee, 194, 198, 199, 200
aruchi, 63
asafoetida paste, 73
ashi points, TCM, 53
Ashrū Agra marma, 94
Ashrū Antara marma, 94
Ashrū Madhya marma, 94
ashtānga yoga, 239
Ashtavidhā Parīkshā, 41
asthi dhātu, 14, 43, 254
    disturbances of, marmāni for, 237
    marmāni of, tissue disturbances of, 63
asthi vaha srotas, 220
    disturbances of, treating, 225
    systems associated with, 255
asthma, 82, 101, 102, 103, 105, 120, 123, 124, 128, 136, 138, 140, 141, 145, 160, 161, 170, 171, 172, 187, 199, **235**
    acute, 232
    bronchial, 137
ati pravrutti, 63
atrial fibrillation and flutter, 161
attachment, 236
attars, 211
attention deficit hyperactive disorder (ADHD), 82, 84, 86, 89, 107, 130, 131, 184, **238**
atyanu srotas, 51
aum sound, 9
auric fields (koshas), **27**, 29
austerities (yama), **239**, 241
avalambaka kapha, 14, 21
avyākta, 7, 37
awareness
    enhancing, 20
    pure, 29
    Sahasrāra chakra for, 29, 258, 259
axillary lymph adenopathy, 173

Ayurvedic Cooking for Self-Healing (Lad, Usha and Lad, Dr. Vasant), 67

B

Bāhū Indrabasta marma, 176
Bāhū Ūrvī marma, 174
Bāhya Kūrpara marma, 179
bāhya mārga, 60, 61
Bāhya Manibandha marma, 181
Bāhya Vartma marma, 97
back
    lower, pain in, 131, 163, 164, 165, 166, 193, 198, 199, **232, 233**
    massage of, 167
    pain in, 160
    upper, pain in, 161, 170, **233**
Baihui acupoint (GV 20), 82
Balāsana (Child's Pose), 250
bala bhramsha, 63
basti, 44, 65
    netra, 95
Basti marma, 22, 66, 152
bed wetting (enuresis), 152, 153, 154, 164
Bell's palsy (facial paralysis), 91, 105, 106, 107, 108, 110, 132, **232, 233**
bhūta agni, 62
Bhaga marma, 66, 153
bhakti, 12, 87, 129, 213
bheda (differentiation stage), 40, 60
bhrājaka pitta, 13, 21
Bhrūh Agra marma, 92
Bhrūh Antara marma, 92
Bhrūh Madhya marma, 92
Bhujangāsana (Cobra Pose), 243
bhūta agni, 66, 147, 181
bi (pain), TCM, 42, 44
bicipital tendonitis, 170, 171
big bang theory, 9
bīja mantra, 67, 70
bile, stagnant, 147, 150
Binao acupoint (LI 14), 172
binding (veshtana), 72
Bitong acupoint, 104
BL 1 (Jingming acupoint), 95, 97
BL 10 (Tianzhu acupoint), 118
BL 13 (Feishu acupoint), 161
BL 14 (Jueyin Shu acupoint), 161
BL 15 (Xinshu acupoint), 161
BL 2 (Zanzhu acupoint), 92, 94
BL 21 (Weishu acupoint), 163
BL 26 (Guanyuanshu acupoint), 164
BL 31 (Shangliao acupoint), 165
BL 35 (Huiyang acupoint), 166
BL 36 (Chengfu acupoint), 193
BL 37 (Yinmen acupoint), 198

BL 40 (Weizhong acupoint), 199
BL 56 (Chengjin acupoint), 202
BL 62 (Shenmai acupoint), 203
bladder
    disorders of, **234**
    functions of, in TCM, 36
    pain in, 152, 164, 165, 204
    stones in, 175
    See also urination
bleeding, recurrent, 118
bliss body (ānandamaya kosha), 27
bliss, Sahasrāra chakra for, 29, 258, 259
blood
    and acupoints, in TCM, 55
    and channels, in TCM, 46, 48
    and pain, in TCM, 42, 46
    relationship to qi, 38, 41
blood (rakta), 38
    See also rakta dhātu
blood pressure
    high, 118, 125, 126, 155, 195, **234**
    low, 125, 126, **234**
bloodletting
    in TCM, 74
bloodletting (rakta moksha), **74**
blurry vision, 118
bodhaka kapha, 13, 21
bodily tissues. See dhātus
body/mind medicine, 26
bone marrow. See majjā dhātu
bone. See asthi dhātu
Bow Pose (Dhanurāsana), 245
brachial plexopathy, 136, 173
bradycardia, 138
Brahmā (deity), 87
brahmī oil, 211, 212, 215
Brahma (avyākta), 7, 37
Brahmarandhra marma, 22, 70, 84–85, 87
breasts
    abscesses, 142, 144, 173
    cysts, 142, 144
    disorders of, general, **235**
    fibrocystic changes in, 136, 142, 144, 173
    lactation, insufficient, 142, 143, 144, 146
    mastitis, 142, 173
    painful or tender, 142, 144, 173
    swelling in, 173
    tissue of, congestion in, 138, 142, 144, 173
breath awareness
    branch of yoga. See prānāyāma
    for practitioner of marma chikitsā, 74
breath body (prānamaya kosha), 27
breathing problems
    asthma. See asthma
    breathlessness, 102, 105
    difficulty breathing, 99, 100, 102, 103, 104, 123, 124, 127, 128, 138, 140, 160, 162, 185

shortness of breath, 136, 137, 161, 170, 187, 205
Bridge Pose (Setu Bandha Sarvāngāsana), 246
bronchial asthma, 137
bronchial congestion, 105
bronchitis, 101, 136, 137, 160, 170, 171, 172
Bruhatī marma, 162
buddhi, 32, 219
buddhi (intellect), 8, 25
Bulang acupoint (KD 22), 138, 142
Burong acupoint (ST 19), 146
bursitis, 136, 170, 171, 172

C

C1 (Huatuojiaji extra points), 118
C2 (Huatuojiaji extra points), 120
C3-C6 (Huatuojiaji extra points), 121
Camel Pose (Ustrāsana), 246
camphor oil, 66, 211, 212, 215
camphor paste, 73
cardiac dysfunction, 195, **235**
    arrhythmia, 124, 125, 126, 127, 137, 138, 140, 141,
        184, 235
    pain, 73, 161, **232**, **233**
    See also angina; palpitations
cardinal symptoms (rūpa), 59
carpal tunnel syndrome, 175, 176, 182, 184, 185, **236**
cells
    awareness and intelligence of, 8, 20
    communication between, 8, 19
    created by kapha, 13
    elements' relationship to, 9
    identity of, 7
    immunity of, 20
    memory of, 62
    metabolism of, 20
    See also anu
cerebral circulation disorders, 234
cerebral ischemia, 107
cerebrovascular accident (CVA), 82, 84, 86, **232**, **233**
cervical dysfunction, 99, 101, 166, **235**
    cervical lymph adenopathy, 125, 126, 127, 131
    cervical lymph node, enlargement of, 121
    pain, 108
cervical spondylosis, 86, 118, 122
chakras, **28–29**
    connection to marmāni, 29
    healing and balancing for, 259
    koshas related to, 29
    marmāni associated with, 29
    properties of, 258
    See also specific chakras
chakshusha nādī, 51
chala, 8
chamomile oil, 212, 215
champa attar, 212, 216

chandan. See sandalwood, 212
channels, **45–52**
    in Āyurveda, 45, 50–52
    in TCM, 45, 46–48
    See also srotāmsi
Charana marmāni, 200
Chengfu acupoint (BL 36), 193
Chengjiang acupoint (CV 24), 108
Chengjin acupoint (BL 56), 202
Chengqi acupoint (ST 1), 97
chest
    energy of (zong qi), TCM, 33
    pain in, 137, 145, 184
    pain in, non-cardiac, 138
Chest/Knee Pose (Pāvanmuktāsana), 243
Chibuka marma, 110
chikitsā (treatment), 65
    See also marma chikitsā
Child's Pose (Balāsana), 250
chitakash, 28
chitta, 25, 32, 219
chromotherapy, **18**, 68, 260
chronic fatigue syndrome, 148, 150, 174, **234**
chronic obstructive pulmonary disease (COPD), 235
Chuchuka marma, 143
cinnamon oil, 212, 215
circulatory conditions, **234**
    poor circulation, 136, 172, 174, 195, 198, 199, 200, 202,
        204
    poor circulation, in lower extremities, 155
clarity, Vishuddhi chakra for, 29, 258, 259
cleansing (shodhana), 65–66
clinical examination, methods of, 41
clove oil, 212, 215
Cobra Pose (Bhujangāsana), 243
coccyx, pain at, 166, 193
cognitive organs, 8
coitus, painful, 153, 154
cold, 207
cold feet, 155
cold hands, 136
colitis, 91
colon dysfunction, 91, 103, 204, **234**
    descending, toxins in, 116
    pain, 106
    toxins in, 121, 150
    See also constipation; diarrhea; flatulence
color blindness, 95
color vision, poor, 96
colors, therapy based on, **18**, 68, 260
coma, 107
Commentary, 175
communication between cells. See prāna
communication, Vishuddhi chakra for, 29, 258, 259
competitive behavior, 100
complications stage (bheda), 40, 60
concentration (dhārana), 239, **240**

concentration, poor, 82, 89, 107, 184, **238**

confusion, 82, 125

consciousness

equilibrated (samādhi), 7, 241

spiritual. See prāna

unbounded, pure (Puruṣha), 7, 37

constipation, 147, 148, 149, 150, 164, 174, 176, 187, 193, 194, 202, 204, **235**

constitution (de), TCM, 39

constitution, in Āyurveda. See prakruti

convulsions, 232

cooking, Āyurvedic, book about, 67

cooling and heating energy (vīrya), 211, 212

coronary artery disease, 235

Corpse Pose (Shavāsana), 250

cosmic intelligence (Mahad), 7, 8, **25–27**

cosmic unity, 37

cough

chronic, 123, 124, 136, 137, 138, 140, 145, 160, 161, 187

dry, 232

Cow Pose (Gomukhāsana), 248

creation

big bang theory, 9

Sānkhya's description of, 7, 8

sound's role in, 9

TCM's description of, 33–36

See also elements, Sānkhya

creativity (Prakruti), 7, 8

cremasteric reflex, testing in paralyzed male patients, 195

Crohn's disease, 176, 202

crown chakra (Sahasrāra), 29, 258, 259

cun, TCM, 53

cupping, TCM, 74

CV 11 (Jianli acupoint), 149

CV 12 (Zhongwan acupoint), 149

CV 15 (Jiuwei acupoint), 141

CV 18 (Yutang acupoint), 140

CV 2 (Qugu acupoint), 153

CV 21 (Xuanji acupoint), 128

CV 22 (Tiantu acupoint), 124

CV 23 (Lianquan acupoint), 123

CV 24 (Chengjiang acupoint), 108

CV 4 (Guanyuan acupoint), 152

CV 5 (Shimen acupoint), 152

CV 8 (Shenque acupoint), 150

cystitis, 152, 163, 165, 175, 198, 204

cysts, breast, 142, 144

D

Dabao acupoint (SP 21), 144

Dadun acupoint (LR 1), 205

Daling acupoint (PC 7), 182

darshana, 28

darshanam (visual examination), 41

dashamūla oil, 86, 138, 148, 182, 195

dashamūla paste, 73

Dazhui acupoint (GV 14), 122

de (constitution), TCM, 39

death by injuries to marmāni, 17

deep connective tissue massage (mardana), 72

deep, dry pressure (pīdana), 72

defective space (khavaigunya), 60, 62

degenerative joint disease (DJD), 170

degrees of vitality for marmāni, 22

dental problems. See temporomandibular joint (TMJ) pain; toothaches

deodara oil, 212, 215

deposition stage (sthāna samshraya), 40, 59

depression, 125, 160, 236

descending colon, toxins in, 116

desires, positive, fulfillment of (kāma), 239

detoxification (shodhana), 65–66

deviated nasal septum, 89

dhārana, 52, 239, **240**

dhātu agni, 62, 225

dhātus (bodily tissues), **14**, 254

āma affecting, 63

disturbances of, marmāni for, 19, 237

relationship to srotāmsi, 219

dhamanī (arteries), 51

Dhanurāsana (Bow Pose), 245

dharma (righteous duty), 239

dhī, 25

dhruti, 25

dhyāna (meditation), 239, **240**

for practitioner of marma chikitsā, 74

methods of, 31

diagnosis

in Āyurveda, 19, 41–42

in TCM, 41, 42

diaphragm, congestion in, 136

diarrhea, 147, 148, 149, 164, 176, 187, 202, **232**, **235**

Dicang acupoint (ST 4), 110

dietary choices, as causes of disease, 58

dietary therapy, 68

differentiation stage (bheda), 40, 60

digestion

impaired, 150

indigestion, 97, 116, 142

post-effect of (vipāka), 211

weak, 110, **235**

See also agni (digestive fire)

dīnāchārya, 66

Diji acupoint (SP 8), 202

disease. See diagnosis; etiology; pathogenesis

disequilibrium, 116, 118

disorientation, 82

diverticulosis, 174, **235**

divine chakras, 29

Divine Mother (Prakruti), 7

dizziness. See vertigo

DJD (degenerative joint disease), 170
doshas, **11–14**
　agni diminished by, 62
　balancing postures specific to, 242–249
　cleansing (shodhana), 66
　compared to TCM elements, 39
　compared to yin and yang, 38
　emotions associated with, 30, 32
　imbalances of, marma therapy for, 19
　marmāni regions associated with, 21
　pacifying with shamana, 66
　pain types associated with, 44
　stages of disease manifested in, 59
　tridoshic balancing postures, 249
Downward Facing Dog Pose (Adhomukha Svānāsana), 248
drig parīkshā, 41
drowsiness, 82
dual doshic prakruti, 14
duality, 37
duhkha, 67
duodenal ulcer, 91, 141
duty, righteous (dharma), 239
dysmenorrhea, 150, 152, 153, 154, 155, 196, 202
dysphagia (difficulty swallowing), 123, 124, 125, 126

E

ear apex point, 131
ear disorders, 106, **233**
　earaches, 130, 131, 132
　middle ear infection, 120
　tinnitus. See tinnitus
earth element (pruthivī), 11, 251
　and gandha, 9
　marmāni regions associated with, 21
earth element, TCM, 263
edema, 73, 155, 203, 204
　of lower extremities, 163, 194, 195, 198, 199, 200, 202,
　　236
　of upper extremities, 236
ego (ahamkāra), 7, 8
Eight Great Marmāni, 22
ejaculation, premature, 182, 196
elbow
　pain in, 175, 178, 179, **232, 233**
　restricted movement of, 178, 179
elements, Sānkhya, **9–11**, 251
　compared to TCM elements, 38
　marmāni regions associated with, 21
elements, TCM (Wu Xing), 33, 36, 263
　compared to doshas, 39
　compared to Sānkhya elements, 38
Elevated Lotus Pose (Ūrdhva Padmāsana), 244
emotional disturbances, 82, 84, 86, 88, 91, 99, 108, 123,
　124, 125, 127, 128, 137, 138, 140, 141, 147, 148, 149,
　161, 163, 172, 176, 180, 182, 184, 202, 203, **236**

aggressiveness, 100
anger, 100
anxiety, 92, 97
competitive behavior, 100
suppressed emotions, 92
emotions, **29–31**
　balancing, 20
　doshas associated with, 30, 32
　leading to disease, 41
　marmāni associated with, 30, 31
　organs associated with, 30, 31, 41
　processing of, 30
　suppression of, 30
　touch accessing, 25
　See also manomaya kosha (mental body)
emphysema, 102, 105
Empty Bowl Meditation, 75
energy
　elements representing types of, 9
　pathways of. See nādīs
　See also tejas; vīrya
　vital life force in TCM. See qi, TCM
　vortexes of. See chakras
energy points. See acupoints; marmāni
enlightenment, 29
　See also Sahasrāra chakra
enuresis (bed wetting), 152, 153, 154, 164
environmental components of imbalance, 57
envy, 236
epicondylitis, 175, 178, 179
epididymis, 198
epigastric pain, 146, 147, 148, 149, **232, 233**
epilepsy, 233
epistaxis (nosebleeds), 82, 100, 102, 103, 104, 105, 107,
　118, **232**
equilibrated consciousness. (samādhi), 7, 241
essence (Jing), TCM
essences, vital. See ojas; prāna; tejas
essential oils, 69, 211
　actions of, 215
　heating or cooling properties of, 212
estrogen, decreased, 153
ether element. See space element
etiology, 40–41, 57–58, 62
eucalyptus oil, 212, 215
examination, methods of, 41
Extra Vital Marmāni, 22
eyelids
　drooping, 92
　lower, puffiness of, 96, 97
　twitching or fluttering of, 97
eyes
　allergic reactions of, 97
　disorders of, general, 91, **233**
　examination of, 41
　eye strain, 89, 95, 96, 127
　hyperacidity of, 95

irritation of, 88, 92, 95
pain in, 127
pressure behind, 92
tearing (lacrimation), excessive, 95, 96, 97
See also glaucoma

F

facial massage, 111–112
facial paralysis (Bell's palsy), 91, 105, 106, 107, 108, 110, 132, **233**
fainting, 116, 125
fallopian tube disorders, 154
fatigue
  mental, 170, 171
  physical, 128
fear, 236
feces, examination of, 41
feelings. See emotions
feet, 207
  cold, 155, 203, 204
  massage of, 208
  pain or tenderness in, 204, 206, 207, **233**
  swelling of, 204
Feishu acupoint (BL 13), 161
Fengfu acupoint (GV 16), 116
Fengshi acupoint (GB 31), 194
fetus, Mūrdhni marma affecting, 83
fever, 232, 234
fibrocystic changes in breasts, 136, 142, 144, 173
fibroid tumors, 152
fields of action, 211
fire element, **10**, 251
  and rūpa, 9
  marmāni regions associated with, 21
  See also agni; tejas
fire element, TCM, 36, 263
first aid therapy (sadyah phaladai chikitsā), 67, 231, 232
Fish Pose (Matsyāsana), 246
fissures
  rectal, 166
Five Element Therapy (Tanmātrā Chikitsā), 211
five elements. See elements, Sānkhya; elements, TCM
flatulence, 174, 176, 187, 195, 202, 204
food or physical body (annamaya kosha), 27
food, energy of (gu qi), 33
forearm
  decreased circulation in, 179
  pain in, 136, 172, 175, 178, 179
Forward Bend Pose (Paschimottānāsana), 244
four goals of life (purushārthas), 239
frontal headaches, 84, 88, 92, 94, 95, 99, 232
Fujie acupoint (SP 14), 150
Full Boat Pose (Paripūrna Nāvāsana), 248
Futu acupoint (LI 18), 126

G

gallbladder
  dysfunction of, 127, 146, 147, 150, **234**
  functions of, in TCM, 36
gallstones, 91
gandha (smell element), 9
  aromatherapy using, 69
  as earth element, 9
gandha chikitsā (aromatherapy), 18, 69, 211
gandhari nādī, 51
Ganesha (deity), 170, 205, 213
garlic paste, 73
gastric dysfunction, 174
gastritis, 91, 140, 141, 172, **235**
gastroesophageal reflux disease (GERD), 91, 123, 124, 128, 140, 141, 146, 149, **235**
gastrointestinal disturbances, 235
gaurava, 63
GB 1 (Tongziliao acupoint), 96, 97
GB 12 (Wangu acupoint), 132
GB 21 (Jianjing acupoint), 170
GB 27 (Wushu acupoint), 155
GB 31 (Fengshi acupoint), 194
GB 34 (Yanglingquan acupoint), 200
genetic predisposition, 62
genital disorders, 194
genitourinary disorders, 235
GERD. See gastroesophageal reflux disease
gharshana, 73
ginger paste, 73
glandular disturbances, 234
glaucoma, 89, 92, 95, 96, 97, 99
gluteal region, pain in, 193
goals of life (purushārthas), 239
goiter, 123, 124, 125, 126, 128
Gomukhāsana (Cow Pose), 248
"great qualities" (maha gunas), 37
greed, 236
grief, 103, 104, 105, 120, 160
Grīvā marma, 121, 22
gross elements (pañcha mahābhūta), 9
ground (universal) mind (vibhu), 26
gu qi, TCM, 33
Guanyuan acupoint (CV 4), 152
Guanyuanshu acupoint (BL 26), 164
Guda marma, 22
guggulu paste, 73
Guilai acupoint (ST 29), 154
Gulpha marmāni, 203
gunas
  of doshas, 11
  maha gunas ("great qualities"), 37
  of Prakruti, 7, 37
GV 14 (Dazhui acupoint), 122
GV 15 (Yamen acupoint), 118

Index

GV 16 (Fengfu acupoint), 116
GV 19 (Houding acupoint), 86
GV 2 (Yaoshu acupoint), 166
GV 20 (Baihui acupoint), 82
GV 22 (Xinhui acupoint), 84
GV 24 (Shenting acupoint), 88
GV 25 (Suliao acupoint), 101
GV 26 (Renzhong acupoint), 107

H

Halāsana (Plow Pose), 244
Half Boat Pose (Ardha Nāvāsana), 245
Half Spinal Twist (Ardha Matsyendrāsana), 247
hands
  arthritis in, 180, 181, 182, 183, 184, 185, **236**
  cold, 172, 174
  massage for, 189
  neuropathy in, 180
  pain in, 180
  tremors of, 136
Hanu marma, 108
haridra (turmeric) paste, 73
Hasta Kshipra marma, 186
hastajihva nādī, 51
hatred, 30, 68, 236
head massage, 111–112, 133
Head Stand (Shīrshāsana), 243
Head To Knee Pose (Jānu Shīrshāsana), 245
Head To Knee Pose (Paschimottānāsana), 244
headaches, 82, 84, 86, 88, 91, 96, 107, 108, 186, 207, **232**
  frontal, 92, 232
  occipital, 116, 118, 120, 121, 170, **232**
  ophthalmic, **232**
  periorbital, 130, 132
  related to cervical spondylosis, 118
  sinus, 73, 92, 103, 104, 180, 186, **232**
  suboccipital, 132
  temporal, 130, 232
  tension, 120
  vertex, 205
health
  definition of, in Āyurveda, 40
  definition of, in TCM, 40
hearing, poor, 132
  See also ears
heart
  Anāhata chakra for, 29, 258, 259
  disorders of, general, 138, **234**
  functions of, in TCM, 36
  See also cardiac dysfunction
heat application (agni karma), 73
heat therapy (svedana), 72
heat, excess, 186
heating or cooling energy (vīrya), 211, 212
Heding acupoint, 199

heel, pain in, 206
Hegu acupoint (LI 4), 180
hemorrhoids, 101, 108, 166, 182, 183, 202, **235**
hepatic dysfunction, 150
hepatic pain, 162
hernia, 82, 154
He-Sea point, 53
hiccups, 84, 123, 124, 127, 128, 137, 141, 145, 170
Hidden Lotus Pose (Supta Padmāsana), 246
hina attar, 212, 213, 215
hina paste, 73
Hinduism, trinity in, marmāni corresponding to, 87
hing (asafoetida) paste, 73
hip
  arthritis of, 194, 195, 198
  pain in, 155, 194, **232**, **233**
hoarseness of voice, 123, 232
holding (veshtana), 72
Holy Basil oil, 212, 214, 217
hormonal imbalance, 82, 89, 108, 205, **235**
Houding acupoint (GV 19), 86
Hrid marmāni, 138
Hridayam marma, 22, 140
HT 1 (Jiquan acupoint), 173
HT 2 (Qingling acupoint), 174
HT 3 (Shaohai acupoint), 176
HT 9 (Shaochong acupoint), 188
HTJJ. See Huatuojiaji extra points
Huatuojiaji extra points (C1), 118
Huatuojiaji extra points (C2), 120
Huatuojiaji extra points (C3-C6), 121
Huatuojiaji extra points (L5), 164
Huatuojiaji extra points (T12), 163
Huatuojiaji extra points (T3-T5), 161
Huatuojiaji extra points, TCM, 264
Huiyang acupoint (BL 35), 166
hyperactivity, 130, 131, 207
hyperglycemia, 174, 207
hypertension, 137
hyperthyroidism, 123, 124, 125, 126, 128
hypocortisolism (adrenal insufficiency), 150, 163
hypoglycemia, 116
hypotension, postural, 116
hypothyroidism, 123, 124, 125, 126, 128
hypoxia, 107

I

I-former (ahamkāra), 7, 8
īdā nādī, 51, 99
imbalance (vikruti), 15, **61–64**, 74
immunity
  disorders of, general, 150, **234**
  low, 128, 148, 185, **234**
  See also prīnana; wei qi, 52
impotence, 153, 154, 165, 166, 198

incisors, lower, pain in, 108
incontinence, 152
index finger, pain, swelling or arthritis in, 187
indigestion, 97, 116, 142
individual mind (anu), 26, 51
Indrabasta marmāni, 202
infections, 73
inflammation, 73
inflammatory bowel disease, 176, 202, **235**
inguinal hernia, 82, 154
inherited energy (yuan qi), TCM, 33
injuries to marmāni, 17, 22
insight, Ājñā chakra for, 29, 258, 259
insomnia, 73, 82, 84, 86, 88, 89, 92, 94, 161, 170, 205, 207, 236, **238**
intellect (buddhi), 8, 25
intelligence
    cosmic (Mahad), 7, 8, **25–27**
    flow of. See prāna
intercostal pain, 145, 146, 162
interscapular pain, 160, 170
intracranial pressure, 84, 86, 116
intuition, Ājñā chakra for, 29, 258, 259
irritable bowel syndrome (IBS), 150, 176, 202, **235**
irritation (trasana), 73

J

jāthara agni, 62, 66, 149, 174, 225
jīvātman, 151
Jānu marmāni, 199
Jānu Shīrshāsana (Head To Knee Pose), 245
jasmine oil, 212, 213, 215
jatamāmsī oil, 212, 213, 215
Jatru marma, 66, 128
jealousy, 236
Jianjing acupoint (GB 21), 170
Jianli acupoint (CV 11), 149
Jianyu acupoint (LI 15), 171
jiaos, TCM, 36
Jiexi acupoint (ST 41), 204
jihva, 221
jihva parīkshā, 41
jīvana, 52
Jimen acupoint (SP 11), 198
Jing (essence), TCM, 38
jing luo qi, TCM, 33
jing luo, TCM, 46
Jingming acupoint (BL 1), 95, 97
Jing-River point, 53
Jing-Well point, 53
Jiquan acupoint (HT 1), 173
Jiuwei acupoint (CV 15), 141
judgment, 236
Jueyin Shu acupoint (BL 14), 161
Jyotis, 90, 241

K

kāma (fulfillment of positive desires), 239
kāya chikitsā, 62
kadamba oil, 212, 213, 215
Kaksha marma, 173
Kakshadhara marma, 70, 136
kalāntara prānahara marmāni, 22
Kanīnaka marma, 70, 95
Kanīshthikā marma, 188
Kantha marma, 22, 123
Kanthanādī marma, 124
Kapāla marma, 88
kapha dosha, 13–14
    āsanas for, 247–250
    balancing, marmāni for, 236
    compared to yin and yang, 38
    congestion associated with, 73
    essential oils for, 211
    marmāni regions associated with, 21
    pain associated with, 44
    stages of disease manifested in, 59
Kapola Madhya marma, 106
Kapola Nāsā marma, 105
Karna Ūrdhva marma, 131
Karnamūla marmāni, 70, 132
Karnapālī marma, 70, 130
Karnapāla marma, 131
Kati marma, 165
KD 1 (Yongquan acupoint), 207
KD 22 (Bulang acupoint), 138, 142
KD 23 (Shenfeng acupoint), 138
KD 24 (Lingxu acupoint), 138
KD 25 (Shencang acupoint), 137
KD 5 (Shuiquan acupoint), 203
kewrā attar, 212, 213, 216
khamala, 224
khavaigunya, 60, 62
khus oil, 66, 212, 213, 216
khus paste, 73
kidneys, 163
    dysfunction of, general, 132, 150, 203, **234**
    functions of, in TCM, 36
    infection of, 132
    left, disorders of, 150
    pain in, 145, 164
    right, disorders of, 150
    stones in, 145, 163, 165
    stressed, 97
klama, 63
kledaka kapha, 14, 21
kloma, 221
kloma agni, 62, 174
Knee/Chest Pose (Pāvanmuktāsana), 243
knees
    arthritis of, 194, 198, 199, 200

Index

limited range of motion, 199, 200
    pain in, 194, **232**, **233**
koshas (auric fields), **27**, 29
Krikātikā marma, 120
kuhu nāḍī, 51
Kukundara marma, 164
kundalinī, 28, 50
kundalinī shakti, 28
Kūrcha marma, 185
Kūrcha Shira marma, 183
Kūrpara marma, 178

L

L5 (Huatuojiaji extra points), 164
lacrimation, excessive, 95, 96, 97
lactation, insufficient, 142, 143, 144, 146
Lad, Usha and Dr. Vasant (Ayurvedic Cooking for Self-Healing), 67
Laogong acupoint (PC 8), 184
large intestine, 36
laryngeal congestion, 121, 127, 128
laryngitis, 124, 128
lavender oil, 212, 213, 216
legs
    massage of, 208
    pain in, **232**, **233**
lepa (pastes), 73
lepana (paste application), 52, 72
lethargy, 236
leukorrhea, 154
LI 1 (Shangyang acupoint), 187
LI 11 (Quchi acupoint), 179
LI 12 (Zhouliao acupoint), 179
LI 14 (Binao acupoint), 172
LI 15 (Jianyu acupoint), 171
LI 17 (Tianding acupoint), 126
LI 18 (Futu acupoint), 126
LI 20 (Yingxiang acupoint), 105
LI 4 (Hegu acupoint), 180
LI 5 (Yangxi acupoint), 181
Lianquan acupoint (CV 23), 123
liberation (moksha), 239
libido, low, 153, 154, 165, 166, 182, 194, 196, 198
light-headedness, 207
Lingxu acupoint (KD 24), 138
Lion Pose (Simhāsana), 247
little finger, pain, swelling or arthritis in, 188
liver
    congestion in, 142, 144, 145
    dysfunction of, general, 127, 146, 147, 162, **234**
    functions of, in TCM, 36
    pain in, 118, 145, 180
    stagnation in, 142, 144
    toxins in, 147, 181
Locust Pose (Salabhāsana), 243

Lohitāksha marma, 195
Lohita marma, 155
loneliness, 236
Lotus Pose (Padmāsana), 249
Lotus Pose With Forward Bend (Yoga Mudrā), 244
love, Anāhata chakra for, 29, 258, 259
lower extremities
    edema of, 198, 199, 200, 202, **236**
    neuropathy of, 193, 194, 195, 198, 199, 200, 202, 207, **236**
    pain in, 193, 194, 195, 198, 199, 200, 202, 207
    poor circulation in, 155
LR 1 (Dadun acupoint), 205
LR 10 (Zuwuli acupoint), 195
LR 13 (Zhangmen acupoint), 145
LR 8 (Ququan acupoint), 200
LU 1 (Zhongfu acupoint), 136
LU 10 (Yuji acupoint), 185
LU 11 (Shaoshang acupoint), 186
lumbar radiculopathy (sciatica), 164, 165, 166, 195, 206
lumbosacral radiculopathy (sciatica), 193, 194, 198, 199, 202
lungs
    congestion in, 102, 136, 172
    disorders of, general, **234**
    functions of, in TCM, 36
lymph adenopathy, 162
lymph nodes
    circulation disorders, **234**
    congestion in, 116, 125, 126, 127, 136, 138, 148, 162, 180
    enlarged, 173
    obstruction of, 155
lymphedema, 172, 174, 175, 176

M

māmsa dhātu, 14, 43, 254
    disturbances of, marmāni for, 237
    marmāni of, tissue disturbances of, 63
māmsa vaha srotas, 220
    disturbances of, treating, 224
    systems associated with, 255
mārga, 51
Madhya Vartma marma, 97
madhyama mārga, 60, 61
Mahānārāyana oil, 72
maha gunas ("great qualities"), 37
Mahad (cosmic intelligence), 7, 8, **25–27**
majjā dhātu, 14, **27**, 43, 254
    disturbances of, marmāni for, 237
    marmāni of, tissue disturbances of, 63
majjā vaha srotas, **27**, 220
    disturbances of, treating, 225–226
    systems associated with, 255
Malāshaya marma, 70

Mala Parīkshā, 41
malabsorption, 106
manas, 32, 40
manas (sensory mind), 25
Manibandha marma, 182
manifestation stage (vyakti), 40, 60
Manipūra chakra, 28, 258, 259
mano vaha srotas, **26–27**, 220
    disturbances of, treating, 228–229
    openings for, 27
    systems associated with, 256
manomaya kosha (mental body), 27
Mantha marma, 125
mantra chikitsā (sound therapy), 67, 70
mantraya, 28
Manyāmūla marma, 116
Manyāmani marma, 122
mardana (deep connective tissue massage), 72
marmāni, **17**
    āsanas, relationship to, 241–242
    acupoints compared to, 52–53
    acupoints corresponding to, 18, 297–298
    chakras associated with, 29
    classification of, 53
    communication between, 18
    communication between cells using, 19
    degrees of vitality for, 22
    diagnostic indicators of, 19
    doshas associated with regions of, 21
    Eight Great Marmāni, 22
    elements associated with regions of, 21
    emotions associated with, 30, 31
    history of, 17
    illustrations of, 269–283
    as khavaigunya, 62
    list of, 291–293
    locations of, organization of, 21
    measurement units for locating, 53
    mechanism of action, 18
    meditation on, 31
    mind connected to. See majjā dhātu; mano vaha srotas
    organs associated with, 22
    pain or sensitivity at, 18, 19
    role in samprapti, 61
    sadyah prānahara marmāni, 22
    selecting for treatment, 43, 74
    Special or Extra Vital Marmāni, 22
    srotāmsi associated with, 22
    therapeutic influences of, 19–20
    translations of, 295–296
    See also specific marmāni
marma, 17
marma agni, 62
marma chikitsā, 15, 25
    clinical knowledge required for, 74
    compared to acupuncture, 42
    forms of, 65

    apunarbhava, 66
    rasāyana, 66
    sadyah phaladai, 67
    shamana, 66
    shodhana, 65–66
    tanmātrā, 67–69
    parallels in TCM, 71
    practitioners of, guidelines for, 74–76
    pressure and touch used for, 68, 75–76
    role of, in Āyurveda, 69
    spiritual aspect of, 25
    techniques for, 71–74
marma gata āma, 63
massage
    arms and hands, 189
    back, 167
    back of head, 133
    head and facial, 111–112
    legs and feet, 208
    mardana (deep connective tissue), 72
    neck, 133
    pīdana (deep, dry pressure), 72
    trunk, 156
    tui na, TCM, 71
    veshtana (binding or holding), 72
    whole body, 284–289
mastitis, 142, 173
mastoid infection, 132
material comfort (artha), 239
Matsyāsana (Fish Pose), 246
Mayūrāsana (Peacock Pose), 249
measurements for locating energy points, 53
meda dhātu, 14, 43, 254
    disturbances of, marmāni for, 237
    marmāni of, tissue disturbances of, 63
meda vaha srotas, 220
    disturbances of, treating, 224–225
    systems associated with, 255
Medhra marma, 196
medical systems. See Āyurveda; modern medicine; Traditional Chinese Medicine
meditation (dhyāna), 239, **240**
    for practitioner of marma chikitsā, 74
    methods of, 31
memory, poor, 82, 84, 86, 89, **238**
Ménière's disease, 91, 120
meningitis, 86
menstruation
    cramps caused by, 176, 202
    disorders of, general, **235**
    irregular, 153, 154, 155
    painful. See dysmenorrhea
    PMS, 202
mental body (manomaya kosha), 27
mental disturbances, **238**
meridians, TCM, 45, 46–48
    direction of flow, 48

energy of (jing luo qi or zhi qi), 33
functions of, 46
list of, 48
organs associated with, 48
pathology of, 46
principal, 265
See also channels
metal element, TCM, 36, 38, 263
migraines, 73, 82, 84, 86, 88, 89, 91, 92, 95, 99, 118, 130, 180, 186, 205, 207, **233**
mind
    calming, 20, 31–32
    connections to. See majjā dhātu; mano vaha srotas
    cosmic and individual, 8
    imbalance caused by, 57
    individual (anu), 26, 51
    intellect (buddhi), 8, 25
    sensory (manas), 25
    universal (vibhu), 26
mind/body medicine, 26
mitti attar, 212, 213, 216
modern medicine
    channels in, 45
    limitations of, 2
moha, 63
moksha (liberation), 239
mono-doshic prakruti, 14
motor organs, 8
movement. See vāta dosha
moxibustion, TCM, 19, 71, 73
    See also agni karma
mukta triveni, 50
mumps (parotitis), 106, 131
muscles
    aches, 73
    cramps, 202
    spasticity, rigidity, flaccidity, 82
    twitching, spasms, 73, 82
    See also māmsa dhātu
musta oil, 212, 213, 216
musta paste, 73
mustard oil, 66
Mūlādhāra chakra, **28**, 258
Mūrdhni marma, 70, 82, 87, 22
mūtra parīkshā, 41
mūtra vaha srotas, 220
    disturbances of, treating, 227
    systems associated with, 255
myalgia, 174

N

Nābhi marmāni, 22, 66, 150
nādī parīkshā, 41
nādīs, 18, 45, **50–51**
    compared to srotāmsi, 50

functions of, 52
list of, 51
organs associated with, 51
See also channels
Nāsā Agra marma, 101
Nāsā Madhya marma, 100
Nāsā Mūla marma, 99
Nāsā Puta marma, 102
nasal disorders, **233**
    congestion, 82, 97, 105
    irritation, 101
    polyps, 89
    See also nose; sinus disorders
nasya, 65, 89, 101, 103
nausea, 82, 127, 141, 142, 147, 149, 174, **235**
neck
    decreased range of motion, 120, 122
    massage for, 133
    pain in, 86, 116, 118, 120, 121, 122, 126, 160, 170, **232**, **233**
    stiffness in, 118, 121, 126, 170
needles, puncturing with. See acupuncture; sūchi bharana
nerve, pinched (radiculopathy), 122, 170, 179
nervous system channel. See majjā vaha srotas
nervous tissue. See majjā dhātu
nervousness, 236
netra basti, 95
netra parīkshā, 41
neurological disorders, 233
neuropathy, 136
    of lower extremities, 155, 193, 194, 195, 198, 199, 200, 202, 207, **236**
    of the hand, 180
    of upper extremities, 172, 174, 175, 176, **236**
night blindness, 95, 97
night vision, poor, 96
nirgundi oil, 212, 213, 216
niyama, **239**, 241
nose
    deviated nasal septum, 89
    dryness of, 97
    itching of, 88
    runny, 99
    See also nasal disorders; sinus disorders
nosebleeds (epistaxis), 82, 100, 102, 103, 104, 105, 107, 118, 232
numbness. See paresthesia
nutmeg oil, 66, 212, 214, 216
nutmeg paste, 73
nutrition (prīnanam), 52
nutritive energy (ying qi), 33

O

observances (niyama), **239**, 241
occipital headaches, 86, 88, 116, 118, 120, 121, 170, **232**

oil massage (abhyanga), 20
oil treatment (snehana), 52, 71–72
oils. See essential oils
ojas
    balancing, marmāni for, 236
    compared to Jing, 38
    imbalances of, marma therapy for, 20
    rejuvenation of, 66
oleation (snehana), 52, 71–72
ophthalmic headaches, **232**
oral mucus congestion, 104
"organ clock", TCM, 47
organs
    cleansing, 66
    cognitive organs, 8
    disturbances of, **234**
    dysfunctions of, marma therapy for, 19
    emotions associated with, 30, 31, 41
    energy of, TCM (zang fu qi), 33
    mantras for, 70
    marmāni associated with, 22
    meridians associated with, 48
    motor organs, 8
    nādīs associated with, 51
    srotāmsi associated with, 51
    yin and yang associations with, 35–36
orgasm, premature, 196
Oshtha marma, 107
Otitis Media, 91
ovarian disorders, 153, 154, 165, **235**
ovaries, pain in, 198, 206
ovulation, pain during, 183, 185

P

pāchaka pitta, 13, 21
Pāda Charana marma, 204
Pāda Kshipra marma, 205
Pāda Madhya marma, 207
Pārshnī marma, 206
Pārshva Sandhi marma, 145
Pārvatī (deity), 51, 170
Pātañjali (founder of yoga), 239
Pāvanmuktāsana (Knee/Chest Pose), 243
Padmāsana (Lotus Pose), 249
pain, **232–233**
    in Āyurveda, 43, 44
    comparing Āyurveda and TCM models of, 42–44
    first aid therapy for (sadyah phaladai chikitsā), 67, 231, 232
    relieving, marma therapy for, 20
    in TCM (bi), 42, 44
    See also specific disorders or areas of the body
palliation therapy (shamana), 66
Palm Tree Pose (Tādāsana), 247
palms, heat or sweating of, 184

palpation, diagnosis using, 41
palpitations, 82, 124, 125, 126, 127, 137, 138, 140, 141, 160, 171, 188, **232, 235**
pañcha mahābhūta (gross elements), 9
pañchakarma, **17**, 65
pancreatic dysfunction, 116, 149, 150, 171, 174, 175, **234**
paralysis from stroke, 232
paramātman, 151
parashabdha vaha srotas, 51
parasthesia (tingling or numbness), 120, 122
    of lower extremities, 155
    of upper extremities, 179
parathyroid dysfunction, 121, 122
Paripūrna Nāvāsana (Full Boat Pose), 248
parotitis (mumps), 106, 131
particular (individual) mind (anu), 26, 51
Paschimottānāsana (Forward Bend/Head To Knee Pose), 244
paste application (lepana), 72
pastes (lepa), 73
patchouli oil, 212, 214, 216
pathogenesis
    in Āyurveda. See samprāpti
    in TCM, 40–41
pathogenic energy (xie qi), 33
PC 3 (Quze acupoint), 175, 176
PC 7 (Daling acupoint), 182
PC 8 (Laogong acupoint), 184
Peacock Pose (Mayūrāsana), 249
pelvic disorders, **235**
    pain, 152, 153, 154, 155, **232, 233**
    pelvic floor, disorders of, 166
pelvic inflammatory disease (PID), 152, 153, 154, 155
peppermint oil, 212, 214, 216
peptic ulcer, 91, 140, 141, 146, 149, 150, **235**
perception, 26, 29
perfectionism, 236
pericardial effusion, 137
pericardium
    functions of, in TCM, 36
    pain in, 140
periorbital headaches, 130, 132
peripheral vascular disease (PVD), 155, 195, 198, 199, 200, 202
pharyngeal congestion, 121
pharyngitis, 128
philosophy embraced by Āyurveda, 7
photophobia, 95
physical components of imbalance, 58
physical or food body.(annamaya kosha), 27
pīdana (deep, dry pressure), 72
pinched nerve (radiculopathy), 122, 170, 179
pingalā nādī, 51, 99
pitta dosha, 12–13
    āsanas for, 245–246
    balancing, marmāni for, 236
    compared to yin and yang, 38

Index

essential oils for, 211
marmāni regions associated with, 21
pain associated with, 44, 73
stages of disease manifested in, 59
pituitary dysfunction, 82, 84, 88, 89, 122, 205, **234**
plantar fasciitis, 206
plasma. See kapha dosha; rasa dhātu
pleural effusion, 137
pleuritic pain, 136, 137, 141, 142, 145, 146, 160, 161, **232**, **233**
plexus, injury of, 173
Plīhā marma, 70, 148
Plow Pose (Halāsana), 244
plum blossoming, TCM, 71, 74
PMS, 202
politics, Manipūra chakra for, 28, 258, 259
positive desires, fulfillment of (kāma), 239
possessiveness, 236
post-digestive effect (vipāka), 211
posterior cranial fossa conditions, 86, 116
postnasal drip, 103, 104
postural hypotension, 116
postures. See āsanas
power, Manipūra chakra for, 28, 258, 259
prājñāparādha, 57
prāna, 8, **18**, **25**
balancing, marmāni for, 236
compared to qi, 38
imbalances of, marma therapy for, 20
rejuvenation of, 66
relationship to blood, 38
prāna vāyu, 12, 21, 27
prāna vaha srotas, 50, 220
disturbances of, treating, 220
nādīs and organs associated with, 51
systems associated with, 255
prāna vahini nādīs, 50
prānāchārya, 68
prānāyāma, 20, 31, 239, **240**, 241
prānamaya kosha (breath body), 27
prāno raktānu dhavati, 38
prajanana (procreation), 52
prakopa (provocation stage), 40, 59
prakruti (constitution), **14–15**
compared to de, 39
determining for yourself, 261
duality with purusha, 37
importance of, for treatment, 74, 76
types of, 14
Prakruti (infinite creative potential), 7, 8
prasara (spreading stage), 40, 59
prashanam (questioning), 41
pratyāhāra, 239, **240**
premature ejaculation, 154
pressure used for marma chikitsā, 75–76
prestige, Manipūra chakra for, 28, 258, 259
preventative care, 20

preventive therapy (apunarbhava chikitsā), 66
prīnanam, 52
principal meridians, TCM, 265
procreation (prajanana), 52
procreation, Svādhishthāna chakra for, 28, 258, 259
prodromal symptoms (pūrva rūpa), 59
prostate dysfunction, 99, 101, 153, 154, 166, **235**
prostate, pain in, 206
prostatitis, 108
protective energy (wei qi), 33
provocation stage (prakopa), 59
Prushtha marmāni, 161
pruthivī (earth element), 11, 251
and gandha, 9
marmāni regions associated with, 21
ptosis, 92
pulmonary congestion, 104, 185, 199
pulse diagnosis, 41, 42
pulse diagram, TCM, 265
punarnava paste, 73
purīsha parīkshā, 41
purīsha vaha srotas, 220
disturbances of, treating, 227
nādīs and organs associated with, 51
systems associated with, 255
purity, Vishuddhi chakra for, 29, 258, 259
purushārthas (goals of life), 239
Purusha, 7, 8, 37
pūrana, 52
pūrva rūpa (prodromal symptoms), 59
PVD. See peripheral vascular disease

Q

qi (energy), TCM, 33
compared to prāna, 38
relationship to blood, 38
types of, 33
Qigong, TCM, 46, 68
qing qi, TCM, 33
Qingling acupoint (HT 2), 174
Qishe acupoint (ST 11), 127
Qiuhou acupoint, 97
quantum physics, 17
Quchi acupoint (LI 11), 179
questioning, as form of diagnosis (prashanam), 41
Qugu acupoint (CV 2), 153
Ququan acupoint (LR 8), 200
Quze acupoint (PC 3), 175, 176

R

radiculopathy (pinched nerve), 120, 121, 122, 170, 179
rajas guna, 7, 9, 37
rakta (blood), 38
rakta dhātu, 14, 43, 254

330

disturbances of, marmāni for, 237
marmāni of, tissue disturbances of, 63
rakta moksha, 65
rakta moksha (bloodletting), **74**
rakta vaha srotas, 220
disturbances of, treating, 223–224
systems associated with, 255
rañjaka pitta, 13, 21
rasa (taste element), 9
as water element, 9
dietary therapy using, 68
rasa (taste), 211
rasa dhātu, 14, 43, 254
disturbances of, marmāni for, 237
marmāni of, tissue disturbances of, 63
rasa vaha srotas, 220
disturbances of, treating, 222–223
nādīs and organs associated with, 51
systems associated with, 255
rasāyana (rejuvenation), 20, 66
re bi, TCM, 44
rectal pain, 166
rectal prolapse, 183
red sandalwood paste, 73
rejuvenation (rasāyana), 20, 66
renal colic, 145, 163, 198, 203
renal infections, 163
Renying acupoint (ST 9), 125
Renzhong acupoint (GV 26), 107
reproductive disorders, 235
reproductive tissue
female. See ārtava dhātu
male. See shukra dhātu
respiratory disorders, **235**
See also breathing problems
respiratory infections, recurrent, 128
rhinitis, 97, 100, 102
righteous duty (dharma), 239
rishis, 18
roma rujā, 63
root chakra (Mūlādhāra), **28, 258**
rose oil or attar, 212, 214, 216
rotator cuff tendonitis, 170, 171, 173
rujakara prānahara marmāni, 22
runny nose, 103, 104
rūpa (cardinal symptoms), 59
rūpa (vision element), 9, 68
rūpa vaha srotas, 51
Ruzhong acupoint (ST 17), 143

S

sādhaka pitta, 12, 21
sākshin, 7
See also Purusha
sāma jihvā, 63

Sānkhya philosophy, **7–9**
compared to TCM, 37–39
duality concept in, 37
unity concept in, 37
sacral area, pain in, 166
sacroiliac joint pain, 165, 166
sadness, unresolved, 103, 104, 105
sadyah phaladai chikitsā, 67, 231, 232
sadyah prānahara marmāni, 22, 66
saffron attar, 212, 214, 216
Sahasrāra chakra, 29, 258, 259
Sakthi Ūrvī marmāni, 198
Salabhāsana (Locust Pose), 243
salivation, excess, 106, 108, 110
samādhi, 7, 239, **241**
samāna vāyu, 12, 21
samprāpti (pathogenesis), 15, **40, 57–61**
role of marmāni in, 61
stages of, 58–60
san jiao, TCM, 36
sañchaya (accumulation stage), 40, 59
sandalwood oil, 66, 212, 214, 217
sandalwood paste, 73
sanga, 63
sarasvati nādī, 51
Sarvāngāsana (Shoulder Stand), 246
sarvanga sāda, 63
sattva guna, 7, 8, 37
sciatica, 131, 163, 164, 165, 166, 193, 194, 195, 198, 199, 202, 206, **232, 233**
"science of life". See Āyurveda
science, parallels in Āyurveda
big bang theory, 9
ever-expanding universe, 7
quantum physics, 17
scoliosis, 122
seizures, 82, 84, 107, 186
self-esteem, Svādhishthāna chakra for, 28, 258, 259
self-realization, Sahasrāra chakra for, 29, 258, 259
senses, withdrawal of (pratyāhāra), 239, **240**–240
sensory mind (manas), 25
Setu Bandha Sarvāngāsana (Bridge Pose), 246
sex, Svādhishthāna chakra for, 28, 258, 259
sexual dysfunction, 108, 110, 182, **235**
shabda (sound element), 9
See also mantra chikitsā (sound therapy)
shabda parīkshā, 41
shabda vaha srotas, 51
shaktipat, 28
shalākā, 72
shamana, 66
Shangliao acupoint (BL 31), 165
Shangyang acupoint (LI 1), 187
Shanka marma, 22, 91
shankhini nādī, 51
Shaochong acupoint (HT 9), 188
Shaohai acupoint (HT 3), 176

Index

Shaoshang acupoint (LU 11), 186

Shavāsana (Corpse Pose), 250

Shen (spirit), TCM, 38

Shencang acupoint (KD 25), 137

Shenfeng acupoint (KD 23), 138

Shenmai acupoint (BL 62), 203

Shenque acupoint (CV 8), 150

Shenting acupoint (GV 24), 88

Shīrshāsana (Head Stand), 243

Shimen acupoint (CV 5), 152

shirodhāra, 66, 89

Shiva (deity), 87

Shiva Svarodaya, 51

Shivarandhra marma, 22, 86, 87

shleshaka kapha, 14, 21

shodhana, 65–66

Shoulder Stand (Sarvāngāsana), 246

shoulders
> frozen (adhesive capsulitis), 136, 170, 171, 172, 173
> pain in, 136, 160, 161, 170, 171, 172, 173, **232**, **233**
> stress and tension in, 118

shringa shunthi paste, 73

Shuiquan acupoint (KD 5), 203

shukra dhātu, 14, 43, 254
> disturbances of, marmāni for, 237
> marmāni of, tissue disturbances of, 63

shukra vaha srotas, 220
> disturbances of, treating, 226–227
> nādīs and organs associated with, 51
> systems associated with, 255

Shu-Stream point, 53

SI 11 (Tianzhong acupoint), 160

SI 5 (Yangu acupoint), 183

siddhi, 101

Simhāsana (Lion Pose), 247

sinus disorders, 89
> congestion, 82, 95, 99, 100, 102, 103, 104, 105, 180
> headaches, 73, 92, 103, 104, 180, 186, **232**
> pain, 103, 104
> See also nasal disorders; nose

sirā (veins), 51

sirā granthi, 63

Sirāmantha marma, 126

Sizhucong acupoint (SJ 23), 92, 94

SJ 17 (Yifeng acupoint), 132

SJ 23 (Sizhucong acupoint), 92, 94

Skandadhara marma, 67, 136

skeletal system. See asthi dhātu

sleep problems
> difficulty falling asleep, 99
> drowsiness, 82
> See also insomnia

small intestine
> disorders of, 150, **234**
> functions of, in TCM, 36

smarana, 28

smell element (gandha), 9, 69

smell, diminished sense of (anosmia), 102, 105

smruti, 25

snehana (oleation), 52, 65, 71–72

snoring, 99, 100, 104

So'Hum meditation, 75

Soul, cosmic and individual, 8

sound element (shabda), 9

sound therapy (mantra chikitsā), 67, 70

SP 1 (Yinbai acupoint), 205

SP 11 (Jimen acupoint), 198

SP 14 (Fujie acupoint), 150

SP 21 (Dabao acupoint), 144

SP 8 (Diji acupoint), 202

space element (ākāsha), 10, 251
> compared to TCM elements, 38
> marmāni regions associated with, 21

sparsha (touch element), 9
> as air element, 9
> marma chikitsā using, 68, 75–76

sparsha chikitsā. See marma chikitsā

sparsha parīkshā, 41

sparshana, 28

sparshanam (palpation), 41

Special or Extra Vital Marmāni, 22

speech disorders, 91, 107, 123, 124, 128, **233**

speech, diagnosis using, 41

spermatorrhea, 154

Sphij marma, 193

spirit (Shen), TCM

spiritual absorption (samādhi), 239

spiritual consciousness. See prāna

spiritual value of touch, 25

spleen
> congestion in, 142, 144, 145, 162, 180
> disorders of, general, 127, 148, 150, 162, **234**
> functions of, in TCM, 36
> pain in, 118, 145, 162, 180
> stagnation in, 142, 144

sprains, 73

spreading stage (prasara), 59

srotāmsi, 45, **51–52**, **219–220**, 255
> āma affecting, 63
> dhātus, relationship to, 219
> disturbances of, 19, 220–229
> functions of, 52
> list of, 51
> marmāni associated with, 22
> nādīs compared to, 50
> organs associated with, 51
> See also channels

sroto mārga, 219

sroto mukha, 219

sroto mūla, 219

sroto rodha, 63

ST 1 (Chengqi acupoint), 97

ST 11 (Qishe acupoint), 127

ST 17 (Ruzhong acupoint), 143

ST 19 (Burong acupoint), 146
ST 23 (Taiya acupoint), 150
ST 29 (Guilai acupoint), 154
ST 4 (Dicang acupoint), 110
ST 41 (Jiexi acupoint), 204
ST 9 (Renying acupoint), 125
stages of disease. See pathogenesis
Stanya Mūla marma, 142
Stanya marma, 143
Stanya Pārshva marma, 144
stanya vaha srotas, 220
    disturbances of, treating, 227
    systems associated with, 256
steam therapy (svedana), 72
sthāna samshraya (deposition stage), 40, 59
Sthapanī marma, 89
stomach
    disorders of, **234**
    functions of, in TCM, 36
stools, loose, 106
stress, mental, 88, 89, 92, 94, 95, 99, 108, 120, 122, 130,
    170, 171, 185, 207, **238**
stroke (cerebrovascular accident), 82, 84, 86, **232**, **233**
suboccipital headaches, 132
subtle elements (tanmātrā), 9
sudation (svedana), 72
sukha, 67
Suliao acupoint (GV 25), 100, 101
supraorbital pain, 92, 94, 96
"Supreme Ultimate" (Tai Ji) symbol, TCM, 33, 34
Supreme Yang acupoint, 91
Supta Padmāsana (Hidden Lotus Pose), 246
survival, Mūlādhāra chakra for, **28**, **258**
Sushruta (surgeon), 17, 22
Sushruta Samhitā, 17
sushumnā nādī, 51, 28
sūchi bharana, 71, 73
Sūrya marma, 70, 149
sūtras, 17
Svādhishthāna chakra, 28, 258, 259
sveda vaha srotas, 220
    disturbances of, treating, 228
    systems associated with, 256
svedana, 65
svedana (sudation), 72
swallowing, difficulty in, 123, 124, 125, 126
sweating
    acidic smell to, 173
    excessive, 173
    lack of (anhidrosis), 173
swelling of upper extremities, 172, 174, 175, 176
symptoms, 59
    See also pathogenesis
syncope, 82, 84, 101, 107, **233**

T12 (Huatuojiaji extra points), 163
T3-T5 (Huatuojiaji extra points), 161
Tādāsana (Palm Tree Pose), 247
tachycardia, 138
tada, 54
Tai Ji ("Supreme Ultimate") symbol, TCM, 33, 34
Taiyang acupoint, 91
Taiyi acupoint (ST 23), 150
Tala Hrida marma, 68, 184
tamas guna, 7, 9, 37
tanmātrā (subtle elements), 9, 67–69
tanmātrā chikitsā, 65
Tanmātrā Chikitsā (Five Element Therapy), 211
tanmātrā nādī, 51
Tao Teh Ching, 33
Tao, TCM, 33, 37
tapasyā, 176
Tarjani marma, 187
tarpaka kapha, 13, 21
taste (rasa), 211
taste element (rasa), 9
    as water element, 9
    dietary therapy using, 68
TCM. See Traditional Chinese Medicine
Tea Tree oil, 217
tea tree oil, 212, 214
tearing (lacrimation), excessive, 95, 96, 97
tejas (subtle fire essence), **10**
    balancing, marmāni for, 236
    compared to Shen, 38
    imbalances of, marma therapy for, 20
    rejuvenation of, 66
temperature sensitivity of marmāni, 18
temporal headaches, 130, 232
temporomandibular joint (TMJ) pain, 91, 108, 110, 131,
    132, **232**, **233**
tendonitis, 206
tennis elbow (epicondylitis), 175, 178, 179
tension headaches, 120
tension, emotional, 95, 171, 185
"the 10,000 things", 39
testicles
    disorders of, general, **235**
    pain in, 108, 185, 198
testosterone, decreased, 153
therapeutic influences of marmāni, 19–20
"third eye" (Ājñā chakra), 29, 258, 259
thoughts. See emotions; mind
three treasures, TCM, 38
throat disorders, 233
thrombophlebitis, 155
thumb
    arthritis in, 186
    pain or swelling in, 181, 186

Index

Thunderbolt Pose (Vajrāsana), 242
thyroid disorders, 121, 122, **234**
Tianding acupoint (LI 17), 126
Tiantu acupoint (CV 22), 124
Tianzhong acupoint (SI 11), 160
Tianzhu acupoint (BL 10), 118
tikta ghrita, 110, 147, 166
tingling. See paresthesia
tinnitus, 86, 91, 120, 130, 131, 132, 171
tissue massage (mardana), 72
tissues of the body. See dhātus
TMJ. See temporomandibular joint
tong bi, TCM, 44
tongue diagnosis, 41, 42
Tongziliao acupoint (GB 1), 96, 97
tonsillitis, 124
tonsils, enlarged, 121
toothaches, 91, 104, 106, 107, 108, 110, 132, **232**, **233**
touch element (sparsha), 9
    as air element, 9
    marma chikitsā using, 68, 75–76
touch, diagnosis using, 41
toxins. See āma
Traditional Chinese Medicine (TCM), **1**
    channels in, 45, 46–48
    compared to Sānkhya philosophy, 37–39
    creation model of, 33–36
    diagnosis in, 41, 42
    duality concept in, 37
    elements of. See elements, TCM
    etiology and pathogenesis, 40–41
    health, definition of, 40
    marma chikitsā, parallels to, 71
    pain (bi), types of, 42, 44
    unity concept in, 37
    yin and yang, 33–36, 37, 38, 265
    See also acupoints
trasana (irritation), 71, 73
treatment (chikitsā), 65
    See also marma chikitsā
Tree Pose (Vriksāsana), 247
tremors, 136, 172, 174, 175, 176
trigeminal neuralgia, 91, 106, 107, 108, 110, 132, **233**
Trik marma, 166
trinity in Hinduism, marmāni corresponding to, 87
Triple Burner or Heater (san jiao), 36
triple doshic prakruti, 14
trunk, massage of, 156
tui na, TCM, 71
Tulsi oil, 217
tulsi oil, 212, 214
tumors, 84, 86
turmeric paste, 73

U

udāna vāyu, **12**, 21
udaka vaha srotas, 220, 221
ulcerative colitis, 106, 176, 202
ulcers
    duodenal, 91, 141
    peptic, 91, 140, 141, 146, 149, 150, **235**
ulnar neuropathy, 183
Unduka marma, 70
unity, cosmic, 37
universal mind (vibhu), 26
upadhātu, 219
upper extremities
    edema of, 236
    neuropathy of, **236**
ureteric pain, 164
urethritis, 152, 153, 154, 163, 164
urinary tract disorders, 150, 235
urinary tract infection (UTI), 152, 163
urination
    difficulty with, 153, 154, 203
    dribbling urine, 203
    excess, 232
    frequent, 152, 153, 154, 164, 166
    incontinence, 175, 198, 203
    infections, 150
    pain during, 152
    retention of, 150, 152, 153, 154, 166, 203
    urgency of, 153, 154
urine, examination of, 41
Ustrāsana (Camel Pose), 246
uterine contractions, difficult, 143
uterine pain, 154
UTI (urinary tract infection), 152, 163
Ūrdhva Ganda marma, 103
Ūrdhva Padmāsana (Elevated Lotus Pose), 244
Ūrdhva Skandha marma, 170
Ūrū marmāni, 70, 194

V

vāta dosha, 11–12
    āsanas for, 242–244
    balancing, marmāni for, 236
    compared to yin and yang, 38
    essential oils for, 211
    marmāni regions associated with, 21
    pain associated with, 44, 73
    stages of disease manifested in, 59
vāyu (air element), 10, 251
    compared to TCM elements, 38
    marmāni regions associated with, 21
vacha oil, 66, 212, 214, 217
vaikalyakāra prānahara marmāni, 22
Vajrāsana (Thunderbolt Pose), 242

vamana, 65

Vankri marma, 146

Vankshana marma, 70, 154

varman, 17
    See also marma

veins (sirā), 51

venous circulation disorders, 234

ventricular dysfunction, 160

vertex headaches, 205

vertigo, 82, 84, 86, 91, 107, 116, 118, 125, 126, 130, 131, 132, 180, 186, 199, 207, **232**, **234**

veshtana (binding or holding), 72

vibhu (universal mind), 26

Vidhuram marma, 118

vīrya (heating or cooling energy), 211, 212

vijñānamaya kosha (wisdom body), 27

vikruti (state of imbalance), 15, **61–64**, 74

vimārga gamanam, 63

vipāka (post-digestive effect), 211

virechana, 44, 65

vishalya prānahara marmāni, 22

Vishnu (deity), 87

Vishuddhi chakra, 29, 258, 259

vision
    blurry, 95, 96, 118, 130
    color blindness, 95
    color vision, poor, 96
    diminution of, 95, 96, 97
    disturbances in, 118
    night blindness, 95, 97
    night vision, poor, 96
    poor, 130
    See also glaucoma

vision element (rūpa), 9, 68

visual examination (darshanam), 41

vital essences. See ojas; prāna; tejas

vital substances, TCM, 35

vitality, degrees of, for marmāni, 22

voice, hoarseness of, 123, 124, 125, 126, 232

Void (Wu), TCM, 33, 37

vomiting, 82, 127, 141, 142, 147, 149, 174, **235**

Vriksāsana (Tree Pose), 247

Vrukka marma, 70, 163

Vrushana marma, 22, 70, 197

vyāna vāyu, 12, 21

vyadhi mārga, 60

vyakti (manifestation stage), 40, 60

W

Wangu acupoint (GB 12), 132

water element (āpas), 9, 11, 21, 251

water element, TCM, 36, 263

weakened site (khavaigunya), 60, 62

wealth (artha), 239

wei qi, TCM, 33

Weishu acupoint (BL 21), 163

Weizhong acupoint (BL 40), 199

Western medicine. See modern medicine

wisdom body (vijñānamaya kosha), 27

wood element, TCM, 36, 38, 263

wrist joint, pain or swelling in, 181, 182, 183, 184, 185

wrist pain, 232, 233

Wu (Void), TCM, 33, 37

Wu Xing (five elements), TCM, 33, 36

Wushu acupoint (GB 27), 155

X

xie qi, TCM, 33

xing bi, TCM, 44

Xinhui acupoint (GV 22), 84

Xinshu acupoint (BL 15), 161

Xiyan acupoint, 199

Xuanji acupoint (CV 21), 128

Y

Yakrut marma, 66, 70, 147

yama, **239**, 241

Yamen acupoint (GV 15), 118

yang, TCM. See yin and yang, TCM

Yanglingquan acupoint (GB 34), 200

Yangu acupoint (SI 5), 183

Yangxi acupoint (LI 5), 181

Yaoshu acupoint (GV 2), 166

Yifeng acupoint (SJ 17), 132

yin and yang, TCM, 33–36
    doshas compared to, 38
    duality of, 37
    gunas compared to, 37
    organs associated with, 35–36, 265
    relationship between, principles of, 34
    symbol for, 33, 34

Yinbai acupoint (SP 1), 205

ying qi, TCM, 33

Ying-Spring point, 53

Yingxiang acupoint (LI 20), 105

Yinmen acupoint (BL 37), 198

Yintang acupoint, 89, 99, 100

yogāsana, 25, 66, 240

yoga, 239–241

Yoga Mudrā (Lotus Pose With Forward Bend), 244

yoga postures. See āsanas

Yoga Sūtras (of Patāñjali), 239

yogic breathing. See prānāyāma, 20

Yongquan acupoint (KD 1), 207

Yoni Jihvā marma, 22, 196

Yoni Oshtha marma, 70, 197

yuan qi, TCM, 33

Yuji acupoint (LU 10), 185

yukta triveni, 50

Index

Yutang acupoint (CV 18), 140
Yuyao acupoint, 92, 94

Z

zang fu qi, TCM, 33
Zanzhu acupoint (BL 2), 92, 94
Zhangmen acupoint (LR 13), 145
zhi qi, TCM, 33
Zhongfu acupoint (LU 1), 136
Zhongwan acupoint (CV 12), 149
Zhoujian acupoint, 178
Zhouliao acupoint (LI 12), 179
zhuo bi, TCM, 44
zong qi, TCM, 33
Zuwuli acupoint (LR 10), 195

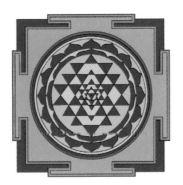

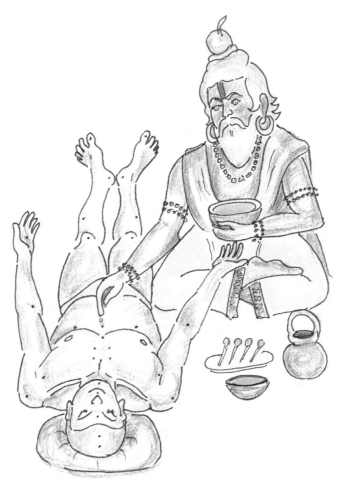

सप्तोत्तरं मर्मशतम् । तानि मर्माणि पञ्चात्मकानि भवन्ति । तद्यथा मांस
मर्माणि सिरामर्माणि सिरामर्माणि स्नायुमर्माणि अस्थिमर्माणि सन्धिमर्माणि
चेति । न खलु मांससिरास्नायुवस्थिसन्धिव्यतिरेकेणान्यानि मर्माणि
भवन्ति यस्मान्नोपलभ्यन्ते ॥२॥

सु. श. अ. ६

Classification of Marmas: There are one hundred and seven Marmas (in the human organism), which may be divided into five classes, such as the Mānsa-Marmas, Sirā-Marmas, Snāyu-Marmas, Asthi-Marmas and the Sandhi-Marmas. Indeed there are no other Marmas (vulnerable or vital parts) to be found in the body than the preceding ones.

Sushruta Samhitā, Shārīrasthāna, Ch. 6, V. 2

Notes

Notes

Notes

Notes

Notes

Notes

Notes

Notes

Notes

"Ayurveda and Chinese medicine are the world's two preeminent systems of holistic health and healing. These two systems, each complete in itself, have been cross-fertilizing for millennia, and will continue to do so for generations to come. This truly timely book, which presents one approach to how each system's concepts might be accurately translated into the idioms of the other, blazes a trail that future efforts can expand into a traditional medicine information highway."

Dr. Robert E. Svoboda, B.A.M.S.
Author, *Ayurveda: Life, Health and Longevity*, the *Aghora* series and others

"This is not your typical book about Ayurveda and yoga. One of the topics the authors write about is based on their personal knowledge of traditional yoga postures. But they also offer insight into the ancient practice of Indian pressure points, or marma, which are stimulated in the body during yoga poses. What is unique is how the authors connect the two practices. Following their suggestions can contribute to your deeper understanding of your body and to enhanced health. Recommended for yoga teachers and students alike."

Judith Hanson Lasater, Ph.D., P.T.
Yoga teacher and author, including *30 Essential Yoga Poses*.

"An excellent and invaluable resource for acupuncturists to enhance their clinical knowledge of acupoints. The authors offer an insightful comparison between Ayurveda and Traditional Chinese Medicine and how both systems have a similar approach to heal body, mind and spirit through treatment of these energy points."

Dr. Qijian Ye
Former Professor and Academic Dean of Southwest Acupuncture College, Albuquerque